The Body Clock Guide
to Better Health

**MICHAEL SMOLENSKY, PH.D.,
AND LYNNE LAMBERG**

The BODY CLOCK GUIDE TO BETTER HEALTH

How to Use Your Body's Natural Clock to Fight Illness and Achieve Maximum Health

AN OWL BOOK

HENRY HOLT AND COMPANY ◆ NEW YORK

Henry Holt and Company, LLC
Publishers since 1866
115 West 18th Street
New York, New York 10011

Henry Holt® is a registered trademark
of Henry Holt and Company, LLC.

Published in Canada by Fitzhenry & Whiteside Ltd.,
195 Allstate Parkway, Markham, Ontario L3R 4T8.

Library of Congress Cataloging-in-Publication Data
Smolensky, Michael H.
    The body clock guide to better health/Michael Smolensky
and Lynne Lamberg—1st ed.
        p.   cm.
    Includes index.
    ISBN 0-8050-5662-9
    1. Health. 2. Biological rhythms. 3. Chronobiology.
I. Lamberg, Lynne.   II. Title.
RA776.59 2000   00-027651
613—dc21   CIP

Henry Holt books are available for special promotions
and premiums. For details contact: Director, Special Markets.

First published in hardcover in 2000 by
Henry Holt and Company

First Owl Books Edition 2001

Designed by Victoria Hartman

Printed in the United States of America

1   3   5   7   9   10   8   6   4   2

A Message to Readers

This book aims to help you monitor and improve your health, but it is not a substitute for a physician's advice and treatment. Do not change the dose or time of a prescribed medication or other activity without first consulting your doctor or other health care professional.

Contents

The Body Clock Guide
to Better Health

It's about TIME

In 1996 the American Medical Association (AMA) asked the Gallup Organization to see if the nation's physicians and the general public knew that symptoms of many common illnesses worsen at predictable times of day or night, and improve at other times. When do heart attacks and asthma attacks occur most often? When are stuffiness, runny nose, sneezing, and other allergy and hay fever symptoms worst? When is blood pressure highest?

- Most physicians got every answer wrong.
- The typical adult flunked, too.
- Even persons with the target illnesses lacked vital facts that could improve their health, and possibly save their lives.
- Both doctors and patients wanted more information about how time of day affects illness and well-being.[1]

This book addresses that quest for knowledge. It starts with this claim: Most of us don't know how to tell time. *Body time.*

We pay more attention to watches we wear on our wrists than to clocks we acquire in the womb.

A wristwatch tells only one kind of time: world time. You must heed world time if you are getting married in the morning, have to catch a train, or want to see the six o'clock news. But no wristwatch tells when you think fastest, add numbers best, or swing a tennis racquet most deftly. A glance at your watch might make you think "time to eat," or "time for bed," even if your stomach isn't rumbling, or you haven't started to yawn. Feeling hungry or sleepy, however, requires a watchful brain, a brain with its own clock. A biological clock. A hard-wired program that ties your daily behavior to the rhythms of our planet and runs in the background of your life, adjusting automatically, as circumstances demand.

Most of us think we run our lives by the world's clock. Indeed, we often protest that this clock runs us, griping, as did Shakespeare's King Richard III, "time is wasting me." Life in the fast track both seduces and enslaves us. At work, we churn out faxes and E-mail, sometimes even to the person in the office next door. We've revved up our pace to Internet Time, fretting at the few seconds' delay signaled by the icon on our computer screens depicting the now obsolete hourglass.

Who has time to visit with friends? To read the books and magazines piled on the nightstand? Where do we find so-called quality time for our partners or children? Some 47 million Americans now work at paid jobs on weekends.

Recognition that nighttime is the right time for sleep has faded with the availability of hundreds of television channels at any hour, and the ease of ordering pizza around the clock even in small towns. If we can't fall asleep or stay asleep, or can't get going in the morning, we grumble about bad sleep, but the real problem may be bad timing. Most people don't know they can fix this broken clock themselves.

While we drive, we gulp coffee, gobble fast-food meals, and gab on the phone. Some cars now boast fax machines. Cats nip the heels of dogs as Americans' favored pets; cats don't need to be walked.[2] A New York woman earns her living as a personal shopper. She picks out clothes for her busy clients . . . from catalogs. We're under the sway of what Stephen Bertman, author of *Hyperculture*, calls "the power of now."[3] We mimic the March hare, constantly complaining, "I'm late. I'm late, for a very important date."

The brain's clock governs whether or not you're crabby before you have your morning coffee, how quickly you can write a letter and how accurately you can proofread it, how long it takes you to bike ten miles, whether or not you fall asleep at the symphony, when your ulcers act up, and more. Like the crocodile in *Peter Pan*, we carry this clock around inside of us. Many of us don't hear it tick.

Sara Discovers Her Body Clock

◆ Sara liked to bound out of bed in the morning, pull on her jogging clothes, and go for an easy run. When her knees and back started hurting, she added ten minutes of warm-ups and cool-downs. The pain, unfortunately, did not go away. To give herself more time to stretch, she put off running until she came home from work. Happily, her pain disappeared. What's more, Sara could run faster and farther. She certainly enjoyed her exercise more.

A specialist in *chronobiology*, the science of body time, could tell Sara why. Peak performance in most sports occurs in late afternoon and early evening, when body temperature reaches its daily high. Respect for this body rhythm may decrease your likelihood of injuries, whether you're a neighborhood jogger or an elite athlete. Training and competition times may influence who wins Olympic games and other high-powered sporting events. Stanford University scientists found that players' biological rhythms predicted winners of Monday Night Football games better than the Las Vegas point spread did.

If Sara wants to maintain or lose weight, or become a partner in her law firm, tuning into her body rhythms can help her achieve those goals more effectively. If she develops a cold, suffers from hay fever, or becomes pregnant, body rhythms will move to center stage in her life.

These findings represent a major leap in scientific understanding: a new way to maintain and optimize health, and to prevent and treat illness. Known as *chronomedicine*, it holds implications for vastly improving all of our lives.

What Chronomedicine Means to You

Chronomedicine can help you cope better with short-lasting illnesses such as colds and flu, episodic ones such as headaches and back pain, and persistent ailments such as arthritis, high blood pressure, heart disease, cancer, and more. This book details important recent advances to help you in your everyday life.

We report evidence from studies at leading medical centers worldwide showing that:

- *Many illnesses disrupt normal body rhythms.* Upsets in the body's most dominant rhythm, the daily wake/sleep cycle, provide an important clue to alert you that something is wrong. Complaints about fatigue and poor sleep trigger visits to the doctor for diseases as diverse as AIDS, diabetes, depression, and multiple sclerosis.
- *The signs and symptoms of many illnesses vary across the twenty-four-hour day, over the month, and around the year.* Some disorders peak in the morning; heart attacks, strokes, cluster headaches, hay fever, and rheumatoid arthritis are some examples. Others flare at night, including asthma, gout, colic in infants, gastric ulcers, and heartburn. Most chronic illnesses in women worsen in the days just before a menstrual period. Over the year, premenopausal women are most likely to discover a cancerous lump in a breast in the springtime, and men to find a testicular cancer in the winter.
- *Time of day patterns help identify causes of many illnesses.* Bringing symptom patterns to your doctor's attention may help your doctor figure out what's wrong faster and more accurately. The predictable morning spurt in blood pressure and clotting of red blood cells, for instance, make heart attacks and strokes peak in the morning, too. Disruptions in the flow of oxygen to the brain in sleep may produce morning headaches.
- *Chronotherapy, or timed treatment, aims to correct these underlying causes or*

reduce their adverse impact. Knowing symptoms' time of origin may enable your doctor to use more precise and effective treatment.

- *Glitches in the body clock itself may undermine health,* making you fall asleep too late, wake up too early, or suffer blue moods. Chronotherapy offers new ways to reset your body clock and resolve such problems.

- *The time of day you take diagnostic tests or undergo medical procedures alters the results.* If you have asthma, for example, your airway function will vary over the day. It probably is best in midafternoon, and poorest in the early morning. If you routinely go for a checkup in the afternoon, your doctor may think your treatment is working fine. But if you routinely go for a checkup first thing in the morning, the severity of your illness will be more apparent.

- *Time-of-day norms are known for many rhythms.* In the majority of the population, persons who stay awake in the daytime and sleep at night, who follow fairly regular schedules, the ups and downs of most daily rhythms prove quite predictable from day to day. Some labs already report findings with a time-of-day correction factor. New ambulatory monitoring devices can show your doctor how your blood pressure, heart rate, activity/rest cycle, and other indicators of your health change around the clock. Computer programs can analyze the data, making its collection and assessment practical.

- *The time you take medicine matters.* Taking the right medicine at the right time for your body and your illness may boost the medicine's efficacy and cut its unwanted side effects. The upshot is that you probably will feel better, be more willing to continue taking the medicine, need to see the doctor less often for symptom flare-ups or adverse drug reactions, and need fewer hospitalizations for chronic illnesses.

- *Nondrug treatments may help correct underlying disturbances in the body clock.* Exposure to sunlight-equivalent light, as one example, is now held to be the treatment of choice for persons with winter depression. Light exposure also benefits elderly persons who sleep poorly and wander at night, as well as shift workers and jet-lagged travelers.

- *How you organize your daily life, with respect to sleep, meals, exercise, and other factors may make symptoms better or worse, and hasten or slow your recovery.* If you have insomnia but stick to a regular wake-up time seven days a week, however bad the night, for instance, you'll probably sleep better in the long run than if you succumb to the impulse to sleep in.

How This Book Can Help You

We will show you

- the time of day, month, and year that symptoms flare in asthma, arthritis, diabetes, headaches, and many other common diseases
- how to observe and chart your personal symptom patterns by using do-it-yourself tests and diaries
- which times are best for many medical tests and procedures
- when to take your medicine to ensure that it works best and causes the fewest unwanted side effects
- how to monitor your own treatment
- which times are best for different types of exercise
- how to instill good sleep habits in young children, why not to hassle your teenagers when they sleep late on weekends, and how to get a good night's sleep yourself
- how to reach and maintain your ideal body weight
- what time of day is best for intercourse if you want to conceive
- how to prevent or minimize jet lag
- how to cope with working outside the traditional 9 to 5 hours

This information has never before been gathered in one place for both doctors and the general public. This book aims to be the first comprehensive guide to chronomedicine and chronotherapy.

What Doctors Don't Know about Health and Body Time

Chronomedicine is a brand-new concept, not only to the average person but also to most doctors. More than half of the 320 primary care physicians surveyed in 1996 for the American Medical Association said they were not familiar with chronobiology. One in four asserted that biological rhythms are not important in diagnosis or treatment.

Most of the doctors—even those who claimed to know something about chronobiology—did not know that some common illnesses predictably flare in the morning, afternoon, evening, or night, or they picked the wrong time. They did not know that blood pressure varies significantly over the day or that labor pains spontaneously start most often at night. They thought that diagnostic tests give the same results whenever they are performed, and that medications and other treatments work equally well, and are equally likely to cause unwanted side effects whenever they are given. They were wrong. We will show you why.

These were experienced physicians in their peak professional years. Most were under age fifty and had been practicing general family medicine or internal medicine for ten years or more. Nearly all saw 400 patients or more each month, persons with all of the illnesses or conditions included in the survey. Yet they knew only slightly more than their patients about the time patterns for high blood pressure, arthritis, respiratory allergies, asthma, chest pain, heart attacks, and migraine headaches.

Only one out of three physicians, most under age forty, said they had learned about chronobiology in medical school. Most of those who had at least some familiarity with the topic said they had gotten their information from reading medical journals. In 1996, the year of the survey, about two thousand articles on chronobiology were published in the world's scientific journals, far more than any one doctor was likely to read, but perhaps still not a critical mass.

Doctors and their patients also learned about chronobiology from news media reports. In recent years, *The New York Times, The Washington Post, The Wall Street Journal, Time, Newsweek,* and many other leading newspapers and magazines have reported advances in chronobiology. All of the television networks have produced stories on such topics as timed treatment for cancer and other illnesses, drowsy driving, the genetics of the biological clock, sleepy teenagers, jet lag's impact on athletes, melatonin, light therapy, and more.

Such stories still may be too infrequent, or too diverse and seemingly unconnected, to reshape attitudes and behavior. Among the general public, even persons who had the illness in question rarely recognized the predictability of its time course.

- Now that you mention it, I do often wake up with a migraine.
- My hay fever is worse in the morning.
- My osteoarthritis acts up in late afternoon. Guess I try to do too much early in the day.
- I just got to work when *wham!* The pain hit me. It's lucky I wasn't driving when I had my heart attack that morning.

What Do You Know about Health and Body Time?

The American Medical Association wanted to know what American physicians and the general public knew about body time. Compare your answers to those from the AMA's 1996 Gallup survey:

What time does this event most often occur?	Right answer	% of 320 physicians who knew the right answer	% of 1,011 members of general public who knew right answer
Heart attacks	Between 6 A.M. and noon	40%	26%
Asthma attacks	Between midnight and 6 A.M.	26%	15%
Highest blood pressure	Between noon and 6 P.M.	Not asked	44%
Stuffiness, sneezing, and other nasal allergy symptoms worst	Between 6 A.M. and noon	24%	34%
Angina (heart pain)	Between 6 A.M. and noon	38%	Not asked
Rapid rise in blood pressure	Between 6 A.M. and noon	45%	Not asked
Migraine headache	Between 6 A.M. and noon	24%	Not asked
Rheumatoid arthritis—worst symptoms	Between 6 A.M. and noon	46%	Not asked
Onset of labor at childbirth	Between midnight and 6 A.M.	33%	Not asked
Onset of menstruation	Between 6 A.M. and noon	14%	Not asked

Same Dose of Medicine Sometimes "Too Much" or "Too Little"

Think how often a doctor has handed you a prescription, saying, "Take this medicine three times a day." By linking pill-taking to mealtimes, the doctor knows you'll be more likely to remember to take your medicine. A "four times a day" prescription adds bedtime to the list. This approach is obsolete.

In prescribing equal doses over the day, your doctor presumes that your need for medication is the same all day, and that a consistent amount of medication confers a uniform benefit at all times. This belief is wrong.

If your symptoms wax and wane over the day, you need proportionately more medication to control them at some times, and less at others. Moreover, the way your body absorbs, uses, and excretes drugs varies over the day. The same dose of medicine may be too much at one time, and too little at another. Medicine that may help you at one time may not work as well at another. It may not even work at all. At some times, it may even be harmful.

Consider aspirin, the staple of the family medicine cabinet and one of the world's most widely used medications. Aspirin has a high safety record, particularly when taken in relatively small doses now and then. The problems come mainly with prolonged use, since aspirin may irritate the lining of the stomach and cause stomach ulcers and bleeding. These effects may occur even with the "baby aspirin" dosage (75 to 100 milligrams) that millions of Americans, particularly those in their forties and older, take once a day to prevent a heart attack or stroke. Taking aspirin at the proper time dramatically lowers your risk of developing stomach irritation and injury. Aspirin is least likely to cause irritation if you take it at night, and most likely to do so if you take it in the morning. Some persons who cannot tolerate aspirin when they take it in the morning have little or no difficulty when they take it at night.[4] (See page 209.)

Asthma attacks are one hundred times more frequent at night than in the day. Persons with severe unstable asthma who live on a conventional awake-in-the-daytime, asleep-at-night schedule get the most relief and greatest protection at night by taking their tablet steroid medication around 3 P.M. If you are a night worker, your doctor will need to synchronize treatment time with your schedule. (See page 220.)

Most medications used to ease peptic ulcers work best when taken once a day, around 6 P.M., with dinner. Taken at this time, they help block the normal late-night peak in daily secretion of stomach acid. (See page 323.)

In cancer, cells are most vulnerable to damage when they are dividing. Anticancer medications attack different stages of the cell reproduction rhythm. Some, such as 5-fluorouracil, which is used to treat cancers of the intestinal tract, are best tolerated and cause the fewest side effects when given by infusion while the patient sleeps at night. Others, including adriamycin and doxorubicin, which are used to treat bladder, ovarian, and other cancers, are best tolerated when given in the morning. When cancer medications are given in a chronobiological manner, that is, according to body rhythms, patients may be able to tolerate higher, more potent doses than would be possible otherwise.[5] (See page 229.)

Monthly Rhythms May Alter Symptoms, Too

In the AMA's 1996 survey, only three out of four doctors agreed that the menstrual cycle is a biological rhythm. *All* doctors should know this is true. Women know it: most recognize that their weight, energy, mood, sleep, cravings for particular foods, interest in sex, skin eruptions, frequency of migraines, asthma attacks, and symptoms of other illnesses predictably wax and wane over the month. Numerous factors, including stress, work, sleep, diet, and even the weather, may make some months more troublesome than others. Some women suffer more intensely than others, a reason some physicians and even some women dismiss or trivialize these symptoms.

Being tuned into these rhythms, however, can afford women a hardy measure of equanimity. A woman who is watching her weight may feel less guilty about nibbling a brownie right before her period starts. For many women, this is "the chocolate time of month," a few days with increased craving for chocolates and other sweets. A female athlete or actor may tolerate slight slips in performance, if she knows it's normal to be less coordinated, less "together," when she's menstruating.

Many women don't know that a routine test for cervical cancer, the Pap smear, gives the most accurate results if performed near ovulation. A woman can boost her odds of having this cancer detected at its earliest, most curable stage simply by scheduling this exam midway between her periods. (See chapter 11: "Time for Sex.")

Many chronic illnesses flare around the time of menstruation. Consider asthma: three out of four adults admitted to the hospital for treatment of life-threatening asthma attacks are female. Their hospital admissions occur four times more often just before or after menstruation than at any other time of month. Knowing that this is a more vulnerable time should heighten women's attention to their symptoms, and prompt physicians to fine-tune treatment. That won't happen until both patients and doctors focus their attention on body clocks. (See chapter 15: "Sickness and Health from A to [nearly] Z.")

The time of month also may influence the success of treatment. Fifteen studies involving more than 5,000 women with breast cancer show that those whose surgery is performed in the early part of the later half of their menstrual cycle live longer on average than women who undergo surgery earlier or later in the month.[6] But many cancer experts still are skeptical about these findings, and most operations for breast cancer are scheduled according to the surgeon's convenience. (See page 233.)

Ancient Cultures Recognized Body Time

"Of themselves, diseases come among men, some by day and some by night" the Greek poet Hesiod wrote in 700 B.C.[7] "Whoever wishes to pursue the science of medicine in a direct manner," the great Greek physician Hippocrates observed three hundred years later, "must first investigate the seasons of the year and what occurs in them."[8] Yet generations of physicians have paid little heed.

Nei Ching, the classic Chinese medical text written in 300 B.C., set forth the notion of health as a balance of opposites: cold and warm, moist and dry, passive and active. *Yin* and *Yang,* moon and sun, night and day, wife and husband, together represent the whole universe. Yin/Yang remains a central concept in Chinese medicine. It is represented pictorially by a circle that shows the moon and sun embracing. The American Academy of Sleep Medicine, the sleep field's leading professional organization, uses this symbol to signify its goal of optimizing both sleep and wakefulness.

Monuments built by ancient civilizations reflect knowledge of body time as well as planetary time. Shadows cast by the sun on the towering slabs at Stonehenge constructed in southwestern England some 4,000 years ago show changes in day length over the year. One circle at Stonehenge holds the correct number of markings to calculate the length of a woman's menstrual cycle or the likelihood of pregnancy, chronobiologist Sue Binkley reports.[9]

Twenty-four baboons carved into the face of a cliff at Abu Simbel 3,200 years ago guard the entrance to a temple to Pharaoh Ramses II. The baboons represent the twenty-four hours of the day, a way of dividing up time the ancient Egyptians devised some 400 years earlier. The baboons symbolize the Pharaoh's round-the-clock rule, gaining this honor by dint of the Egyptians' belief that they urinated once an hour: an overstatement, researchers who specialize in baboon behavior today say.

The words of Ecclesiastes remind us that our ancestors took rhythmic behavior for granted: "To every thing there is a season, and a time to every purpose under the heaven." The list includes "a time to be born, and a time to die," as well as "a time to heal."

Even the notion of body clocks is not brand new. The English writer Robert Burton observed, in the seventeenth century, "Our body is like a clock; if one wheel be amiss, all the rest are disordered, the whole fabric suffers: with such admirable art and harmony is a man composed."[10]

Early in the twentieth century, most physicians in the United States attended to all sorts of ills. When called in the late evening, they could predict their patient might have a flare of a peptic ulcer. If roused closer to dawn, they could anticipate seeing a patient with an asthma attack or a woman about to give birth. The morning brought heart attacks. Today, a person with stomach ulcers might see a gastroenterologist; one having trouble breathing, an allergist or lung specialist; and one with chest pain, a cardiologist. Births more often are induced, typically at the convenience of mother and doctor, and in the daytime. Only the sickest patients go to hospitals, where activity around the clock blurs the distinction between night and day. The present-day lack of appreciation for body time thus is a relatively recent phenomenon. The rise of specialization in medicine has eroded physicians' recognition of the ubiquity and significance of daily rhythms for health and disease.

The history of medicine is studded with facts that were known, lost, and later rediscovered. Body rhythms are "hot" again today. Some formidable hurdles, however, still stand in the way of their widespread acceptance.

Your Body Is a
Time Machine

In 1925 one in four Americans lived on farms. People rose with the sun and worked in the daytime. When it was dark, they slept. They planted seeds in the spring, tended crops in summer, and harvested in the fall. The natural cycles of the day and year shaped daily life and even determined the nine-month school calendar we still use.

That same year, 1925, the great physiologist Walter Cannon of Harvard Medical School introduced the principle of *homeostasis*, or steady state. Cannon drew on the work of the French physiologist Claude Bernard, who suggested in 1885 that the body strives to maintain constancy in its *milieu interieur*, its internal environment. Cannon asserted that the body continually fine-tunes itself to adapt to demands placed upon it, maintaining equilibrium. When thirsty, we drink. When hot, we sweat. So far, so good. The notion of health as equilibrium goes back to ancient times. The work of Cannon quickly became part of "the canon," the body of principles that guide medical practice. Homeostasis still dominates medical school teaching today. Its overarching reach is the key reason doctors overlook rhythmicity.

Constancy Is an Illusion

Here is the problem with homeostasis: it is incomplete. As an explanation of how the body works, it tells the truth, but not the whole truth. In any one person, in all of us, body temperature, blood pressure, pulse and breathing rates, concentrations of hormones in the blood, hand dexterity, sensitivity to pain, and all other bodily functions differ markedly over the twenty-four-hour day. These variations are not random. They occur in synchrony with our habitual daily pattern of activity and rest. (See the chart, "The Best of Times," page 15.) Variations also occur in women across the menstrual cycle, and in both sexes over the year. Age brings about further changes.[1]

These changes do not simply reflect a fine-tuning process. More than a thousand rhythmic bodily functions, the musicians in the body's orchestra, each have a role as distinct from the others as that of a violin from a tuba. They play softer or louder, faster or slower, as the score dictates. All follow their own music, sometimes rearranged as circumstances require. Harmony ensues only when all work together. A simple example: your brain anticipates your usual lunchtime, making you think about food. Your stomach might rumble. Secretion of digestive juices starts, readying your stomach for the cheese sandwich you just ordered. Before you take your first bite, your pancreas starts to manufacture the hormones insulin and glucagon, which you will need to derive energy from the food you eat.

Cannon recorded some variations in bodily activities, including ups and downs in body temperature and blood pressure. But he thought these variations were akin to static on a radio dial, noise caused by interference from sleep, activity, or diet. He did not see their time-of-day patterns, and he viewed the differences as meaningful only when they strayed far afield, outside a range he categorized as "normal."

Certainly, large variations are important. Body temperature of 104° Fahrenheit (F), for example, indicates disease. But the widely held belief that normal body temperature is 98.6° F is wrong. This reading is simply an average. Body temperature ranges from about 96° F to about 100° F over the day. It is lowest two to three hours before you habitually awaken, about 4 A.M. to 5 A.M. in someone who sleeps at night and arises around 7 A.M. It starts rising before the normal wake-up time, plateaus in early afternoon, dips a fraction of a degree in midafternoon, and then inches up slightly, hitting its high at about 7 P.M. At 4 A.M., a reading of 98.6° F in such a person would not be normal at all. It would reveal a fever. What's more, recent studies using improved thermometers and taking repeated measurements across the day, show that the daily average for young adults is 98.2° F. You can see your own pattern by taking your temperature every two hours, starting when you wake up and before you get out of bed.

The daily pattern of body temperature is the most commonly measured rhythm in chronobiology studies. It offers a useful way to tell what time it is on the body clock, and offers an easy reference point for comparisons with other rhythmic body functions.

In Cannon's day, the technology necessary to easily make round-the-clock measurements did not exist. It took a pint of blood to determine hormone levels then. Today, a drop of blood will suffice. Scientists now know, for example, that people typically secrete ten to twenty times more of the stress hormone cortisol in the morning, at their habitual wake-up time, than they do at night. Night workers who regularly sleep in the daytime secrete their highest amount of cortisol in the afternoon, when they usually arise.

Blood pressure similarly varies over the day. It often is 20 percent higher in the late afternoon than in the morning. Suppose you have been told that you

THE BEST OF TIMES

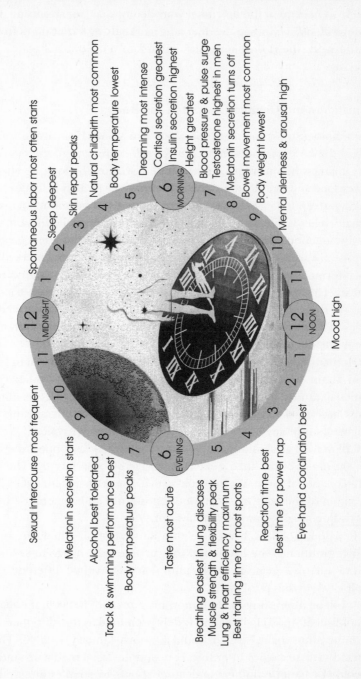

12 MIDNIGHT
1 Spontaneous labor most often starts
2 Sleep deepest
3 Skin repair peaks
4 Natural childbirth most common — Body temperature lowest
5 Dreaming most intense
6 MORNING — Cortisol secretion greatest — Insulin secretion highest — Height greatest
7 Blood pressure & pulse surge — Testosterone highest in men
8 Melatonin secretion turns off
9 Bowel movement most common — Body weight lowest
10 Mental alertness & arousal high
11
12 NOON — Mood high

1
2
3 Reaction time best — Best time for power nap — Eye-hand coordination best
4
5 Breathing easiest in lung diseases — Muscle strength & flexibility peak — Lung & heart efficiency maximum — Best training time for most sports
6 EVENING — Taste most acute
7 Body temperature peaks
8 Track & swimming performance best — Alcohol best tolerated — Melatonin secretion starts
9
10 Sexual intercourse most frequent
11

have high blood pressure. If you routinely go for a checkup in the afternoon, your doctor may think your problem is worse than it really is. If you routinely go for a checkup in the morning, your doctor may not appreciate the severity of your illness. If you see the doctor at markedly different times from one visit to the next, the doctor may find it hard to tell how well your treatment is working.

Constancy and Change Coexist in the Body

Both homeostasis and chronobiology are valid. Homeostatic mechanisms reveal the body's impressive facility for self-correction in the face of momentary changes in our internal environment. Chronobiologic mechanisms help us respond successfully to predictable variations in daily activities triggered by waking, sleeping, eating, and, in women, shifts in hormones across the menstrual cycle. While temperature, blood pressure, cell division, and other bodily functions display set points, sometimes called *normal limits*, these set points vary across the day, menstrual cycle, and year, often markedly.

In formulating the concept of homeostasis, Cannon concentrated on daily activity. He neglected longer time periods, such as the menstrual cycle. He also overlooked annual rhythms, easily seen in animals that breed at certain times of year and grow thicker, darker coats in winter, changes related to seasonal fluctuations in daylight exposure.

Humans display annual rhythms, too. More babies are born in late summer than at any other time of year in the United States and other countries of similar latitude. In the more than sixty years that U.S. government statisticians have tracked dates of birth, more babies were born in this country in August than in any other month. July and September typically vie for second place and occasionally come in first. In 1998, July topped the chart, with 47,000 more births than February, the least busy month. The birth rates reflect seasonal variations in sexual activity, most likely spurred by heightened secretion of the male sex hormone testosterone in late autumn, possibly triggered by changing amounts of daylight.[2]

Religious holidays, harvest celebrations, vacation schedules, and personal choices influence the likelihood that people will engage in sexual behavior. But despite the great variety of cultural and individual differences, the yearly biological rhythm persists.

It will be interesting to see if monthly rates shift in 2000, the year this book is published. April 11, 1999, was widely promoted as the ideal date to conceive a "millennium baby," which would be born January 1, 2000. The Internet buzzed with strategies to ensure conception. News media around the world provided romantic dinners and hotel rooms to couples attempting to produce the first baby of the year and promised extravagant gifts for the lucky arrival.

Being born in the summer once played a bigger role in enhancing the newborn's survival than it does today. Plentiful supplies of food meant nursing mothers could eat well. Warm weather eliminated dangers of exposure to frigid air. Fewer viruses float around in summer than in winter. Even today, babies born in the summer and fall tend to be slightly heavier than those born in other seasons, giving them a head start on a healthy life.

Male babies born in the spring, curiously, tend to be a tiny bit taller as adults than those born in the fall. The difference is only one-quarter inch, or 0.6 centimeters, but it's interesting because it points to yearly variations in hormones critical for growth. The findings come from a study of records collected on more than 500,000 Austrian men at age eighteen, at the time of their compulsory entrance into the army. Spring babies are conceived in summer months, when hours of daylight in Austria are greatest. It is not clear how sunlight might affect height. Increased sunlight simply may bring a more bountiful supply of fresh fruits and vegetables than at other times of year, improving women's nutrition in the first months of their pregnancy.[3]

There are seasonal variations in illnesses, too. The risk of developing schizophrenia, for example, is highest for persons born in February and March, and lowest for those born in August and September. Danish researchers reached this conclusion after reviewing records of 1.75 million persons born to Danish mothers between 1935 and 1978, and charting birth dates of the 2,700 who developed schizophrenia. Many factors that affect brain development are believed to play a role in triggering schizophrenia: some, the most critical, are genetic, and thus run in families. But these do not account for all cases of the illness. Other triggers may originate in the environment, including increased exposure to influenza viruses in winter months. There also may be an innate annual rhythm of increased susceptibility to such viruses at that time of year.[4]

A Half-Century of Studies Shows That Body Time Matters

Animal research, starting in the 1950s, showed the importance of timing in treatment. In 1959 Franz Halberg and his colleagues at the University of Minnesota discovered that nearly all the mice given a potential poison at one time of day died. None or only a few of those receiving the same dose of the same chemical twelve hours later did so. Further, the researchers found that almost all of a group of mice exposed to abnormally loud noise at 10 P.M., when they were in their daily activity span, developed seizures. Another group of mice, hearing the same noise at noon, in their rest span, suffered no or minor ill effects. The adverse effects of X rays and other physical and chemical stresses varied across the day in similar fashion.

Time Tells

♦ Mice and men and women and children prove to be strikingly similar. All respond differently to the same treatment at different times of day. Michael Smolensky learned this lesson as a graduate student in Halberg's chronobiology laboratories in the 1960s.

"Halberg had embraced with missionary-like fervor the critical, though tedious, task of assessing different medications at different times of day. I decided to study corticosteroids, a synthetic form of the hormone cortisol used to reduce inflammation in severe flare-ups of asthma, arthritis, and other illnesses.

"The body produces cortisol on a regular schedule. Peak secretion occurs around the time we normally awaken, at the start of our daily activity span. I wondered if giving corticosteroids at that time, when the body was prepared for that hormonal surge, would lessen their adverse side effects.

"In one study, I planned to inject groups of young laboratory mice at different times around the clock with either a commonly prescribed corticosteroid medication called *methylprednisolone* or an inactive saltwater solution. Since graduate students don't have assistants to help them, I had to camp out in the laboratory. I couldn't take the chance of missing even one injection time. I collected bread, peanut butter, jelly, apples, Snickers bars, and instant coffee, the staples of a student's diet, grabbed my sleeping bag, and moved in with my mice.

"Each day, I injected methylprednisolone into different groups of mice at midnight, 4 A.M., 8 A.M., noon, 4 P.M., and 8 P.M. In between, I washed and sterilized my instruments, prepared for the next round of injections, and, when I could, grabbed a few minutes of rest. After twenty-one days, I was foggy and cranky from lack of sleep. I was twelve pounds thinner. My clothes had acquired a rodent smell that clung to them through several washings. But the results thrilled me: the mice did well when injected with the medication just after the start of their activity period. They suffered the most side effects when they received the medication just before or in their rest period."[5]

Most Drug Testing Ignores Time of Day

In more recent studies, researchers around the world have seen the same results with methylprednisolone and other medications in numerous human illnesses. But some of their peers regard these findings more as curiosities than as guidelines for standard practice.

About 95 percent of modern drug-development studies use laboratory mice and rats, both nocturnal animals. The humans who conduct the studies work mainly in the daytime. "How much time, effort and money have been wasted in this way, we shall probably never know," railed chronobiologist Josephine Arendt of the University of Surrey. "It is almost unbelievable that drugs should be first tested in the middle of the rat's night," she said, "when they are mostly destined to be used in the human day."[6]

The implications are unsettling. Can we trust our current drug safety tests? Some chemicals found to be likely carcinogens in these tests may have been considered safe had they been given at the appropriate biological time. Some that looked harmless may prove dangerous if given at a different time.

Even when medications reach the stage in which doctors evaluate their safety and efficacy in humans, time of day often gets little or no attention. Most scientists assume, as the theory of homeostasis claims, that drugs will act the same way and carry the same risk of side effects whenever they are taken. Drug studies typically are conducted in the daytime for the convenience of both scientists and subjects. Tests often begin early in the morning so they can be completed by the end of the normal workday. Ludicrous as it may seem, even some sleeping pills undergo testing this way.

Daily rhythms in the acidity, blood flow, and muscular activity of the stomach alter the rate and even the amount of medication released into the body. Daily rhythms in blood flow to the heart, brain, lungs, and other organs, and in the uptake of drugs by cells and tissues, affect how quickly drugs go to work throughout the body. Daily rhythms in the liver, kidneys, and other organs affect how fast the body uses medications and how long medications stay in the body. All of these rhythms collectively determine how long the medication continues to exert its therapeutic effect. These rhythms also influence interactions between drugs, particularly important in persons with chronic illnesses, who may take two, three, or more medications several times a day.

The only way to find out how a drug will act around the clock is to test it around the clock. Such studies are highly labor intensive. Volunteers must agree to be tested at different times under highly controlled conditions. Subjects sometimes must agree to stay awake for twenty-four hours or longer to avoid the rhythm changes induced by sleep. They may have to sleep at certain times, with periodic awakenings for testing. In medication studies, subjects typically eat standardized meals for breakfast, lunch, and dinner, timed not to interfere with the behavior of the drug they are taking. They must permit frequent blood samples and cooperate in measurements of body temperature, urine output, and other functions. Researchers in turn must assess whether the absorption, metabolism, and other effects of medications differ over the day. Investigators themselves usually have to forgo sleep to follow their subjects.

Few pharmaceutical companies test their products for possible differences related to the time they are taken. The U.S. Food and Drug Administration does not require such testing.

This situation could change, with wider use of ambulatory monitors to collect round-the-clock data, and computer programs to analyze the results. Such devices, already in use to study blood pressure, heart rate, and other bodily functions, enable physicians to see in their own patients that both these functions and symptoms of disease vary over the day as well as over longer time periods.

New Drug Design Exploits Body Rhythms

Synchronizing treatment with body rhythms, or *chronotherapy*, may simply involve judicious scheduling of conventional medicines. You are using chronotherapy now if you take aspirin in the afternoon to relieve evening osteoarthritis pain, an acid-blocking drug at supper time for your stomach ulcer, or an antihistamine at bedtime to relieve morning allergy symptoms.

Chronotherapy also may involve taking unequal amounts of medication at different times. Persons with diabetes already do this, testing their blood and using insulin as needed.

The first use of chronotherapy in modern medicine occurred in the United States in the 1960s. Researchers at the National Institutes of Health showed that persons with asthma, arthritis, and other inflammatory diseases who took the cortisol-like drug Medrol at the same time their bodies produced this hormone naturally, that is, in the morning, got better faster, with fewer unwanted side effects, than those who took the same amount of the same drug at other times.[7] The introduction of this drug, manufactured by the Upjohn Company, strengthened chronotherapy's credibility. Doctors saw it worked better and became more attentive to the concept of timed dosing.

The first chronobiologically designed American medication, Uniphyl, a theophylline medication for asthma, was introduced in this country by Purdue Pharma in 1989. Taken once daily in the early evening, it delivers its maximal amount of asthma-fighting medication in the middle of the night when the risk of an asthma attack is greatest.

A medication for high blood pressure and heart disease, Covera-HS, introduced in the United States by Searle in 1996, utilizes an even more sophisticated chronobiological design. The "HS" in its name is a Latin abbreviation that tells you this medication is taken at the hour of sleep, that is, at bedtime. The medication has an outer shell that dissolves slowly, delaying its release until just before the user awakens. Most of the drug is released in normal waking hours. The dose tapers down in the evening and overnight, when users of such medication normally need less of it.

Some pharmaceutical manufacturers have latched onto chronobiology as the "next new thing." They have a clear economic incentive to produce more effective and safer drugs. They have not only a vested interest in boosting physicians' awareness of body time, but also deep pockets to support their commitment. Medical journals are full of four-page, full-color advertisements for once-a-day medications. Some ads misuse the term *chrono*. Some allege the products provide "24-hour control," a claim that displays lack of knowledge of chronotherapy. Most of these medications are simply slow-release products, not aligned with daily rhythms. True chronotherapies consist of medication that kicks in only when needed, and in the amount needed.

New drug-delivery technology will make chronotherapy more practical in the future. "Smart" drugs that can be taken when convenient will permit release of the appropriate dose at a designated time.

Chronomedicine Fosters Research on Gender

The chronomedicine revolution accompanies another major area of ferment in medicine: changing attitudes toward gender. Research in both animals and humans up to nearly the end of the twentieth century was mainly "male-only" turf. Scientists felt the normal, cyclic changes induced by female reproductive hormones would add unwanted complexity to the collection of data. To reproduce results easily, they needed a uniform study population. They rarely included females in their research, except in studies of the reproductive system itself. They maintained that results obtained in men applied to everyone.

As a result, major studies neglected half the human population. A nation-wide federally supported study in the 1980s, for example, explored whether changing diet, exercise, and other behaviors could help prevent heart disease. This study involved 360,000 men, but no women. Its name reflected this bias: it was called the Multiple Risk Factor Intervention Trial, or MRFIT for short. Only today are doctors starting to appreciate that symptoms of heart disease may be quite different in men and in women. Some women who suffer heart attacks delay seeking treatment, or aren't taken seriously by their doctors, because they don't show the "classic" symptoms. Crushing chest pain, for example, now is increasingly regarded as a "male" symptom. (See "Heart Disease," in chapter 15, page 276.) The National Institute on Aging (NIA) published its report on the Baltimore Longitudinal Study of Aging in 1984, using data derived only from men. The NIA called the report *Normal Human Aging*.[8]

Health activists of both sexes recognized the shortsightedness of this approach and lobbied to change it. In 1990 the National Institutes of Health (NIH) established its Office of Research on Women's Health. The NIH Revitalization Act, signed into law by President Bill Clinton in 1993, requires that both women and minorities be included in all NIH-funded clinical research. It even specifies that cost is not an acceptable reason for excluding these groups.

If you are female, chronomedicine may hold special appeal, not only because women previously were barred from medical study but because your biology constantly reminds you of the body's natural cycles. If you are male, you may be surprised to learn how much a creature of rhythms you are, too, with every function of your life—sleeping, waking, working, and working out—governed by your body clock.

Chronomedicine: It's Not a "Some Day" Science

The evidence is solid and growing, but physicians, like the rest of us, resist change. There is no active conspiracy against chronomedicine. The biggest barrier is simply inertia. No one wants to be the first to say the emperor has no clothes.

To embrace chronomedicine, physicians will need to abandon many of their current practices. They will need to throw out many "norms" by which they now evaluate patients. They will need to write in their charts not only what signs and symptoms they find, but when they find them. They will need to pay attention to the time of day they draw blood, and when they collect urine and other bodily tissues for diagnostic tests. They may even need to schedule tests at specific times of day or night. They will need to instruct patients not only what medicine to take but also when to take it. And they will need to give more credibility to the impact of time of day on their own judgment and performance, and pay more attention to patterns in their own levels of alertness and fatigue.

These are big obstacles, but they are not insurmountable. The history of medicine, indeed of all fields, abounds in examples of those who initially proposed changes and met considerable derision, even outright rejection. Then, one or two forward-thinking practitioners voiced interest, still demanding proof. As evidence mounted, their numbers grew. Eventually, the new ideas caught on. Doctors ridiculed the stethoscope when it was first introduced in France two hundred years ago. For centuries, surgeons washed their hands only after they performed operations, not before. The chronomedicine revolution has begun. We hope this book will help raze the barricades.

The Discovery of
Inner Clocks

It may have begun as an idle thought.

Sipping his coffee that summer morning, he may have noticed the plant by the window stretching its leaves and branches toward the sun. "My plant and I are waking up at the same time," he might have mused.

For most of us, this rumination might go no further. But Jean Jacques Dortous de Mairan, an astronomer and mathematician living in Paris in the early 1720s, probably toyed with the idea a bit. Was the plant simply responding to sunlight? Did humans do that as well? Why then do people awaken about the same time even in winter darkness? What would the plant do if it could not see the sun?

By then, his coffee most likely was cold. While de Mairan's thoughts are conjecture, what he did is on record. He stepped to the window, picked up the plant, and carried it to a dark cabinet. He shut it inside, hidden from daylight.

When de Mairan returned to the closet that evening, candle in hand, he saw the plant's leaves folded down, its stems drooping. He may have wondered if the plant's state reflected jostling on the way to the closet. Known as "a sensitive," the plant took its name from its dramatic collapse both at sunset and when touched. De Mairan's plant probably was a *Mimosa pudica*, botanists say, using the Latin name first assigned by the great Swedish naturalist Carolus Linnaeus in 1735.

The next morning, de Mairan discovered the plant's fernlike leaves unfurled, reaching upward. Observing the plant for several days, he found that it continued to raise its leaves in the morning, lower them in the evening, and stay this way all night.

De Mairan repeated his experiment with other sensitive plants and saw that all followed suit. He told his friend Marchant about his findings, but resisted Marchant's entreaties to write up the results to present to colleagues. The fifty-one-year-old de Mairan pleaded other, more pressing demands: he had a major study of the aurora borealis, or northern lights, then in progress. Perhaps he thought the behavior of his household plants a mere *curiosité*.

Science Prompts "The Buzz"

In the early 1700s, interest in scientific information by the literate classes of France was burgeoning. From the sophisticated *salons* of Paris to provincial towns, and even at court, both scientific and pseudoscientific subjects were among the favorite topics of conversation. Natural history was particularly popular, science historian Roger Hahn of the University of California at Berkeley reports. People found it easy to understand. The general public was seized with a mania for collecting. Those who could afford to do so, Hahn relates, could dazzle their friends with their expertise by buying a "cabinet," and showing off amazing novelties they had amassed, much as those who collect seashells or dinosaur bones do today. Botany became fashionable, too. Pharmacists seeking information on medicinal herbs flocked to talks on the topic. General audiences, the forerunners of today's horticultural societies and garden clubs, mushroomed, prompting the need for increasingly larger lecture spaces.[1]

In this receptive climate, it is no surprise that Marchant decided to present de Mairan's work himself at a scientific meeting. This was not an unusual practice, for scientists of the day often shared results of their own work and that of their colleagues in prolific exchanges of letters. Marchant's report, *Observation Botanique*, or *Botanical Observation*, appears on a single soft linen page in the telephone-book-sized *Mémoires de l'Académie des Sciences* (The Proceedings of the Academy of Sciences), published in Paris in 1729.[2]

"We know that the Sensitive is heliotrope, that is, that the leaves and branches always reach in the direction of the greatest light intensity," Marchant wrote. "We also know that in addition to this property that it shares with other plants, it has one that is more particular, it is sensitive with regard to the sun or daylight; the leaves and their stems fold and contract toward sunset, just as they do when the plant is touched or shaken.

"But Monsieur de Mairan," he reported, "observes that this reaction can be observed even if the plant is not in the sunlight or outdoors. The phenomenon is only slightly less marked when the plant is kept inside a dark place. It does not open quite as much during the day and it regularly folds or closes in the evening for the whole night. The experiment was done at the end of the summer and properly repeated."

De Mairan's scrupulous observation merits respect. At a time when many notions about scientific matters rested solely on untested theories, de Mairan not only detailed his findings but repeated his experiments to be sure his results did not occur by chance. Scientific discovery, he asserted in one of his many publications, requires us to proceed slowly and methodically from what we know to what we do not know and would like to know. "His reputation as an experimenter is unassailable," says Ellen McNiven Hine of York University, in Toronto, Canada, who has studied scientific networking in the eighteenth century. "There is little doubt," she writes, "that he regards experiment and observation as the linchpins of scientific methodology."[3]

No Sun Worshipers Here

The plant's behavior, as de Mairan discovered, was not a passive response to the presence or absence of sunlight, an idea that had persisted for centuries. Androsthenes, a scribe who chronicled the expedition of Alexander the Great to India two thousand years earlier, for example, reported that the tamarind tree raised its leaves in the morning and lowered them at night. The tree, he wrote, appeared to be worshiping the sun. De Mairan's careful observation did away with this romantic sentiment. Even in the dark, the plant raised and lowered its leaves at the same times of day. It knew when to be active and when to sleep.

"So the Sensitive feels the sun without in any way seeing it," Marchant wrote. This supposition is wrong. Had de Mairan observed his plants for weeks instead of days—a task no one pursued until a hundred years later—he would have seen that the plant's leaf raising and lowering, while predictable, followed a schedule twenty-two to twenty-three hours long. This pattern confirms that the plant's behavior originates within the plant, that no mysterious signal from the sun directs it. If the sun controlled it, twenty-four-hour cycles would be the rule.

The beat goes on, as de Mairan discovered, even in the absence of sunlight. Sunlight serves a critical function, however: it synchronizes the biological clock with planetary time. De Mairan's plant did not extend its leaves as far in the dark as it did when it sat by the window. Synchronizing, also called *entraining*, establishes predictability and promotes survival, not just in de Mairan's plant but in all plants and animals, including humans. All living things occupy a special niche in time. All display their highest energy levels when their food sources are most available. All punch highly specific time clocks. Plants' flowers need to be open when the insects that pollinate them are buzzing. Bats and frogs need to be out and about at the same time as the mosquitoes and other insects they devour. And we humans, too, see better, feel most alert, and function better in the daytime than at night.

De Mairan, or perhaps Marchant, made a conceptual leap, linking plant and human behavior and acknowledging their shared rhythmicity. The plant's activity, as noted in *Observation Botanique*, "seems to be related to the delicate sensitivity by which invalids confined to their sickbeds perceive the difference between day and night."

This is a brilliant insight. An internal timing mechanism, a built-in clock, a biological clock, tells the plant on your windowsill, your cat, and you, when to be active, and when to sleep. Even if you remain indoors, even if you stay in bed, even if you volunteer as a research subject and live for weeks or months in windowless rooms, with no clocks and no knowledge of the hour of day, you still will stay awake and be active about two-thirds of the time and sleep for the rest.

In windowless research apartments cut off from time, however, humans lose touch with the external day and night. They generally go to sleep a little later each day, unknowingly following a day length that ranges from slightly more than twenty-four hours to about twenty-five hours. Thus, if they participate in such research for several weeks, they will go to sleep and wake up all around the clock. When told that the study is over, they often think it is ending early, that is, that they'd spent fewer days than expected in the lab.

In contrast to the earth's twenty-four-hour rotation, living creatures have some built-in flexibility. This makes it possible to function at different latitudes, and to adapt easily to changing day lengths over the year.

Cinderella Has a Message for You

The practical benefit of having a clock that runs longer than the planetary day is that it is easy for us to stay up late if we wish. Indeed, most of us are pretty casual about bedtimes. Few of us go to sleep at exactly the same time every night, even though we typically get up around the same time most days. For most of us, the difference from one night to the next is minutes more often than hours. The Cinderella story reminds us that we pay a price for staying too late at the ball. If we change our schedules drastically—jetting across several time zones, or switching work hours from days to nights, for example—we no longer feel our best. Our internal timing system balks at change and adapts slowly, often causing havoc such as difficulty falling asleep or staying alert on our new schedule, or feeling hungry when it's not normally time to eat.

Rhythms that are close to but not exactly twenty-four hours long are termed *circadian,* a term created in 1959 by the American chronobiologist Franz Halberg from the Latin words *circa,* meaning "about," and *dies,* "a day." In humans, as in plants, the most obvious circadian rhythm is the daily alternation of activity and rest, waking and sleeping. There are hundreds of other circadian rhythms, covering every bodily function that has ever been studied, from cell division to hormone release to mental and physical performance. "Everything is rhythmic unless proved otherwise," asserts the British chronobiologist Josephine Arendt. Some rhythms peak while we are active, and others while we are at rest. Their sheer number suggests they are essential for our overall health and well-being. Circadian rhythms also govern the predictable appearance of symptoms in many illnesses at particular times of day, and the body's response to medications.

While circadian rhythms are the most prominent in our lives, we also experience internal cycles both shorter and longer than a day. Our pulse rate and the firing of nerve cells in the brain, for example, cycle in minutes and seconds. Among longer cycles, men display a weekly rhythm of beard growth, and women have monthly menstrual cycles.

After describing de Mairan's experiments, Marchant proposed several additional ones. "It would be interesting to see if other plants, whose leaves or flowers open in the day and close at night," he wrote, "conserve this property when kept in dark places as does the Sensitive." He wondered about the impact of temperature. "It would be interesting to see if one could use ovens to give a warmer or cooler temperature and artificially make day and night that they would sense, if in this way, one could reverse the order of phenomena of true day and true night, etc."

De Mairan had no plans to pursue these studies, nor, evidently, did Marchant. "The customary occupations of Monsieur de Mairan," Marchant wrote, "did not allow him to carry his experiments to that point." There is some irony here. De Mairan is the author of numerous publications, including a major treatise on the formation of ice. He traveled in intellectually and socially prominent circles. He was a prolific letter writer, and his correspondence, Hine tells us, is "a treasure house of information on personalities, ideas and controversies of crucial importance to the international scientific community of his time." Voltaire called him one of the five most outstanding scientists and mathematicians of the eighteenth century. Yet in the fields that were his primary life's work, he is credited with no original discovery. Instead, it was his simple observation of one type of plant in his own home, a study he did not deem important enough to write up himself, for which he is best known today.

There is more. Since de Mairan did not intend to look further at plant behavior, "he had to be content," Marchant said, "to invite botanists and physicians, who themselves may have other things to do."

De Mairan's perception of the need for physicians to attend to rhythmic behavior again was prophetic. Physicians of the eighteenth century, the Age of Enlightenment, did not explore the possibilities. A German physician living in the 1800s, however, deserves to be called the "patron saint" of chronobiology, according to a leading twentieth-century chronobiologist, Colin Pittendrigh of Princeton University. "The 24-hour period which is imparted to all inhabitants of the terrestrial body by its uniform rotation is especially distinct in the physical economy of man," Christoph Wilhelm Hufeland noted in 1823. "In all diseases this regular period makes its appearance," Hufeland wrote. "It is, so to speak, the unit of our natural chronology."[4]

This prescient notion, however, did not change medical practice in Hufeland's lifetime. Even today, at the dawn of the twenty-first century, many physicians remain in the dark about what inner rhythms are, and how they influence human health. Marchant, presumably speaking for de Mairan, recognized the rigors of scientific research. "The progress of true Physics [meaning Science], which is experimental," he said, "must necessarily be slow."

Seminal Discovery Set Off No Fireworks

It was not until thirty years later that the French botanist Henri-Louis Duhamel decided to repeat de Mairan's experiment. Wondering whether de Mairan truly had sequestered his plants from light, Duhamel took his plants to a wine cave and set them far in the back where no light penetrated. In another experiment, he put plants in a large leather trunk covered with wool blankets and then shut the trunk in a closet. He invariably obtained the same results as did de Mairan. Duhamel also explored the effects of temperature, finding that the daily cycle persisted even in a hothouse. "One can conclude from these experiments," he wrote, "that the movements of the sensitive plant are dependent neither on light nor on heat."[5]

Linnaeus, too, had noted plants' daily rhythms. In 1754, he created a clock in his garden to tell the time from dawn to dusk, with beds of flowers that opened at different hours, from the morning glory to the evening primrose, all behaving in the same way as de Mairan's sensitive plant. Such clocks continue to delight visitors to botanical gardens.

Interest in how plants tell time languished until the next century. One hundred years after de Mairan's discovery, in 1832, Augustin Pyrame de Candolle, a Swiss botanist, reported that plants kept in constant light displayed a cycle of leaf opening and closing about twenty-two to twenty-three hours long. This pattern, still close to the planetary day, shows that plants have a built-in ability to adapt to seasonal changes in hours of daylight. De Candolle also reversed day and night for his plants, using banks of lamps to mimic natural daylight. When the schedule changed, the plants at first seemed confused. They needed a few days to adjust to their new regime,[6] an experience that will be familiar to contemporary shift workers and jet travelers.

Evidence that leaf raising and lowering enables the plant's survival came from the great biologist Charles Darwin. In the last years of his life, Darwin and his son Francis conducted hundreds of studies, exposing plants to different amounts of light coming from different directions, at different times. Father and son concluded that the daytime leaf position maximized exposure to sunlight essential for growth, and that the nighttime leaf position minimized exposure to cold, keeping the plant's temperature from dropping too low in the absence of sunlight. These findings, reported in their book, *The Power of Movement in Plants,* published in 1881,[7] resonate with those of contemporary scientists who believe that conservation of body temperature is one of the key functions of sleep in humans. (See chapter 7: "A Good Night's Sleep.")

The twentieth century sparked new interest in many types of predictable behavior, well documented by careful observers of plants and animals, including humans. Many more decades would pass, however, before scientists figured out how they all tell time.

4

How Your Body Clock Works

In the film *Groundhog Day*, Bill Murray's character gets trapped in a time warp, where every day is exactly the same. His alarm clock wakes him at the same time each morning. The radio blares the same news as the day before.

This fantasy rests on a central truth: this *is* how life works. Our days and nights, viewed at a distance, are pretty much alike. Their routine nature makes life manageable. We wake, we sleep, we wake, we sleep, tumbling incessantly from one state to the other. This cycle provides the scaffolding that supports hundreds of other daily rhythms.

Every day, before you wake up, your body temperature and blood pressure rise, your heart beats faster, and numerous glands squirt out pulses of cortisol and other hormones you'll need to get going. Every night, before you go to sleep, temperature, heart rate, and blood pressure fall, and the body produces a nighttime hormone, melatonin.

Architects say the house of the future will be a "smart" house, envisioning computerized sensors that will learn from your habits, turning on lights and the radio before you usually enter the kitchen in the morning, making the coffee, adjusting heat and air-conditioning, and saving you from having to remember to attend to numerous chores.

You already live in a very smart house, smarter than any computer will ever be. Its controller, your internal time-sensor, the body's biological clock, is a twin cluster of nerve cells roughly the size and shape of a letter V on this page. These twin islands each contain about 50,000 of the estimated 30 to 50 billion nerve cells that make up the entire human brain.

How Your Brain's Brain Does Its Job

Collectively, these nerve cells are called the suprachiasmatic nucleus, or SCN. The SCN takes its name from its location, which is supra (meaning "above") the optic chiasm, a major junction for nerves that transmit information from the eyes to the brain. The SCN resides within the bean-sized hypothalamus, sometimes called the body's master gland, because it helps regulate breathing and heart rate, body temperature, blood pressure, hormone production, and other vital bodily functions.

The body's biological time system works like a real-world company, with the SCN as chief executive officer. At Body Rhythms, Inc., nerve connections from the eyes tell the SCN what levels of light are available. The SCN interprets this message and delegates tasks to vice presidents in the hypothalamus and nearby pituitary gland. They in turn issue commands to mid-level managers elsewhere in the brain and in organs throughout the body, all the way down to the individual cells making up the round-the-clock workforce. Reports from the field filter their way back up to the SCN, which constantly processes and modifies job assignments.

Some peculiarly human behaviors, such as flying to distant spots across time zones, or working on different shifts, upset the staff. They get orders from two bosses at the same time, the day manager and the night manager. Some workers pay attention to one, and others, to the other. Their internal mix-ups vex travelers as jet lag, and shift workers as trouble adapting to new hours for waking and sleeping. The SCN straightens things out, though this job may take several days to several weeks.

The Search for Master Clock Spanned Decades

Researchers suspected that some type of internal pacemaker existed long before they found it. After watching rats run around their cages, rest, and start up again back in the 1920s, Curt Richter of the Johns Hopkins University School of Medicine wondered what controlled this self-organizing behavior. He and others observed once-a-day patterns like those of de Mairan's plant throughout the entire animal kingdom, from the one-celled paramecium to humans. They observed shorter and longer cycles, too.

In the 1960s, Richter found that destroying a tiny sliver of the hypothalamus in rats made his animals sleep, wake, run, eat, and drink at odd hours.[1] People with tumors that involve their hypothalamus often find their daily routines break down in the same way.

The surgical techniques available to Richter weren't quite precise enough to pinpoint the SCN. In 1972, two independent teams of researchers led by Irving Zucker at the University of California at Berkeley and Robert Moore at the University of Chicago zeroed in on it by following electrical[2] and hormonal[3] signals. Their discovery fostered a host of discoveries that expanded understanding of what it means to be well, how illness upsets cyclic behavior, and how breakdowns of regular rhythms may cause some types of illness.

To confirm that the SCN was the body's master clock, researchers first destroyed it and saw that an animal's rhythmic behavior disappeared. They then transplanted SCN tissue from another animal into the first animal and found that the cyclic behavior returned.

A Rare Hamster Opens New Doors

A curious hamster, the rodent equivalent of a black sheep, showed that genes regulate SCN rhythms. One of a hundred hamsters Martin Ralph of the University of Oregon purchased from a breeding lab had a twenty-hour rest/activity cycle, about four hours shorter than those of all its companions. Hamsters normally start running when put in darkness, but this animal defied the rules and ran on its own schedule.

Ralph bred it, and found its short cycle to be the result of a genetic mutation. When he removed the SCN from a hamster with a twenty-four-hour cycle and replaced it with SCN tissue from one of the twenty-hour crowd, the recipient animal adopted the short cycle.[4] Ralph, now at the University of Toronto, found transplants in the opposite direction worked the same way, showing that our rhythm patterns are "factory-installed" in our brains.[5]

Individual SCN cells keep time even outside the body, waking up and sleeping in a laboratory dish according to their usual cycle. Researchers are just starting to localize subregions within the SCN and to assess their differential influence. They also have found genes that regulate rhythms, spawning something of a "name that gene" game among competing labs. Recent entrants include the aptly named *CLOCK*, along with *TIM* (time), *PER* (period), and *NOCTURNIN*, which turns on only in the early part of the night.

Light Signals Set the Clock

Sunlight keeps most of us synchronized with the local twenty-four-hour day, just as it did de Mairan's mimosa plant. Until the 1980s, many scientists doubted the primacy of light for people. Humans, after all, figured out how to use fire and invented electricity. Researchers believed people organized their lives using social cues such as mealtimes, work hours, or school bells.

Many early studies involved observing how animals behaved in constant light or constant dark, or on unusual light/dark schedules. These studies led to general recognition that control of rhythms comes from within but responds to time cues in the environment, most notably light. Some rodents shift rhythms after exposure to a pulse of light only a fraction of a second long. Animals living outside the laboratory rely on changes in day length over the year to tell them when to breed, migrate, and hibernate. In the 1950s, Colin Pittendrigh of Princeton University showed that animals use light rather than temperature to set rhythms, because light is more consistent. December may have hot days and July cool ones, but the sun still rises and sets at predictable times.

The eclipse of the sun on August 11, 1999, provided a good demonstration of light's rule over much of the animal kingdom: birds, horses, and many other creatures living in the path of total darkness went to sleep in the middle of the day. Humans merely banged on drums.

Early studies of humans in windowless time-isolation laboratories in the 1960s appeared to confirm that people relied more on social cues than light to set their body clocks. At the Max Planck Institute in Munich, Germany, subjects never saw clocks. They went to sleep and got up when their bodies said "it's time," a state called free-running, and typically lived on days lasting about twenty-five hours. In an attempt to control subjects' inner clocks, some studies imposed a twenty-four-hour light/dark cycle. Researchers Jürgen Aschoff and Rütger Wever turned ceiling lights on in the period designated as "morning" and then off at "night." They also sounded a gong periodically to tell subjects to provide urine samples.

At first it seemed that subjects responded to the lights. They lived on twenty-four-hour days. Then, soon after the start of one study, the gong system broke down. The subjects soon slipped back into their natural, longer internal cycles. When queried afterward by Wever, they said they had viewed the gongs as personal calls from the researchers. They had anchored their behavior to this social contact rather than to the lights. They also had used the gongs to organize their day, mentally marking off "day gongs 1 to 6" and "one night gong."[6]

Later analysis of these results revealed a surprising fact: when the overhead lights were turned off, the subjects still used their desk lights and other lamps. They simply didn't get strong enough day or night signals. Researchers at the Albert Einstein College of Medicine in New York repeated these studies in 1980, using cyclic alternation of light and total darkness, controlled at some times by the researchers, and at other times by the subjects themselves. Charles Czeisler and his colleagues discovered that body clocks in humans respond to light cues just as those in other animals do.[7] Around the same time, Alfred Lewy of the National Institute of Mental Health and his colleagues found that lights five to ten times brighter than ordinary room lights, the equivalent of natural sunlight just after dawn, could reset human rhythms.[8] These findings meant researchers could start to use light to fix clocks in people with disordered cycles. In more recent studies, Lewy, now at Oregon Health Sciences University; Czeisler, now at Harvard Medical School; and others have found that both the timing and intensity of exposure to the light signal is crucial.

Why You Need a Night-Light

The time at which the body is most sensitive to light comes when body temperature is lowest, around 4 A.M. to 5 A.M. in most people. Light exposure soon after your lowest daily temperature makes your SCN act as if sunrise comes earlier. Light exposure right before your temperature low point makes your SCN act as if sunrise comes later. The further you are from your lowest body temperature, the less impact light has.[9]

Even ordinary room light may have a potent effect when body temperature is lowest. If you awaken at 5 A.M., say, and get out of bed, but plan to return to sleep, it's wise to use a night-light. Flipping on room lights at this time may trick your SCN into thinking you are seeing the sunrise. You may find yourself waking up at 5 A.M. the next morning. If you must get up early for a meeting or a trip, use lights to foster alertness.

Researchers let animals free-run in constant darkness, exposed them briefly to light pulses at different times of day, and plotted their responses. They later did similar studies in humans to assess the effects of different intensities and lengths of light exposure at different times. This information now helps *jet travelers* (see page 143), *shift workers* (see page 164), persons with some *mood disorders* (see page 296), and those with *circadian rhythm sleep disorders* (see page 339).

The importance of light to human health is one of those facts that everyone once knew and then somehow forgot. Florence Nightingale, the foremother of modern nursing, asserted that patients' faces should be turned toward the light. She campaigned for sunrooms and open windows in hospitals.[10] Researchers at the University of Alberta in Edmonton, Canada, recently affirmed Nightingale's bright idea. They found that getting a sunny room rather than a dull one boosts odds of survival in persons admitted to the hospital after suffering heart attacks.[11] It also helps those with depression recover sooner.[12]

Most of us get surprisingly little natural light exposure. In San Diego, one of the nation's sunniest cities, middle-aged adults averaged only fifty-eight minutes of outdoor light a day even in the summer, mostly while going to and from work, researchers at the University of California at San Diego found.[13] UCSD studies suggest people need three to eight hours of bright light exposure to maximally synchronize circadian rhythms.

Light awareness is making a big comeback today, with new attention to providing large windows in hospitals, schools, workplaces, and homes. The tie between light exposure and moods is increasingly well accepted. In Germany, weather reports may proclaim, "Sunny day, expect an elevated mood."[14] Added appreciation for light comes from recent recognition of problems common in blind persons. Even those who use alarm clocks, work regular hours, eat meals at the same time each day, and have other stable habits often still report trouble with sleep and alertness. Alarm clocks and other external time cues literally don't hold a candle to natural daylight.

Social cues do help anchor rhythms, however. This is easy to see while on vacation, when you let go of daily time constraints and allow yourself to stay up late, sleep late, and eat at odd hours. In ordinary life, you can use regular times for meals, medications, and exercise, to help assure a good night's sleep (see page 77), stay on a diet (page 106), improve sports performance (see page 92), and cope better with illness (see page 201).

Signals from the eyes travel on two pathways to the brain in humans and other animals. Conscious vision travels by one route, and circadian vision, the other.[15] Some seemingly sightless animals, such as the blind mole rat, still have normal circadian rhythms. Some blind people also function well on a twenty-four-hour day. They may not consciously recognize light but still may receive circadian clock-setting light information, Elizabeth Klerman and her colleagues at Harvard Medical School found, by measuring the ability of light pulses to alter daily hormonal rhythms in these persons. This finding has made eye surgeons more aware of the need to assess their patients' circadian patterns, and to preserve light-sensitive tissue if possible when they have to remove eyes damaged by injury or disease.

Do We Need Eyes to See Light?

◆ In 1998 researchers at the New York Hospital–Cornell Medical Center astonished colleagues with their report that shining daylight-equivalent bright light on the back of the knee could reset the clock as many as three hours forward or backward.

Scott Campbell and Patricia Murphy chose the back of the knee for their experiment because of its distance from the eye and because blood vessels in the area are close to the skin's surface. Their subjects stayed in a dimly lit suite where they sat periodically in a reclining chair with a lighting device strapped to their blanket-covered legs. The subjects did not know whether or not the light was on.[16]

How the light signal might get from the knee to the brain is not clear. One theory is that light might cause a chemical change transmitted through the blood. Or humans may be more similar than previously believed to other species, such as fruit flies, whose bodies have multiple light receptors that are not involved in vision.

The journal *Science* highlighted these recent findings about biological clocks in its 1998 top ten list of "discoveries that transform ideas about the natural world and also offer potential benefits to society."

Ways to convey light signals to the brain without using the eyes could benefit blind persons, persons with glaucoma or detached retinas who may not be able to use conventional light treatment, and even sighted persons who require light therapy. Much more research will be needed to see if that is possible.

Melatonin Is the Hormone of Darkness, Not of Sleep

Light tells us it is daytime. The hormone melatonin tells us it is night. Both day- and night-active species secrete melatonin mainly in the dark. Melatonin directs humans to get ready for sleep, and nocturnal animals to get ready for activity. Melatonin is not the hormone of sleep. If it were, people wouldn't be able to sleep in the daytime or animals to stay awake at night.

"Melatonin is the time-keeping hormone," explains Alfred Lewy, who has studied it for more than twenty years. It helps reset body rhythms each day, switching our bodies and minds between day mode and night mode. People sleep best when they go to sleep two to three hours after natural melatonin secretion starts, about 9 P.M. Melatonin release peaks around 2 A.M., and starts to shut down before the time we usually awaken.

Melatonin is produced by the pea-sized pineal gland just behind the hypothalamus. Dusk tells the SCN to tell the pineal to turn melatonin secretion on, and at dawn to turn it off. We secrete melatonin longer in the long nights of winter, and for a shorter time in the short nights of summer. Changes from day to day alert animals that days are growing shorter or longer and, if they breed only in certain seasons, that it is the right or wrong time to breed. Melatonin may play a role in human reproduction, too.[17]

Young adults typically secrete a tiny amount of melatonin each day, a quantity that would fit in the period at the end of this sentence, about 5 to 25 micrograms. The smallest doses of melatonin currently sold to consumers, 0.3 and 0.5 milligrams, produce a level in the bloodstream similar to that of natural melatonin. The more widely available 3-milligram dose produces a blood level ten to thirty times higher. Because plants make melatonin, it is a constituent of some foods. But you would have to consume 120 bananas or thirty large bowls of rice at once in order to ingest a 3-milligram dose, according to Richard Wurtman of the Massachusetts Institute of Technology.

The Time Melatonin Is Taken Governs Its Impact

Lewy and others have charted the effects of taking melatonin orally at different times of day, much as they plotted the effects of light exposure around the clock. Since light comes from outside the body, and melatonin from within, these two time cues work together to keep us in sync with the earth's light/dark cycle. The discovery that exposure to light turns off melatonin secretion provides evidence of their interactive relationship.

While light rocks the body clock most in the middle of the night, melatonin in pill form has its greatest impact in the middle of the day. Their complementary relationship has practical importance: jet-lagged travelers, shift workers, and persons with some sleep disorders may be able to use melatonin instead of light, or in addition to it, to reset rhythms.

In the early 1990s, a melatonin craze swept the world, with extravagant claims made that melatonin could help you live longer, cure cancer, improve your sex life, lower cholesterol, and more. Scientists voiced many concerns about potential dangers from its long-term use. Melatonin is a hormone, after all, and hormones have wide-ranging effects throughout the body that may not become apparent for years. Further, many users take amounts that produce much higher blood levels than normally occur in the body. Great Britain, Canada, and many European countries banned melatonin, or made it available only by prescription.

A quirk in U.S. law permits melatonin to be sold directly to consumers. Because melatonin appears in some foods, it's classified as a dietary supplement. The stringent U.S. Food and Drug Administration (FDA) regulations that apply to medications do not apply to food supplements. Unlike manufacturers of medications, makers of melatonin do not have to demonstrate that their products are safe and effective or to monitor their use. By law, the FDA would have to show that melatonin posed "an imminent hazard to public health or safety" to regulate its use.

By the century's end, many scientists' worries had eased. "One doesn't want to be premature about safety," said melatonin researcher Robert Sack of Oregon Health Sciences University, "but millions of people have taken it, and we haven't seen any major adverse side effects." Minor side effects include occasional daytime sleepiness, headaches, and nightmares. Children and teenagers should not take melatonin, as it may delay normal sexual maturation. Melatonin may not be appropriate for you if you have certain illnesses, including depression, migraine headaches, and some eye diseases. If you are considering using melatonin, seek your doctor's guidance first.

Be a Scientist: Study Your Own Body Rhythms

Around the year 1600, the Italian physician Sanctorius built a room-sized scale in his home. He often ate, worked, and slept there, studying changes in his body weight in relation to food consumed and wastes excreted. Sanctorius found that he weighed less in the morning and more at night. He also found that his weight varied over the month. A woodcut from the era shows him dining at a cloth-covered table on his giant scale, nattily dressed in a well-tailored jacket, knee breeches, stockings, and buckled ankle boots.[18]

It's a lot easier today to study your own body rhythms. You can step on a bathroom scale, monitor your diet, chart how many laps you swim or miles you run, and more. Self-measurement is a good way to monitor your health, and to pick up clues early if something goes wrong.

Chronobiologist Robert Sothern takes his temperature and blood pressure, counts his pulse, measures his breathing rate for two minutes, checks his hand-grip strength and dexterity, rates his mood and vigor, and more, five times a day. He also records when he goes to bed and wakes up, and he weighs himself every morning. He has been doing all this every day for more than thirty years.

Sothern was twenty years old in 1967 when he started this process. For the first seventeen years, he also collected urine samples each day, but he now does that only periodically. He records his results in a daily diary and later enters them into a computer, which enable him to analyze his body rhythms.

A student job in a chronobiology laboratory at the University of Minnesota evolved into a lifetime career for Sothern. His data gathering has generated scientific-journal articles, with titles such as "Circadian and Circannual Characteristics of Blood Pressure Self-Measured for 25 Years by a Clinically-Healthy Man." In this article, he reported that his blood pressure maintained consistent daily highs and lows over the years, with modest elevations in spring and fall.[19] Doctors can relate such findings to those in their patients and may, as a result, have less concern about daily or seasonal variations.

There's been a payoff on a personal level. "If I see my temperature is high in the morning, I know something's wrong. If it's high at midnight, I know I won't be able to fall asleep," Sothern said. "When I go to meetings, my blood pressure is always up. It's a reaction to stress, whether real or perceived."

Sothern persuaded his parents to take their own blood pressure twice a day. After reviewing the results, his mother's doctor cut her high blood pressure medication dose in half. Sothern also teaches self-measurement to students, some quite young, to inspire interest in preventive health practices. In one study, ten children aged nine to fourteen successfully measured daily rhythms in their own blood pressure, temperature, mood, ability to add and estimate time, and more, for three weeks in two consecutive years.[20]

Physician William Bean kept tabs on the growth of his left thumbnail for more than thirty-five years, observing its rhythmic growth patterns. On the first of each month, he made a mark on the thumbnail at the free margin of the cuticle. He then calculated how many days it took for the mark to arrive at the free edge of the nail. Early in his studies, he found that measuring one nail allowed the growth rate to be calculated for all. In some 450 months, he forgot to mark the nail only twice.

His nail grew at a steady state, with no seasonal differences. The thumbnail took 146 days to grow out in 1973, nearly five months, and just seven days more in 1977, a modest slow-down with age. Having mumps slowed growth down, but a compensatory speed-up occurred after he had recovered.

Bean, who died in 1989 after practicing in Iowa City for many years, also charted nail growth rhythms in others. He found that nails grow faster in children than in adults, and faster in warm weather than in cold. Biting fingernails makes them grow 20 percent faster, probably because the activity stimulates growth centers in the nail root. Wearing a cast on an arm or leg slows down growth of nails on that hand or foot. A cast on a single finger or toe slows nail growth only on the affected part. Pregnancy makes growth speed up by one-third. In the illness psoriasis, skin cells turn over more rapidly than is normal, and nails grow faster, too. In persons with disorders that constrict blood vessels, nail growth slows down.

Biologist Sue Binkley wanted to see how the environment affects rhythms in people living in the world, not in a laboratory. To examine her own cycles, she wore a small movement-activated recording device on her left wrist for a year. She then plugged the data into a computer.[21]

Binkley's bedroom had a skylight. She kept her windows uncovered and artificial lights turned off. Because of their work schedules, she and her husband set an alarm for between 5 A.M. and 6 A.M. The alarm served merely as a safety net, however, as they usually awakened before it went off, in the dark before dawn, even on weekends.

In her Philadelphia, Pennsylvania, laboratory, Binkley studied sparrows she kept in cages near the windows. The sparrows began their activity with sunrise and stopped at sunset around the year. Binkley's habits, by contrast, changed minimally with the six-hour annual shift in length of daylight.

She awakened about an hour later on average in winter than in summer. Her bedtimes varied more than her wake-up times, as most people's do. Bedtimes varied more in the summer than in the winter, but not nearly as much as in some college students she also monitored, who had shifted their sleep by six to ten hours between weekdays and weekends.

She thought of herself as a morning person, and her records affirmed this, with her most active hours running from about 7:30 A.M. to 2 P.M. Like many people, she got a later start on weekends, though by only about an hour, and followed a more leisurely schedule then.

Aged forty-six at the start of the study, Binkley still had menstrual periods, and did not use contraceptive drugs, chemicals, or devices. Despite her ongoing exposure to the night sky, the phase of the moon had no influence on her menstrual cycles. The day she ovulated usually proved a slow day, with a later wake-up time and less activity than usual.

While the activity monitor Binkley wore is used mainly for academic studies, you can begin to explore rhythmic aspects of your own life with nothing more than paper and pen. The next chapter includes a test to help you figure out how much of a morning or an evening person you are and tells how this particular characteristic may have a more potent influence on your life than you may now suspect.

Are You a Lark, an Owl,
or a Hummingbird?

One in ten of us is an up-at-dawn, raring-to-go early bird, or lark. About two in ten are owls, who enjoy staying up long past midnight. The rest of us, those in the middle, whom we call hummingbirds, may be ready for action both early and late. Some hummingbirds are more larkish and others more owlish.

Animal studies suggest that being a morning person or an evening person may be built into our genes, like having red hair or blue eyes. This may explain why those of us who are early-to-bed, early-to-rise types, or late-to-bed, late-to-rise types, find it so hard to change our behavior.

The *Octodon degu*, a frisky laboratory rodent whose name comes from its curious back teeth, which resemble the number eight when you look down on them, is helping to clarify the role heredity plays in our daily time sense. Degus are rapidly scampering up the research-animal popularity chart because they run around, eat, and socialize in the daytime. This fact appeals to scientists who investigate biological clocks, as they typically work the day shift, too.

Degus love their running wheels and spend hours working out. Some degus run mainly in the morning, others favor the evening, and the rest show no special preference, Susan Labyak of the University of North Carolina and her colleagues found. They were the first to document morning and evening traits in the laboratory in day-active rodents, not specially bred for these characteristics.

Of the forty-nine degus Labyak's group studied, about one in ten was a distinct morning type, its activity peaking around 7 A.M. About two in ten were distinct evening types, most active around 9 P.M. The rest fell somewhere in between. Just like us.

What Type of Bird Are You?

If you like to linger over your coffee to read the morning paper, you're probably more of a lark. Owls often skip breakfast, and they're always rushing to get to work in the morning. Think of Dagwood Bumstead perennially colliding with the hapless mailman as he races out the door, an act so etched in the public consciousness that it is featured on a U.S. postage stamp. If you do laundry or surf the Internet at midnight, you're probably an owl. If you occasionally get up at dawn to go fishing, and sometimes stay up long past your usual bedtime at parties, you're a happy hummingbird.

Some of us think of ourselves as night people, but humans can't truly claim the night as home territory. We are programmed to function best in the daytime. We can't see in the dark. Even if we insist on flip-flopping our schedules to work at night, Mother Nature isn't fooled. Night is still the down time on the body clock. Morningness and eveningness are as far apart as humans get.

Artist Edward Hopper often portrayed these extremes. In *Cape Cod Morning*, a woman already dressed for the day gazes out her living room window at trees bathed in dawn light. In *Nighthawks*, a man and woman in evening clothes sip coffee in an all-night diner.

Lark and owl traits influence many aspects of daily life, including when we feel most alert and when we sleep best. These traits determine when we most enjoy meals, exercise, sex, and other activities. They also affect when we choose to work, or would, if we could.

If you're a lark, you probably wouldn't enjoy a job as a nighttime bartender. If you're an owl, you'd have to struggle to report the morning news. Lark/owl traits may play a bigger role in job choice than most of us suspect. Emergency-room physicians, for example, spend more time working at night throughout their lives than physicians in other specialties. It's no mere coincidence that ER doctors prove to be owls more often than larks. Researchers asked every emergency-medicine resident in the United States taking an annual exam in 1995 to answer a morningness/eveningness survey. Mark Steele and his colleagues at the University of Missouri–Kansas City School of Medicine handed out 2,600 surveys, and got close to 2,000 back. More of the residents tended toward eveningness than is true for the general population.[1]

Most of us adapt pretty well to life's demands. Cartoonist Scott Adams started *Dilbert* while holding a full-time job, penning it between 5 A.M. and 7 A.M. before going to work. Since he made it easy for readers to contact him, putting his E-mail address right on the strip, we wrote him in 1995, shortly after he left Pacific Bell to work on *Dilbert* full-time.

"I'm quite tuned into my rhythms," Adams replied. "I never try to do any creating past noon. And I only exercise in late afternoon. I do the strip from 6 A.M. to 7 A.M. Then I write for a few hours. I only ink the strip afternoons or evenings when my hand is steady. I can't ink in the morning."

"I created my second career," he claimed, "by 'discovering' the morning."

In 1999, *Dilbert* made its television debut. We wrote Adams again to see whether his life had changed. "My schedule is completely reversed now, because of working with Hollywood," he reported. "They're night owls. So I sleep until 7 A.M. and work off and on until midnight most nights. But I still don't do creative work in midafternoon. I do my mindless stuff, like inking or scanning then."[2]

Like Adams, most of us view our schedules as a compromise between what we have to do and what we would like to do. Most people say they would like to sleep later, for example. College students who seldom go to bed before 2 A.M. almost certainly will turn off the lights earlier after they graduate and enter the daytime workforce, and they will become even more larkish after they become parents. They might complain, but most will manage. By the time they are in their sixties and older, most will be comfortable going to sleep and getting up earlier than they did when younger. All of us might feel and function better, though, if we could synchronize more of our required activities with our natural rhythms throughout our lives.

Indeed, the recent rise of flextime schedules in the workplace, allowing workers to start and stop as much as two or three hours earlier or later, as they wish, is a positive step in this direction. One in five full-time American workers now has flexible hours. (See chapter 13: "Clockwatching at Work.")

A gene may govern owlish behavior in humans. Daniel Katzenberg of Stanford University and his colleagues assessed morningness/eveningness traits in 410 randomly sampled adults with a questionnaire. They also drew blood samples from the respondents and examined the makeup of a gene called *Clock* known to exert influence over biological rhythms. Comparing results from the two tests, they estimated that the owls lagged ten to forty-four minutes behind larks in their preferred times for various activities and for sleep, a significant difference. Moreover, a particular pattern consistently appeared in part of the *Clock* gene in owls, but not in larks.[3] Genetic studies such as this may prove a two-edged sword. Potentially, they could help workers decide which jobs suit them best. But they also could be used to discriminate against workers whose genetic traits do not correspond to an employer's criteria. That would be unfortunate, because lark/owl tendencies do not rule most people's lives. High motivation for all but extreme larks and owls probably has a much bigger impact on job success.

THE OWL/LARK SELF-TEST

Take the test below to discover what type of bird you are. Answer according to your preferences on your days off, regardless of the shift on which you currently are working.

Instructions:

- Answer all questions in numerical order.
- Answer each question independently of others. Do not go back and check your answers.
- Select one answer only. Some questions have a scale. Place a mark at the appropriate point along the scale.

1. Considering only your own "feeling best" rhythm, at what time would you get up if you were entirely free to plan your day?

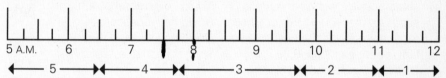

2. Considering only your own "feeling best" rhythm, at what time would you go to bed if you were entirely free to plan your evening?

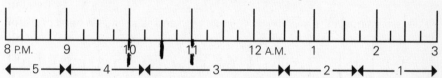

3. If there is a specific time at which you have to get up in the morning, to what extent are you dependent on being woken up by an alarm clock?

Not at all dependent. . . . . ☐ 4
Slightly dependent. . . . . ☐ 3
Fairly dependent. . . . . ☒ 2
Very dependent. . . . . ☐ 1

4. Assuming adequate environmental conditions, how easy do you find getting up in the mornings?

Not at all easy. . . . . ☐ 1
Not very easy. . . . . ☐ 2
Fairly easy. . . . . ☒ 3
Very easy. . . . . ☐ 4

5. How alert do you feel during the first half hour after having woken in the mornings?

Not at all alert. . . . . ☐ 1
Slightly alert. . . . . ☐ 2
Fairly alert. . . . . ☒ 3
Very alert. . . . . ☐ 4

6. How is your appetite during the first half hour after having woken in the mornings?

- Very poor. . . . . ☐ 1
- Fairly poor. . . . . ☐ 2
- Fairly good. . . . . ☒ 3
- Very good. . . . . ☐ 4

7. During the first half hour after having woken in the morning, how tired do you feel?

- Very tired. . . . . ☐ 1
- Fairly Tired. . . . . ☐ 2
- Fairly refreshed. . . . . ☒ 3
- Very refreshed. . . . . ☐ 4

8. When you have no commitments the next day, at what time do you go to bed compared to your usual bedtime?

- Seldom or never later. . . . . ☐ 4
- Less than one hour later. . . . . . ☐ 3
- 1–2 hours later. . . . . ☒ 2
- More than two hours later. . . . . ☐ 1

9. You have decided to engage in some physical exercise. A friend suggests that you do this one hour twice a week and the best time for him is between 7:00–8:00 A.M. Bearing in mind nothing else but your own "feeling best" rhythm, how do you think you would perform?

- Would be in good form. . . . . . . ☐ 4
- Would be in reasonable form. . . ☒ 3
- Would find it difficult. . . . . ☐ 2
- Would find it very difficult. . . . . ☐ 1

10. At what time in the evening do you feel tired and as a result in need of sleep?

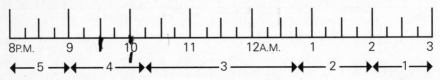

11. You wish to be at your peak performance for a test which you know is going to be mentally exhausting and lasting for two hours. You are entirely free to plan your day and considering only your own "feeling best" rhythm, which ONE of the four testing times would you choose?

- 8:00–10:00 A.M. . . . . ☒ 6
- 11:00 A.M.–1:00 P.M. . . . . ☒ 4
- 3:00–5:00 P.M. . . . . ☐ 2
- 7:00–9:00 P.M. . . . . ☐ 0

12. If you went to bed at 11:00 P.M., at what level of tiredness would you be?

- Not at all tired. . . . . ☐ 0
- A little tired. . . . . ☐ 2
- Fairly tired. . . . . ☒ 3
- Very tired. . . . . ☐ 5

13. For some reason you have gone to bed several hours later than usual, but there is no need to get up at any particular time the next morning. Which ONE of the following events are you most likely to experience?

Will wake up at usual time and will NOT fall asleep again. . . . ☐ 4
Will wake up at usual time and will doze thereafter. . . . . ☒ 3
Will wake up at usual time but will fall asleep again. . . . . . . ☒ 2
Will NOT wake up until later than usual. . . . . ☐ 1

14. One night you have to remain awake between 4:00 and 6:00 A.M. in order to carry out a night watch. You have no commitments the next day. Which ONE of the following alternatives will suit you best?

Would NOT go to bed until watch was over. . . . . ☐ 1
Would take a nap before and sleep after. . . . . ☐ 2
Would take a good sleep before and nap after. . . . . ☒ 3
Would take ALL sleep before watch. . . . . ☐ 4

15. You have to do two hours of hard physical work. You are entirely free to plan your day and considering only your own "feeling best" rhythm, which ONE of the following times would you choose?

8:00–10:00 A.M. . . . . ☒ 4
11:00 A.M.–1:00 P.M. . . . . ☒ 3
3:00–5:00 P.M. . . . . ☐ 2
7:00–9:00 P.M. . . . . ☐ 1

16. You have decided to engage in hard physical exercise. A friend suggests that you do this for one hour twice a week and the best time for him is between 10:00–11:00 P.M. Bearing in mind nothing else but your own "feeling best" rhythm, how well do you think you would perform?

Would be in good form. . . . . ☐ 1
Would be in reasonable form. . . ☐ 2
Would find it difficult. . . . . ☐ 3
Would find it very difficult. . . . . . ☒ 4

17. Suppose that you can choose your own work hours. Assume that you worked a FIVE-hour day (including breaks) and that your job was interesting and paid by results. Which FIVE CONSECUTIVE HOURS would you select?

12 1 2 3 4 5 6 7 8 9 10 11 12 1 2 3 4 5 6 7 8 9 10 11 12
MIDNIGHT   NOON   MIDNIGHT

← 1 →◄► 5 → 4 ← 3 →◄► 2 →◄► 1 →

18. At what time of the day do you think that you reach your "feeling best" peak?

| | | | | | | | | | | | ■■■ | | | | | | | | | | | | |

12 1 2 3 4 5 6 7 8 9 10 11 12 1 2 3 4 5 6 7 8 9 10 11 12
MIDNIGHT   NOON   MIDNIGHT

←— 1 —►◄—5—►◄—4—►◄————3————►◄—2—►◄—1—→

19. One hears about "morning" and "evening" types of people. Which ONE of these types do you consider yourself to be?

Definitely a "morning" type?. . .☐ 6
Rather more a "morning" than an "evening" type. . . . .☒ 4
Rather more an "evening" than a "morning" type. . . . . .☐ 2
Definitely an "evening" type. . . .☐ 0

Scoring:
- The score for each response is beside the answer box or in a range below the scale. For question 17, use the most extreme mark on the right-hand side to find your score on the range below.
- Total your scores and compare them to the scale below.

Definitely Morning Type	70–86
★ Moderately Morning Type	59–69
Neither Type	42–58
Moderately Evening Type	31–41
Definitely Evening Type	16–30

Adapted from "A Self-Assessment Questionnaire to Determine Morningness-Eveningness in Human Circadian Rhythms," by James Horne and Olov Ostberg. *International Journal of Chronobiology*. London, England: Gordon and Breach Science Publishers Ltd., 1976:4:97–110. (Reprinted with permission.)

Punch Your Own Time Clock

Media magnate Michael Bloomberg gets going early. His larkish habits, he claims, gave him a leg up when he was just starting out. One summer while in business school, he worked for a real estate company in Cambridge, Massachusetts. Students would come to town seeking apartments for the fall, get up early to check the ads, and call for appointments to see the rentals. Bloomberg, who went to work at 6:30 A.M., was the only one in the office at the time and captured the lion's share of the student market.

After graduating, he landed a job at Salomon Brothers, the Wall Street investment house. "I came in every morning at 7 A.M., getting there before everyone else except [managing partner] Billy Salomon," Bloomberg relates in his autobiography. "When he needed to borrow a match or talk sports, I was the only other person in the trading room and he talked to me. At age twenty-six," Bloomberg said, "I became a buddy of the managing partner."[4]

Microsoft founder Bill Gates is a legendary night owl. While still a student at Harvard in 1975, Gates and his friend Paul Allen wrote their first recipe for software, working at a frenzied round-the-clock pace for five weeks. "We'd fall asleep on the terminal sometimes," Gates told Barbara Walters on *20/20*. "We were totally focused on getting this done."[5]

Late hours are the norm in Silicon Valley, where even computer stores sell food, aspirin, and other necessities, so techies don't have to leave their monitors for long. Journalist Katie Hafner called her book about the advent of the Internet *Where Wizards Stay Up Late.*[6]

Advice columnist Ann Landers, another owl, reports she takes the phone off the hook in her sleeping hours, 1 A.M. to 10 A.M. "No one's going to call me," she asserts, "until I'm ready."[7] Writer Henry Miller assessed the impact of time of day on his work: "I prefer the morning now, and just for two or three hours," he wrote. "In the beginning I used to work after midnight until dawn, but that was at the very beginning. Even after I got to Paris I found it was much better working in the morning."[8] The freelance life suits Washington, D.C., area writer Pat McNees. "I fall asleep right on the dot of 2 A.M. most nights. Given no reason to do otherwise, I wake up at 10 A.M. or a few minutes before," she reports. "My office answering machine says that my office hours begin at 10, which is true; I will have just walked the twenty feet from my bed to my office in my nightgown."[9]

"My formative years were spent in a job that demanded long hours and great discipline," relates Greg Howard, creator of the comic strip *Sally Forth*. He practiced law for ten years before embarking on his second career. "By the time I quit to take a fling at cartooning, my work habits had apparently been etched somewhere deep in my cerebellum. Try as I might," Howard said, "I have not been able to adopt the unconventional schedule people seem to expect of cartoonists. Acquaintances are routinely disappointed to learn that

I do not work in all-night bursts of right-brain frenzy." His work hours, Howard said, are "from 8 A.M. to when I'm done."[10]

Dozens of academic studies affirm that differences between persons at the extremes of the morningness/eveningness scale are not trivial. Going beyond questionnaires, chronobiologists now often use a technique they call "constant routines." Subjects stay awake for twenty-four to thirty-six hours in dim light. They rest comfortably in recliners, eat small identical meals at hourly intervals, and are taken to the bathroom in a wheelchair roughly every three hours. The aim of these studies is to strip away the effects of sleep, physical activity, and light, and to equalize the influence of meals, effectively distributing body rhythms evenly across the circadian cycle. Such studies act like a colored highlighter on a printed page, making the natural rhythms of the body stand out from daily behavior.

In a study at Leiden University in the Netherlands, Hans Van Dongen followed students who showed pronounced lark or owl traits in both their normal daily lives and in a constant routine study. University students are popular as research subjects for such studies because they can organize their days pretty much as they wish.

Van Dongen found that the larks and owls were as different as, well, day and night. The differences are part of each person's makeup, he said, not simply a reflection of daily activity.[11] We've combined findings from Van Dongen's and other researchers' studies[12] to show the many ways in which larks and owls differ.

How Larks and Owls Differ

Characteristic	Larks	Owls
Most alert (self-report)	Around noon	Around 6 P.M.
Most productive (self-report)	Late morning	Late morning and late evening
Most active	Around 2:30 P.M.	Around 5:30 P.M.
Best mood	Between 9 A.M. and 4 P.M.	Steady rise from about 8 A.M. to 10 P.M.
Temperature highest	Around 3:30 P.M.	Around 8 P.M.
Age	Most persons over age 60	Most college students and twentysomethings
Bedtime	Go to bed two hours earlier than owls; fall asleep faster	More variable bedtimes; stay up later on weekends and holidays
Waketime	Awaken at desired time	Awaken about same time as larks on workdays, 1–2 hours later on days off

Characteristic	Larks	Owls
Use of alarm clock	Don't need it	Need multiple alarms
Temperature lowest	Around 3:30 A.M.	Around 6 A.M.
Quality of sleep	Lifelong: sleep more soundly; wake up more refreshed, usually 3.4 hours after temperature minimum, daily low point on body clock	Lifelong: get less sleep wake up sleepier, usually 2.5 hours after temperature minimum
Nap	Rarely	Take more and longer naps; fall asleep more easily in daytime
Mid-sleep time	Around 3:30 A.M.	Around 6 A.M.
Favorite exercise time	Morning	Evening
Peak heart rate	Around 11 A.M.	Around 6 P.M.
Lowest heart rate	Around 3 A.M.	Around 7 A.M.
Mood	Mood declines slightly over day	Mood rises substantially over day
Morning behavior	Chatty	Bearish
Evening behavior	Out of steam	Full of energy
Mealtimes	Eat breakfast 1–2 hours earlier than owls	Often skip breakfast; eat other meals at same times as larks on workdays, 90 minutes later on days off
Favorite meal	Breakfast	Dinner
Daily caffeine use	Cups	Pots
Personality	More introverted? (Still debated)	More extroverted? (Still debated)
Shift-work adaptability	Work best on day shifts	Work best on evening shifts; tolerate night and rotating shift work better
Travel	More jet lag	Adapt faster to time-zone changes, particularly going west
Partner's report (If well-matched)	We like to get an early start	We are the last to go home
Partner complaint (If mismatched)	He/she stays up too late	She/he won't let me sleep late on weekends
Peak melatonin secretion	About 3:30 A.M.	About 5:30 A.M.

Can Larks and Owls Happily Share a Nest?

In the comic strip *Sally Forth*, Sally, a night owl, and husband Ted, a lark, often bump into each other's circadian rhythms. In one strip, Sally leans over the sink, still in her bathrobe, her hair frowzy from sleep. Ted chatters away: "It's so nice this morning. I even exercised in the backyard, even ate breakfast out there, read the paper. The market's up ten points. Did you hear about the Twins' game last night? It was great! Bottom of the ninth, runners at . . ." Sally interrupts: "You morning people should wear warning labels so we night people can tell who you are before we marry you."

Greg Howard, *Sally Forth*'s creator, acknowledges that he deliberately imbued Sally and Ted with disparate body rhythms. "I did not pattern them after my wife, Joanne, and me," he told us. "*Sally Forth* is, as Joanne must constantly remind her coworkers, a work of fiction. I like the owl/lark tension in the strip but do not live it myself."

Howard reports that he and his wife "have, virtually every day of our thirty-three years as yokemates, gotten up within ten or fifteen minutes of each other. And, if you don't count Joanne's occasional evening snoozes on the couch, we go to sleep at the same time every night. We got married young and have more or less grown up together. As often happens with longtime couples, our habits have melded so that we can no longer even recall who conformed to whom along the way.

"You're probably thinking, 'How dreadfully drab,' " Howard adds. "The only thing I can offer in our defense is that we have not yet succumbed to his-and-her outfits."[13]

Most couples in which one partner is a lark and the other an owl are not this compatible. Human resources specialist and self-described night owl Carolyn Schur surveyed more than 400 persons for her book *Birds of a Different Feather: Early Birds and Night Owls Talk about Their Characteristic Behaviors.* Owl/lark differences can wreak havoc on a marriage, Schur suggests, if a spouse ascribes motives to the other's behavior. "You don't love me because you won't get up to have breakfast with me," a lark might say. "If you were really interested in what I like doing," an owl might assert, "you would come with me this evening." Thriving couples, she found, accepted each other's differences and found ways to adapt. They might tape television shows, for example, and watch them together at a mutually satisfactory time.[14]

If a couple differs about how to celebrate religious holidays, Schur said, it's an issue once a year. If money is the problem, partners may argue once a week or once a month. But if daily body rhythms and schedules don't mesh, couples may clash many times a day, over issues as different as mealtimes, bedtimes, shopping, and child care.

"We have a baby," one woman told Schur. "At 9 P.M., my husband will say,

'Let's go to a movie.' 'What are we going to do with the baby?' I ask. 'Take her with us,' he'll say. 'Over my dead body' is my response."

Others report: "My husband gets to the store before it opens, so he can get started with his planned chores as soon as possible." "My wife is a grouch in the morning." "I've never been to brunch with my husband. He's not up early enough."

Couples with mismatched body rhythms, some studies show, rate their marriages as less satisfactory than do those who are well matched. Brigham Young University psychologist Jeffry Larson and his colleagues surveyed 150 middle-class couples in three states about their lark/owl preferences. Most were in their late twenties, had been married about six years on average, and had two children. Most had at least some college education.

Eighty-two of the couples were mismatched in their morningness and eveningness, Larson's team found. Of this group, one couple in three reported difficulties in their marriage, arguing more often each week than well-matched couples did. Among the sixty-eight well-matched couples, only one in twelve reported marital troubles. The matched couples spent nearly an hour a day on serious conversation, about fifteen minutes more than the mismatched couples. The matched couples spent nearly seven hours a week on shared activities, while mismatched couples spent less than three hours doing things together.

The couples in which both partners were larks had sexual intercourse more often in the morning, and couples in which both partners were owls favored the night. Overall, however, both lark and owl couples had sex more often at night than in the morning, twice a week, on average. Choice of the nighttime, Larson notes, may reflect social norms about the "right" time for sex or lack of privacy in the morning common to parents with young children, or perhaps just a need to get to work on time. The mismatched couples had sex slightly less frequently than the matched couples.

Since married couples generally expect shared activity and communication, Larson says, being matched generally increases marital adjustment and satisfaction. Partners in matched couples still need to find time for themselves, while mismatched couples need to find ways to create togetherness, so that neither spouse feels lonely. A preference for morning or nighttime activities may be the consequence as well as the cause of problems in a marriage. One spouse may go to bed early—or stay up late—to avoid the other.

Mismatched couples who reported happy marriages, Larson's group found, reported more flexibility in problem solving than matched couples did. "Perhaps only very committed and otherwise well-matched couples with good problem-solving skills," Larson suggests, "can handle the problems their mismatched rhythms cause in the marriage."[15]

A study at the University of Amsterdam also affirms the benefits of compromise. Couples who went to sleep and got up at the same times, even if this required some adjustment, expressed more affection, were more satisfied with their relationship, shared more common activities, were more adept at solving problems, and were more satisfied with their sexual relationship, Alfred Lange and his colleagues found, than couples who kept different schedules.[16]

These findings suggest that couples contemplating long-term relationships need to explore the "goodness of fit" of their body rhythms, in the same way they might address issues of religion, work, and child rearing. Treating a troubled marriage by reconciling differences in partners' lark or owl natures gives an additional meaning to the term *chronotherapy.*

Mismatched couples may claim some advantages, particularly in child rearing. One parent may read bedtime stories, while the other prepares breakfast and drives the morning school carpool. On trips, one partner may drive early in the day, and the other later on.

Lark/Owl Traits Affect Family Life

Our lark/owl tendencies may show up in early childhood, further evidence that *chronotypes* are part of our inborn biological makeup. The toddler who is a lark may drag her blanket around early in the evening, showing she is ready for sleep. According to sleep specialist Richard Ferber of Children's Hospital in Boston, this same child may bounce out of bed early in the morning, "too early," her parents wail. A two-year-old owl may balk at going to bed. Another game, another story, another drink: he resists settling down. He needs a regular schedule, Ferber says, with dependable, quiet bedtime rituals. Travel, illness, and visitors in the house often disrupt sleep in little owls—and in older ones, too.

Preadolescent children tend to be more larkish than their parents, while teenagers are notorious owls. The elementary school lark will go to the kitchen to make her own breakfast, while an owl the same age is apt to read under the covers with a flashlight. Parents of a young lark may need to set out breakfast cereal the night before, instruct the child in how to use the microwave oven, toaster, and knives, and issue stern warnings about not venturing out of the house. Parents of a young owl may need to help pick out the next day's clothes the night before, pack up books and papers and leave them by the door, and patiently issue repeated wake-up calls in the morning.

Like well-matched couples, families in which parents and children have similar morningness or eveningness traits report more joint family activities and less friction than families with greater differences.

Researchers at the University of Utah identified thirty-one persons in two families who were extreme larks. They included young children, teenagers, and middle-aged and older adults who went to sleep around 7 P.M. and got up around 3 A.M. This wasn't just a habit. Most had attempted, without success, to change their sleep patterns.

The lark trait was passed from one generation to the next in an autosomal dominant pattern, meaning that either a father or mother with the trait likely would pass it on to half of his or her children. Members of the same families who lacked this inherited trait observed more traditional schedules.

Some of the larks liked getting up early, according to neurologist Christopher Jones, who profiled the family members, while others stressed that they missed being able to participate in social events in the evening.[17]

Are Larks Healthier and Wealthier?

Think of Benjamin Franklin's axiom: "Early to bed, early to rise, makes a man healthy, wealthy, and wise."

This comes from the man who discovered how to harness electricity, making it easy for us to stay up as late as we want. Franklin also reputedly was a bon vivant who was fond of late-night partying. It may not matter that he did not practice what he preached. But was he right?

A team of British researchers decided they would try to find out. In 1996 they examined records from a government study conducted in 1973 and 1974. More than 1,200 persons sixty-five and older had participated in this study, which evaluated their sleep patterns, health, socioeconomic status, and cognitive function. Most then were followed for the rest of their lives. Twenty-three years after the study began, about sixty were still alive.[18]

About three out of ten persons in the original group met the researchers' criteria for larks: to bed before 11 P.M. and up before 8 A.M. Nearly the same number were owls who went to bed at or after 11 P.M., and got up at or after 8 A.M. The rest kept less regular hours. Both the lark and owl groups contained a similar proportion of men and women. The larks proved no healthier at the time of the initial study than persons with other sleeping habits. As the years passed, this fact did not change.

Catharine Gale and Christopher Martyn of Southampton University also found no evidence that larks were richer than owls or persons with more varied sleeping patterns. The owls, in fact, made more money.

Whether larks or owls are wiser is still an open question. Both groups earned comparable scores on a mental performance test given at the study's start. This short test, the researchers conceded, probably doesn't embody the full meaning of the word "wise."

The bottom line: Franklin's pithy advice, while easy to say, lacks evidence to support it.

Timewise Tips

Larks who want to live more like owls and owls who want to live more like larks can take advantage of recent research on the biological clock to ease that task. These tips won't change your basic makeup—that's not possible—but they can help you adapt more comfortably to situational demands. (See also Timewise Tips for Good Sleep, page 77.)

If you are a lark:
Spend time outside in the afternoon or early evening. This tactic should help you stay up later, and may help you sleep later in the morning, too. It's especially helpful to older persons, who often go to bed as early as 8 P.M. and find themselves awake, with nothing to do, at 3 A.M.

Increase evening activity. A walk or light stretching will promote alertness. Socializing is more energizing than reading or watching TV.

Sleep with blinds or curtains closed. Consider purchasing "black-out" drapes. Darkness tells your brain it's nighttime, the right time for sleep.

Leave a dim night-light on in hallways or a bathroom in case you have to get up at night.

See a doctor if you can't stay awake in the evening until a reasonable "social" bedtime, at least 9 P.M., and if you always awaken around 3 A.M. or 4 A.M. and are unable to return to sleep. If this habit developed over the years, particularly late in life, you may have a condition called the Advanced Sleep Phase Syndrome. (See Sleep Disorders, page 344.)

If you are an owl:
Sleep with blinds or curtains open, and let daylight awaken you naturally. It's a gentle process and much easier to take than the annoying bleat of an alarm clock. Set the alarm anyway. Hey, set two alarms, for safety's sake.

Walk outside as soon as possible after waking up. Exposure to daylight in the morning can make you more alert earlier in the day. One sleep specialist tells his patients, "Take your dental floss and step outside." Since owls often leave things to the last minute, it may be hard to get up in time to have breakfast outdoors or to take a twenty-minute walk. Trick yourself by setting the clock a few minutes fast. Close your eyes when you do it, so you won't know if the clock is five minutes or fifteen minutes fast. When rushing in the morning, you'll have a small safety net, but not enough to start making allowances for it. If you can't go outside immediately, have your morning coffee by the sunniest window in your home or use a lighting device that provides artificial light of daylight intensity.

Get up at the same time every day, including weekends and holidays. This tactic will anchor your biological clock at the desired time. If you go to sleep late one night, don't sleep in the next morning. Compensate for missed sleep with a twenty-minute midafternoon nap unless you find naps leave you foggy. In that case, go to bed fifteen minutes earlier the next night.

Do as much as you can the night before. Select the next day's clothes, put cereal boxes on the breakfast table, prepare school lunches. A morning routine helps owls function smoothly without having to think about what they're doing. If you're sleepy, rote behavior fills time until you're more alert.

Keep evenings quiet. Don't exercise, start new projects, or look at TV "for just a few minutes" late at night. Reading, listening to music, and similar activities are good preludes to sleep. Have a regular bedtime snack such as milk or fruit. This ritual also helps program your body for bed.

Use dim lights at night in the bathroom to avoid giving yourself a middle-of-the-night wake-up call the next night.

See a doctor if you can't fall asleep before 3 A.M. or 4 A.M., and if you could sleep until noon or later if permitted to do so. You may have a condition called the Delayed Sleep Phase Syndrome. (See Sleep Disorders, page 342.)

Tips for couples and families:

Civility is the key to getting along despite individual differences, according to Judith Martin, who writes the popular syndicated *Miss Manners* column. "Miss Manners never excuses rudeness at any hour or under any circumstances," she says. But she excuses evening people from sociability until they have had their coffee. "Everybody who is ambulatory," she maintains, "is required to say, 'Good morning,' and to pass the sugar when asked and to reply to comments and questions addressed to them. . . . Being excused from sociability means that they may reply only by making 'Umm' and 'Uh' noises with the mouth closed, and need not offer conversational encouragement."[19]

Summing Up

If you are right-handed, you may be able to learn to use your left hand. A Type A personality may learn to relax. An overweight person can slim down. In the same way, most larks and owls can manage most schedules as their jobs, families, or social lives demand. Some will feel more dissonance than others when they try to follow clocks at variance with their natural proclivities. Extreme larks and owls report the most problems. They may find it difficult, if not impossible, to function in some situations. They are not sick. They are not lazy. They are not lacking in motivation. Happily, in our increasingly twenty-four-hour world, there are plenty of spots where most larks, owls, and hummingbirds can find a secure perch.

Your Mind at Work

At your daily highs, you're fully alert. You feel confident and energetic. At your daily lows, you may perform as poorly as you would after drinking three or four glasses of wine, or after getting only three hours' sleep. Your mental ability on some tasks varies over the twenty-four-hour day by 20 to 30 percent.

This difference from high to low might make or break a sale, put muscle on limp prose or leave it flaccid. If you're a student, it might swing a test grade from a B to a C. The ease with which you perform specific tasks reflects not only your knowledge or skills but also daily rhythms of alertness and sleepiness, which wax and wane in predictable fashion around the clock.

Since research on the biological clock began in earnest in the twentieth century, scientists have measured many skills needed in everyday intellectual tasks. Studies asked: Is there a best time to write a report, plan an event, hold a meeting? When is it easiest to study math? Is this different from the best time to study languages or literature? When is the best time to balance your checkbook? To ask your boss for a raise?

Most studies targeted the usual daytime hours for school and work, mainly 9 A.M. to 6 P.M. Some produced practical advice, suggesting that mornings are best for writing, for example, or that 11 A.M. is the ideal time to hold meetings. These findings reflect experiences of about eight in ten people who work on the traditional daytime schedule, but may not apply to those working evenings and nights. With more and more people working outside the daytime hours, researchers are beginning to explore peak performance times around the clock.

Science Yields New Spin on "Best Times"

The latest findings offer a new and more empowering perspective. Instead of focusing on specific clock hours, today's answer to "When is the best time for . . . ?" is "It depends." The big message now is, "Don't worry about societal averages. Do what you want to do, when it is convenient to do it," asserts Hans Van Dongen of the University of Pennsylvania.

Van Dongen and other researchers say you can do most mental tasks equally well over most of your waking day, provided you expend the necessary effort, and that you got a decent amount of sleep the night before. There's quite a large window for optimal performance of mental tasks. It's open from about 10 A.M. to 10 P.M. for most people, starting about two to three hours after you wake up, when the fogginess of sleep wears off. It winds down a couple of hours before you usually go to sleep. It starts and ends a little earlier for extreme larks, and starts and ends a little later for extreme owls.

Within this window, Van Dongen asserts, alertness is high. The "best" time to do most tasks depends less on the type of task than on your being able to create optimal conditions for doing the task.

If you work a 9 to 5 schedule in a busy office where phones ring nonstop in the morning, and people constantly interrupt you with queries related to their own projects, don't try to analyze a complex report at that time. Wait until later, when things quiet down, assuming that they *do* quiet down. You may need to stay after 5 P.M. to create prime thinking time. If you're an extreme morning-type person, you might come in early, before the others show up. Ideally, you'd find a way to protect yourself from interruptions in the workday, but we all know that's often not feasible. If your task requires resources at a bank or a library, you'll have to tailor your schedule to their hours.

Early researchers thought body temperature and alertness worked in tandem, that is, that alertness was highest when temperature is highest. Some proposed that people's fitness for work could be assessed simply by taking their temperature. But temperature recordings from large numbers of people showed that temperature typically is highest around 7 P.M. or 8 P.M., not the time when most of us report feeling our sharpest. Most people say their peak alertness comes around noon. Even extreme owls report peak alertness around 6 P.M.

It's only when people stay awake at night that the low point of performance and temperature coincide.[1] People think more slowly then. If you work at night, anticipate that performance on comparable tasks will fall below that achieved in the daytime. In a study at the University of Pittsburgh, Timothy Monk and Julie Carrier gave young adults a test of reasoning skill every two hours around the clock for thirty-six hours. One test presented positive or negative statements in random order. The participants had to tell whether each statement was correct. "C is before M—CM," is true, for example, while "M is not before C—MC" is false. The computer recorded the speed and accuracy of their answers.

On the first day, the subjects took about three seconds to respond to the positive sentences, but about four seconds to answer the negative ones, which were both longer and trickier. That night, the subjects needed only a fraction of a second more to handle the positive statements but an extra second to respond to the negative ones. On the second day, after more than twenty-four hours without sleep, the subjects responded more slowly than they did the previous day. But they still solved the problems faster than they did the night before.[2]

This study adds to a great body of evidence showing that night is the "down" time on the body's biological clock. It's still not clear whether the brain takes longer to handle complex problems at night or simply uses a different strategy then.

Most of us know from personal experience that we are more alert in the daytime and sleepier at night. In college, for instance, we stayed up all night to finish a paper. In the predawn hours, we kept nodding off, but when morning came we perked up. The rest of that day, we felt more alert than we did in the middle of the previous night, despite going many hours longer without sleep. The biological clock controls this rhythm. Had we stayed awake a second night, we probably would have been nearly overwhelmed by sleep. Had we managed to stay up, we would have regained some alertness the next morning.

In times of emergency, such as earthquakes or hurricanes, rescue workers, doctors, firefighters, police, and many others, often thousands of workers in all, pull all-nighters, and may not stop for sleep for two or even three days. Their work is physically demanding, dangerous, and emotionally draining, and alertness and good judgment are paramount. Such situations require good management of schedules, and have benefited from recent advances in understanding how body time alters performance. (See chapter 13: "Clock-watching at Work.")

Effort Determines Mental Performance

Despite these findings, it's clear that the biological clock is not the only determinant of daytime mental performance. It is not even the most critical one, Monk says. If trying your hardest, he says, you'll likely do better than if your zeal is halfhearted. Outside influences affect resolve, too. When given feedback, people work harder, a tactic smart bosses, teachers, parents, and athletic coaches often put to good use.

Motivation combined with effort interacts with the alertness and sleepiness rhythm this way: alertness typically heightens the drive to perform a task, while sleepiness dampens it. If you have ever put off paying bills or other mental chores until late in the evening, you know that sleepiness makes it easy to postpone the job. On the other hand, you can be highly motivated and highly alert, yet in a supercharged state that makes simple tasks daunting. Consider how hard it is to unlock your car door or dial a phone in an emergency.

Testing Is Tricky

Many research studies test the same people at different times of day. But this approach raises concerns about the impact of practice. If subjects remember lists of words better in the afternoon than in the morning, is their biological clock responsible, or have they just become better test-takers?

You may think that after reaching a certain level of expertise, people don't continue to improve. Chess masters, golfers, and musicians among others would take exception to that. Even for ordinary folks, it may take a long time to reach a personal "best," longer than most test situations permit.

In one study, a man living in a time-isolation laboratory had to perform a relatively simple test of decision making: to sort a deck of ninety-six playing cards into hearts, clubs, spades, and diamonds. The man lived in the laboratory for six months, and he sorted cards six times a day every day. Four months passed before he reached his top speed. By then, he had sorted the cards more than 750 times.[3]

Researchers sometimes give tests at different times of day but switch the order in which they give the tests. Some persons might take a test first in the morning, and others first in the afternoon or evening. In some studies, researchers also switch subjects' sleep schedules, so that a person might sleep, for example, from 7 A.M. to 3 P.M. For that person, 3 P.M. would feel like morning.

Fatigue alters test results. When weary, whatever the time of day, we often persist in trying clearly useless tactics. You might keep hitting your computer's "escape" key when the screen freezes, for example, instead of trying another key combination.

Researchers also run into the "Hawthorne effect." In the 1920s, scientists installed different intensity lights at Western Electric's Hawthorne Works plant in Cicero, Illinois. In some instances, they merely replaced the lights with identical lights. But every time they fiddled with the lights, workers' productivity went up. The workers responded positively to what they perceived as management's interest in improving their working conditions. The term "Hawthorne effect" lives on as shorthand for saying that any aspect of a research situation may alter its outcome: actual time of day, biological time, mood, interest, fatigue, the heat, the humidity, what people had for lunch, and even the researcher's own preconceptions about the results.

Memory Skills Change over the Day

You look up a number in the phone book and dial. You get a busy signal. Can you redial without looking at the phone book again? You pull into a gas station to get directions. "Third light, turn right. Second light, turn left." How well can you retain what you hear? You meet new people at a party. Can you recall their names a few minutes later? These tasks demand *immediate* or *short-term memory*, holding onto information long enough to use it. We need this mental skill dozens of times every day.

Now suppose you want to understand a legal ruling so you can make use of it in an upcoming trial, read a book and discuss it later, or learn a new language. Retaining these tasks requires *long-term memory*.

Early studies suggested both that you may have better immediate recall for material you learn in the morning, and that you may retain longer in your memory bank material you learn in the afternoon.

In an often-cited 1977 classroom study, British researchers read a story to one group of schoolchildren at 9 A.M., and to another group at 3 P.M. They then tested the children's memory for details of the story. When tested immediately, the morning group did best. When tested a week later, the afternoon group remembered more, Simon Folkard of the University of Wales and his colleagues found.[4]

Later research added new complexity to this picture. The strategies for learning that people bring to the table may change over the day. In another study, Folkard found that people retain words with similar meaning, such as "large," "big," and "huge," better in the morning, but remember lists of words that sound alike, such as "mad," "man," "map," better in the evening.[5]

Time of day is only one consideration. How good you feel, how awake you feel, what you have to do, how well you think you can do it, how well you really can do it, how fast you can do it. . . . There are many factors affecting mental performance that people lump together, Monk notes, but probably should not.

Factors that affect how well you'll remember a phone number, for example, may include who you are calling and why, whether you're in a hurry or not, how much sleep you got last night, what mood you are in, whether you encounter distractions while you make the call, even what sequence the numbers are in (1-2-3 is easier than the reverse), and more.[6]

Age also makes a big difference in how receptive people are to learning at different times of day. Preadolescent children are wide awake and fully alert in the morning, but teenagers are drowsy. Adolescents, in fact, may not reach full alertness until the hours after which the school day normally ends. Some school systems are addressing this issue by starting high schools later, and by using complicated class schedules that rotate all subjects through all hours of the school day. Older persons in one study remembered how much medicine to take and when to see the doctor better in the morning. Researchers postulated they had fewer distractions then.[7]

What about burning the midnight oil? Late-night cramming, Monk found, may help people do better on a test the next morning. This sounds like good news for procrastinators, but it is deceptive. Information acquired between midnight and dawn evaporates more quickly than that learned at other times of day. If you're a student studying for a midterm exam, you'll likely have to relearn many facts you acquire through cramming. If it's a final exam, a multiple choice test, late-night and early-morning review may help you a little. But if the test also will include essay questions, or others that demand reasoning skills, you'll likely do better with less cramming and more sleep beforehand. Sleep deprivation seriously undermines creative thinking.[8]

Don't Let the Post-Lunch Dip Get You Down

Many people experience transient sleepiness in midafternoon. No one knows what causes it, or why some people feel it more intensely than others. The so-called post-lunch dip may occur regardless of when, or even whether, you have lunch. Eating lunch, though, may make you more foggy.

In one study, Gary Zammit of St. Luke's–Roosevelt Hospital Center in New York and his colleagues compared young men who ate a thousand-calorie lunch, a three-hundred-calorie lunch, or skipped lunch. Both lunches were high in carbohydrates, shown in previous research to induce sleepiness. When given the opportunity to nap soon afterward, nearly all of the lunch eaters did so, regardless of whether they ate a big or small meal. They slept ninety minutes on average. Most of those who skipped lunch also took naps, but they slept for only about thirty minutes. Skipping lunch is not a recommended tactic; regular mealtimes are important for overall good health. But if midday sleepiness bothers you, eat only a light lunch, Zammit suggests, and avoid carbohydrates.[9] (See chapter 10: "Time to Eat.")

The best way to minimize midday drowsiness is to get enough sleep the night before. Some people are more susceptible to this down time than others, but anyone can try to avoid boring and sedentary tasks then. "What you are doing matters," says David Dinges of the University of Pennsylvania. "If engaged in an interesting project, you may cross the siesta phase without noticing it."[10] In a typical office setting, you can cruise through this time most easily by interacting with other people, making phone calls, or doing physical tasks, such as filing.

Speakers at midafternoon meetings know they have to work harder to interest their audience than they would earlier or later in the day. Speakers themselves probably won't feel a midday dip. Having to perform before a crowd usually prompts an energizing burst of adrenaline. If you're on the road in midafternoon, you need to exert extra caution. Daytime single-vehicle accidents, those most likely to stem from lapses in attention, peak at this time, particularly in drivers aged forty-five and older.[11]

Most people are programmed to nap in midafternoon, research by Roger Broughton of the University of Ottawa, shows. For most of us, having a long sleep at night and a short one at midday truly is doing what comes naturally.[12] While siestas have long been traditional in warm climates, where afternoon heat interacts with the biological clock to intensify languor, the siesta custom is dying. It's a casualty of our "time is money" world with its increasingly global economy. Before 1999, Mexican government offices stayed open from 10 A.M. to 3 P.M., shut down until 6 P.M., and then reopened until 9 P.M. Under a schedule started that year, offices now stay open from 7 A.M. to 6 P.M. Government employees work their entire eight-hour shift in those hours, getting a one-hour lunch break. In announcing the change, the Mexican government estimated it would save $192 million in electric bills a year and claimed the new schedules would benefit family life.[13]

Some of Mexico's largest companies abandoned siestas even before the North American Free Trade Agreement went into effect in 1994. In other former siesta cultures, such as those of Spain and Brazil, many businesses and government offices now also follow the Western workday.

Such moves come at a time when American industry is starting to endorse napping *at* the job, to combat napping *on* the job. The notion is still a novelty: work sites with nap rooms frequently prompt news stories. But many workers are forced to nap in their cars, at their desks, and even in bathroom stalls, Camille and Bill Anthony report in their lighthearted "how-to" book, *The Art of Napping at Work*.[14] Sleep specialists endorse nap breaks at work, noting that naps enhance both alertness and productivity in most people and cut on-the-job errors.

Moods Change over the Day

Whether you are a lark or an owl may affect your daily mood pattern. In one study, Gerard Kerkhof of Leiden University asked larks and owls to rate their moods on a five-point scale ranging from good to bad five or six times a day for two weeks. The morning-types reported their best moods occurred between 9 A.M. and 4 P.M. The evening-types reported their moods gradually brightened over the day.[15]

Varying the times you sleep, even modest amounts, may alter your mood, too. Diane Boivin of Harvard Medical School and her colleagues analyzed findings from subjects who lived in a time-isolation laboratory on twenty-eight or thirty-hour "days." On such schedules, body rhythms such as temperature chug along at their own pace, distinct from cycles of sleeping and waking, and researchers can assess the impact of sleeping at different times on daily rhythms.

In this study, the volunteers rated their moods from sad to happy as often as every twenty minutes when awake. They ranked their moods highest when body temperature highs occurred in the middle of their waking day, equivalent to 2 P.M. to 10 P.M. in ordinary life. They ranked moods lowest when body temperature lows, which normally occur in sleep, came about eight hours after they awakened. These findings may explain why people who change their sleep times, such as jet travelers and shift workers, commonly report transient feelings of depression. The temporary disruption of body rhythms may upset their mood cycles.[16]

Psychologist Robert Thayer of California State University at Long Beach identifies two key daily rhythms: energy and tension. They may run in tandem or in opposite directions, producing different mood states. The state he calls "calm-energy" is one to which many people aspire. You might be at work, say, focused fully on the task at hand, yet not driven by urgency. You're enjoying what you're doing. Later on, perhaps near bedtime, when you are reading for pleasure, winding down, you might feel "calm-tiredness."

Now imagine a day in which you're a news reporter on deadline. You've got a great story, but you've got to finish it in two hours. You might feel charged up but you're also jittery, concentrating while keeping an eye on the clock. The muscles in your jaws, shoulders, neck, and back are tense. This state Thayer calls "tense-energy."

Suppose things don't go well with this assignment. You can't reach people you need to talk to. The fax machine jams. You have to skip lunch. You can feel a headache coming on. You question your ability to do this job—any job. This is "tense-tiredness." Insignificant hassles or minor stressors, Thayer asserts, may have their greatest impact at tense-tired times. The minor problem with the fax machine, for example, may explode into a crisis of "everything's going wrong around here." This is the mood people most often try to escape, sometimes choosing positive strategies such as exercise, and sometimes negative ones, such as eating, smoking, drinking, or abusing drugs.

You don't necessarily cycle through all four of these states every day. As we discussed earlier, doing tasks when it's convenient to do them helps assure that you'll give them your fullest attention and best effort. Nonetheless, since you probably follow a fairly similar schedule from day to day, your moods probably also follow a fairly predictable pattern, partially tied to your daily cycle of alertness. Anything that disrupts your usual routine likely will alter mood states, too.

Most people awaken with slight feelings of depression. The blahs typically abate within an hour or two. But until they do, you're likely to find activities that demand speed and alertness more stressful than you would later on. These include routine events such as packing school lunches, catching a bus or train, or driving in rush-hour traffic.

You can't avoid this morning down time, but you can minimize its negative impact by advance planning, doing what you can to get ready the night before. It helps to remember the fog will soon lift. If you tune into your early-morning mood every fifteen minutes or so, you'll discover that you keep feeling better and better: more alert, more energetic, more optimistic, with increasing confidence that you can handle the tasks that lie ahead for the day.

By mid- to late-morning, alertness is high. This is the time of day, according to Thayer, when you are most likely to experience calm-energy. Thus, this can be a good time for demanding tasks, if circumstances permit. It's a good time for meetings, too, as sociability is high. In some work situations, or on some days, this also is a peak time for tense-energy.

Midafternoon, around the midday dip, is a time of tense-tiredness. Tempers may flare. This is not a good time to think about personal problems. Save such thoughts for early evening, a time of calm-tiredness. A half hour or so of "worry time" then can move you toward solutions, and may keep qualms from racing through your mind at bedtime. Early- to mid-evening is a good time to read and to socialize. Interacting with others, incidentally, is alerting, and may make you feel more alert than you really are. This is the reason you may feel wide awake at a party, but have a hard time staying awake at the wheel on the ride home.

Thayer once asked volunteers with different personal problems, such as marital distress, family conflict, or excess weight, to rate the seriousness of the problem five times a day for ten days. The times included just after awakening, in the late morning or early afternoon, in late afternoon, just before sleep, and after a brisk ten-minute walk at least ninety minutes from the other ratings. He asked each volunteer to think only about the problem and his or her mood at the time of the rating. The subjects almost always rated the problem as more serious in the afternoon than in the late morning, when they viewed it as least serious, he reports in his book *The Origin of Everyday Moods*.[17] At all times of day, they rated the problem as more serious when they felt tense and tired, and as less serious when they felt calm and energetic. Although these problems had no easy solutions, the subjects' assessed their difficulties less realistically, in Thayer's estimation, when they were tense and tired.

The impact of energy levels on moods may lead to a catch-22 situation. If you plan future tasks when you are tired, he suggests, you may decide you lack the energy to accomplish them. If you plan tasks when feeling energetic, you may be overoptimistic about your odds of success.

Ideally, you'd reserve demanding, potentially stressful tasks, tackling some major work assignment, for example, for times of high energy and clarity. Starting a big project in midafternoon would be a mistake for most of us. Bedtime probably is not a good time to discuss overdue bills or problems with the children with your spouse, or even to plan a vacation trip. Sensitive and difficult discussions demand attentive concern and high energy, a weekend morning, perhaps. Vacation planning doesn't usually require your sharpest decision making, unless, possibly, you are a travel agent, so the upbeat early evening hours, when you are both calm and energetic, may work well.

Timewise Tips

Tune into your own "feeling best" times, the tasks you have to do, and the demands of the environment in which you have to do them. Your convenience is the key determinant of your personal best time.

Try active strategies to improve your mood. You have more power to do this than you may suspect. Stand up and stretch, or take a short walk; you'll feel less tense. Do knee bends; you'll feel more energized. Pick up the phone and call your best friend; you'll feel more cheerful. Eat your next meal slowly; you'll feel calmer.

If you are a student:

Study subjects with details you need to retain, such as history and languages, in the afternoon.

Study subjects that require you to process information quickly, such as mathematics, in the morning.

Get enough sleep the night before your test.

On test days, review your notes in the morning.

In the workplace:

If giving a talk, review your notes that morning.

Schedule training sessions in the early afternoon, before the post-lunch dip, when feasible. If the audience is highly motivated, time of day is less important. Nonetheless, even highly motivated people decline in their ability to pay attention after many hours at work.

A Good Night's Sleep

Some people bemoan sleep as a waste of time. Others side with Shakespeare, who called sleep "nature's soft nurse."[1] Sleep, he wrote, "knits up the ravell'd sleave of care," and is the "chief nourisher in life's feast."[2]

Where you stand in this debate probably influences how much you sleep and when you choose to do it. Your choices control a drove of daily biological rhythms. Sleep holds the reins of your body temperature, blood pressure, secretion of many hormones, and numerous other functions of mind and body.

It is increasingly clear that good sleep, and enough of it, is critical for both mental and physical health. Too little sleep has wide-ranging ill effects.

Going without two to three hours' sleep every night for as little as a week seriously undermines mood, alertness, and performance in the typical adult, David Dinges of the University of Pennsylvania and his colleagues confirmed. In their study, sixteen men and women who normally averaged about 7.5 hours of sleep per night agreed to cut back to about five hours for a week. The volunteers took a battery of tests to measure attention, memory, math ability, moods, and more, several times a day. They showed deficits in virtually every aspect of functioning. After completing the study, the subjects needed two nights with about eight hours of sleep to get back to normal.[3]

Chronic sleep loss may hasten the onset of diabetes, high blood pressure, and memory loss, and make these conditions worse, research at the University of Chicago suggests. This dramatic finding counters the widespread belief that missing sleep has no long-term adverse consequences for physical health. Eve Van Cauter and her colleagues studied eleven healthy young men in the laboratory, controlling the length of time the men stayed in bed, and thus how much sleep they got. On the first three nights, the men spent eight hours in bed. The next six nights, they stayed in bed only four hours. Finally, they had six nights with twelve hours in bed to assure they were fully rested.

When sleep-deprived, the men's ability to make insulin and use glucose, the body's chief source of fuel, fell by about one-third. These problems are early markers of diabetes. They also raise blood pressure and undermine critical thinking. Although the men were all under age thirty, their glucose response pattern was comparable to that of people aged sixty and older. In the sleep-debt state, the men's cortisol levels rose too high in the afternoon and stayed too high through the evening, a possible trigger for memory problems. They also showed disturbances in thyroid function that put people at risk of gaining weight.

The good news coming from this study is that all the symptoms of premature aging disappeared after the six recovery nights, when the men averaged nine hours of sleep per night.[4]

Such studies clarify common everyday experiences. After missing sleep, we often feel muscle aches and pains the next day, and we are cranky and moody. Missing sleep lowers the body's production of natural killer cells, an important part of our self-defense system. People often report they develop colds, flu, or worsening of chronic diseases after sleep loss. To fight infections, we produce chemicals called *cytokines* that make us feel sleepy.[5] We may develop a fever, which makes us sleep more, or more erratically. Sleep may play a vital role in helping our bodies not only to conserve energy but also to ward off infections. Studies in mice injected with flu virus support this theory: after three days, those allowed to sleep normally no longer had the virus in their lungs, but those deprived of sleep still did.[6]

Learning how sleep benefits us brings doctors closer to developing effective treatment for persons with disorders that rob them of sleep. It also suggests strategies for coping with lost sleep, a critical concern as our society moves increasingly into a twenty-four-hour world, where more and more of us miss sleep both because of occupational demands and because there are so many things many of us find more appealing to do than sleep.

How Much Sleep Do People Need?

Sleep need is like fingerprints. No two people are exactly alike. Yet we're not all that different either. In studies at the National Institute of Mental Health, adults encouraged to sleep as much as possible, and given the opportunity to do so, averaged eight hours and fifteen minutes of sleep each night.[7] Chronobiologist Thomas Wehr, who directed the study, suggests this may be the amount most people need.

The notion that eight is the magic number goes way back. "The day and the night equal twenty-four hours. It is enough for a person to sleep one third of them, that is eight hours," the philosopher and physician Maimonides wrote in the twelfth century. Maimonides knew sleep is best at night. "These hours should be at the end of the night so that from the beginning of sleep until the sun rises will be eight hours," he wrote. "Thus, the person will arise from his bed before the sun rises."[8]

While some healthy people sleep less or more than that, both extremely short and extremely long sleep may be hazardous to your health. Daniel Kripke of the University of California, San Diego (UCSD), reviewed records of 1,064,004 men and women collected by the American Cancer Society. Persons aged forty-five and older who said they typically slept less than four hours or more than ten hours per night generally died sooner than those who averaged seven to eight hours.[9] Sleep needs change over the lifetime. (See chapter 8: "The Growing Years.") Certain life experiences, such as pregnancy, may temporarily increase the need for sleep. Many illnesses rob people of sleep. Older adults typically sleep less than younger adults, but it may be their ability to sleep—not need for sleep—that wanes with age, according to Sonia Ancoli-Israel, also at UCSD. Objective tests of daytime sleepiness show that persons sixty-five and older are sleepier in the daytime than are younger adults. These results imply, she said, that they do not get enough sleep.[10]

One in five American adults thinks you can't be successful in your career and get enough sleep, a National Sleep Foundation survey found.[11] Until recently, top executives and politicians bragged about how little sleep they got. The pendulum now may be swinging the other way. Major corporate leaders confidently assert they get all the sleep they need. *The Wall Street Journal* suggested sleep is the new status symbol. Jeff Bezos, chief executive of Amazon.com, and Marc Andreesen, cofounder of Netscape Communications Corp., both get eight hours of sleep each night. "Sleep is a perk of the truly successful," Nancy Ann Jeffrey wrote, "a privilege of membership in that elite stratosphere of people secure in the knowledge that the show can't start until they arrive."[12] Corporate America may be waking up to the benefits of sleep. In a preview of likely trends in the year 2000, published on December 31, 1999, the *Journal* declared, "Even sleep has become a priority, as successful people fight for more shut-eye and for more quality time when awake."[13]

Sleepless in Seattle, New York, and Your Town, Too

Sufficient sleep, by definition, is "the amount that permits optimal daytime functioning," a state that involves quick thinking, high energy, an upbeat mood, and a sense of physical well-being. These feelings are hard to quantify but easy to recognize when you feel them, especially if you haven't felt that terrific for a while.

There's plenty of evidence that most people today need more sleep than they get. Contemporary Americans complain that they feel tired and lack energy more often than did people in the 1930s, Donald Bliwise of Emory University Medical School found. He compared healthy adults who completed a standard mental health questionnaire in the 1930s with a similar group who answered the same questionnaire in the 1980s. While complaints about insomnia did not rise over the fifty-year interval, the 1980s crowd reported more trouble "getting going" and lack of stamina, strong hints of insufficient sleep.[14]

The typical American adult sleeps just under seven hours per night during the workweek, and about forty minutes longer on weekends, according to a 1999 survey for the National Sleep Foundation.[15] This is about ninety minutes less than people got a century ago, before electric lights made it easier to postpone bedtime. Women aged thirty to sixty are the most sleep-deprived, averaging 6.7 hours of sleep on weeknights, and 7.3 hours on weekends.[16]

A standard test of daytime sleepiness shows most American adults are chronically sleepy, nearly as sleepy as persons with serious sleep disorders. This test involves lying down in a darkened room and trying to fall asleep every two hours starting soon after they wake up in the morning, and continuing into the evening. People are awakened as soon as they fall asleep, so as not to influence later assessments. While taking this test, known as the Multiple Sleep Latency Test (MSLT), the typical American adult falls asleep in ten minutes on average. Persons with medical disorders that undermine alertness, such as sleep apnea and narcolepsy, fall asleep in five minutes or less. By contrast, preadolescent children, who are optimally alert, seldom fall asleep at all. The effects of lost sleep night after night build up, William Dement and Christopher Vaughan write in *The Promise of Sleep*.[17] People become clumsy and "stupid," they assert. This lasts until you pay back your sleep debt, which usually requires several nights of extended sleep.

Getting an hour more sleep makes sleepy people more alert and those who already function at a high level are even sharper, extensive research on sleep extension at Henry Ford Hospital in Detroit shows. In one study, Timothy Roehrs and his colleagues recruited twenty-four healthy men who usually slept either seven or eight hours a night. Using the MSLT, the researchers selected men who fell asleep on average in either less than six minutes or more than sixteen minutes. The seven-hour sleepers generally were sleepier in the daytime than the eight-hour sleepers. When the men spent ten hours in bed in the dark, all slept about an hour longer than usual. The extra hour boosted everyone's reaction time and sharpened attention and vigilance skills important in driving and in workplace activities such as monitoring industrial control panels.[18]

Falling asleep at the wheel is a gruesome barometer of sleep deprivation. The U.S. National Highway Traffic Safety Administration estimates that driver drowsiness and fatigue cause at least 100,000 crashes per year in this country and kill more than 1,550 people. More than half of a thousand randomly selected licensed drivers in one survey admitted driving while drowsy in the previous year. One in four had fallen asleep at the wheel, and one in twenty blamed a crash on drowsiness.[19] Public perception of the dangers of drowsy driving, safety experts say, lags about twenty years behind that for drinking and driving. Some contend that DWS, driving while sleepy, is just as much a crime as DWI, driving while intoxicated.

Don't overlook sleep deprivation's chilling impact on sex, suggested by this vignette: A young doctor making hospital rounds after a night on call found one of his patients reading *Playboy*. "Look at this!" said the patient, flashing a photo of a beautiful nude woman lying on rumpled sheets. "My first thought," the doctor said, "was how comfortable that bed looked."

Learn How to Unlock Your Personal Sleep "Gates"

Wakefulness and sleepiness engage in a tug of war across the twenty-four-hour day. The longer you go without sleep, the easier it is to fall asleep. But you don't steadily get sleepier and sleepier as the day progresses. Your biological clock won't let that happen, explains Dale Edgar of Stanford University.[20] In the daytime, it actively promotes wakefulness, fights the building pressure to fall asleep, and usually wins. The push-pull battle makes you feel more awake at certain times of the day, and more sleepy at others. At night, the pressure to sleep shows its muscle power.

If you've ever fallen asleep on the couch, dragged yourself to bed, and then found yourself wide awake, you can appreciate the intrusion of sleepiness into wakefulness, and of alertness into sleep. Most people experience midafternoon drowsiness. Even more dramatic is the "second wind," or feeling of heightened alertness that most of us get roughly between 8 P.M. and 10 P.M. This is the forbidden zone for sleep, Peretz Lavie of the Technion-Israel Institute of Technology found. It is virtually impossible for most people to sleep at this time. Just an hour or two later, Lavie reports, the gate to sleep swings open, and sleep comes easily.[21]

Sleep gates open and shut roughly every 90 to 120 minutes, Lavie found when he asked people to try to go to sleep or to stay awake every twenty minutes around the clock. Sleep gates explain why you may find it hard to fall asleep if you go to bed early. In this instance, you show up at the gate before opening time.

If engaged in a good book, surfing the Internet, or some other demanding activity, you may keep going until after the sleep gate closes. Even though it's past your usual bedtime then, you may find it hard to fall asleep. You may have to wait for the next gate to open.

What Happens When We Sleep?

Sleep is not "time out." Going to sleep and waking up are not like flipping the ignition switch in your car. You don't park your brain when you go to sleep.

You simply shift to a different gear. Even in sleep, the brain maintains its sentinel functions. A mother who may sleep through a thunderstorm or jet planes flying overhead likely will be roused by her baby's whimpers.

Sleep, however, is a world unto itself. Two distinct states alternate in approximately ninety-minute cycles. They're called quiet and active sleep, according to the relative bustle of nerve cells in the brain at each time. You start out in quiet sleep, descending gradually in three stages, from which it becomes increasingly harder to awaken. In Stage 1, thoughts wander and you may have brief, dreamlike fantasies. If asked, "Are you asleep?" you'd probably say no. Stage 2, or light sleep, comes next. It settles into Stage 3-4, the deepest and most restful sleep, once thought separate stages, now combined. As you sink into quiet sleep, your breathing and heart rate become slow and steady, your body temperature and blood pressure fall, you lie still, and your muscles relax.

After about ninety minutes, your brain abruptly revs up for active sleep. Eyes dart behind closed lids, giving this state its name, rapid eye movement, or REM sleep. Most vivid dreams occur in REM sleep. At this time, skeletal muscles lie virtually paralyzed, perhaps to keep you from fleeing your bed to act out dreams. Your heart beats faster and more irregularly, blood pressure fluctuates, breathing quickens, and temperature regulation switches off, making it likely that you will awaken if your bedroom is too warm or too cool. Males of all ages, from babies to the elderly, experience a partial or full erection. Females have a comparable response: the clitoris engorges, and vaginal pulse and lubrication increase. These responses don't necessarily reveal "sexy" dreams. They always occur in REM sleep.

After a few minutes in REM sleep, you return to quiet sleep, tamely called non-REM or NREM sleep. In NREM sleep, your brain idles, and your thinking resembles your waking daydreams. NREM sleep also is the time of peak secretion of growth hormone, necessary throughout life for tissue repair.

As sleep continues, its ninety-minute cycles repeat, but you spend more time in quiet sleep in the first half of the night, and more time in active sleep in the second half. The first REM episode of the night lasts about ten minutes. The last one may fill an hour. Dream stories thus move from previews, to shorts, to full-length feature films. The typical young adult spends about three-quarters of sleep in NREM sleep and the rest in REM sleep. Even good sleepers awaken now and then, but usually for too short a time to remember later.

New brain imaging technologies show the brain is as active in REM sleep as when we are awake, sometimes even more active. Further, activity jumps in brain areas responsible for emotions and falls in those involved with logical thinking, a possible cause of strong feelings and a certain irrationality in dreams. The brain sinks below the level of wakefulness only in the deepest part of NREM sleep, about 20 percent of sleep overall.

Spontaneous awakenings usually occur in REM sleep, leading to the notion that one function of REM sleep is to prepare us for wakefulness. If you awaken from REM sleep, you may recall your last dream clearly. Think how often you've recounted a dream story over breakfast, ending it with "and then I woke up."

Few of us jump out of bed in the morning, raring to go: more proof that there is no simple off/on switch that governs sleeping and waking. Think of sleep as a sedative drug: its effects wear off slowly. It may take five or ten minutes to shrug off grogginess, and as long as two hours to become fully alert. Sleep experts call this muzzy feeling *sleep inertia*, or more graphically, sleep drunkenness. In one study, volunteers routed from deep sleep by a 75-decibel fire alarm got only half as many answers right when they took a test within three minutes of awakening as they did on the same test in the daytime.[22] Sleep inertia may be a big problem for firefighters, doctors on call, and others required to act fast.

You may feel sleep inertia even after a good night's sleep. You'll feel it more, though, if you haven't gotten all the sleep you need, and were roused suddenly, by, for example, a ringing phone or the blare of your alarm clock. Sleep inertia accounts for wooziness after daytime naps that last long enough for you to sink into deep sleep. This is the reason sleep experts generally suggest not napping longer than thirty minutes.

The way people typically sleep—in one long bout—differs from the way other animals sleep. Cats actually take catnaps, for example, waking and sleeping many times throughout the day. Our sleep patterns may be more a function of our lifestyle, however, than nature's design. Thomas Wehr's studies at the National Institute of Mental Health sought to mimic the long nights of winter in a world without electricity. Volunteers went to bed at 6 P.M. every night and spent fourteen hours in the dark for up to fifteen weeks. They typically got their eight hours and fifteen minutes of sleep in two bouts, one at the beginning and the other at the end of the period. They spent the intervening wake time in quiet meditation, often reviewing their dreams. This sleep pattern, which historical studies suggest was common in preindustrial times, Wehr said, may help explain the importance accorded to dreams through the ages.[23]

Put Your Internal Alarm Clock to Work

One alarm clock looks like a baseball: you turn it off by throwing it against a wall. Another crows like a rooster. Some alarm clocks bring biological-rhythms research to your bedroom: they simulate dawn, with light that ramps up gradually, starting thirty minutes before your chosen wake-up time.

You may not need an alarm clock at all if you program your inner clock to

A Normal Night's Sleep

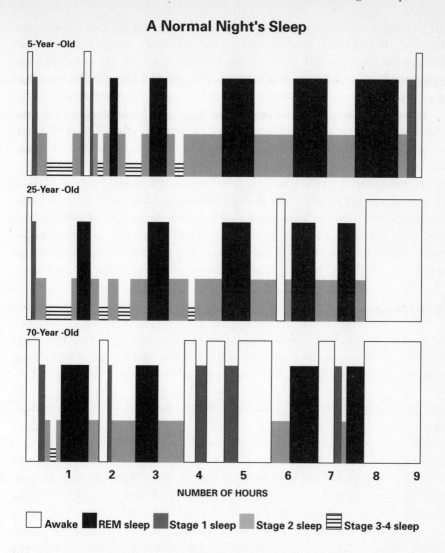

Rapid eye movement sleep (REM) and non-rapid eye movement sleep (NREM) alternate about every ninety minutes through the night. We dream most vividly in REM sleep, and sleep most restfully in NREM sleep. As sleep progresses, REM sleep episodes lengthen, and NREM sleep lightens. As we become older, we experience less deep sleep, more light sleep, and spend more of our time in bed awake.

summon you from slumber. This is easier than it sounds, and more common than you may think. In one study of self-awakening, three-quarters of nearly 300 randomly surveyed adults reported that they never used an alarm.[24] The secret is to get up at approximately the same time every day.

Assuming that you live on a traditional active-in-the-daytime, asleep-at-night schedule, this habit prompts consistent exposure to morning light, the body's most powerful time cue. Because humans naturally run on a longer than twenty-four-hour day, morning light exposure snaps your internal rhythms back in line with those of the outside world. It also helps set your body-temperature clock, so that temperature rises through the day, peaks in the early evening, and starts to fall well before bedtime, easing you into sleep.

You sleep most restfully when temperature is low. When you follow a regular schedule, temperature bottoms out about two hours before you usually awaken, and then starts to rise, making sleep lighter. You awaken at about the same time each day.

The temperature clock is not one you can shut off at will. That can make it a nuisance on weekends. Even though you don't have to go to work then, your body insists at the usual hour that "it's time to get up." If you change your sleep schedule, your temperature clock will adjust, although it may take a few days to do so. That's why shift workers and jet travelers who try to sleep at hours in which they previously were awake often sleep poorly for a few days.

How Do People Cope with Extreme Sleep Loss?

To find out what functions a bodily organ or behavior serves, the time-honored scientific technique is to take it away. You can manage fine without your appendix, and with only one lung or kidney. You'll die without your liver, heart, or brain. Without food or water, other bodily tissues serve as sources of energy, but death comes within several weeks. What happens when you go totally without sleep?

Over the years, there have been some dramatic demonstrations of the human ability to miss sleep for days at a time. Think of the dance marathons popular in the 1930s and '40s. In 1964 high school student Randy Gardner stayed awake for 264 hours for a science-fair project. Sleep specialist William Dement volunteered to provide medical supervision. "A serious problem I did not foresee," Dement relates, "was that I soon became very sleep-deprived myself. On day 5, I turned the wrong way onto a one-way street and almost crashed head-on into a police car." Dement also forgot to pay his fine.[25] He and other researchers now think the seventeen-year-old Randy probably got a few brief snatches of sleep, or "microsleeps," that went unrecognized at the time. But the *Guinness Book of World Records* still lists Randy as the one who went without sleep the longest.

Academic researchers probably could not participate in a similar study today, Dement notes. Human subjects' research committees would deem it unethical. Extreme sleep deprivation has been used and continues to be used today in some countries to torture prisoners, in clear violation of worldwide human rights' conventions.

Most scientific studies of long-term sleep loss have been conducted by military researchers. Their pressing concern is to help troops manage best in field conditions after partial sleep loss. Battlefields once quieted down after dark, but no longer. Night vision technology that came into wide use in the 1980s allows wars to rage around the clock, pushing the limits of human performance, says Col. David Penetar of the U.S. Army Research Institute of Environmental Medicine. The risk of trouble with attention, decision making, and other mental tasks is highest when troops who have missed some sleep must work at night. Jet lag, and the disruption in body clocks that it brings, adds another complication. Troops newly dispatched to the Mideast from the United States, for example, would likely have jet lag for a few days. They would get some sleep, but possibly not as much as they need to function at their best, and some would have to work at night.

Good sleep management is critical in extreme situations in civilian life, too, in the aftermath of hurricanes or earthquakes, for example, and in everyday life for doctors on call, pilots, and some industrial workers. It's also important in extreme sports such as around-the-world solo yacht racing. The perils of this voyage are legion: gales, whales, icebergs near the South Pole, broken masts, lightning, fog, potential collisions with other ships in heavy traffic waters, utter blackness at night. When do sailors dare to sleep? How can they dare not to?

Claudio Stampi, of the Chronobiology Research Institute in Boston, a physician and solo sailor himself, designed a unique program to help participants in the 1998–99 Around Alone race, an eight-month adventure in four legs, with brief breaks for boat repairs. He taught the sailors to sleep at down times on their biological clock, and to adjust sleep length to maximize deep restful sleep, yet awaken without feeling foggy, tactics that can benefit all of us. Adept management of biological clocks, Stampi said, probably helped Italian skipper Giovanni Soldini come in first. Soldini had the most flexible sleep pattern and slept for as little as twenty minutes, and as long as five to six hours, mostly at night. Soldini broke the previous record by nearly five days, completing the 27,000-mile voyage in just under 117 days.

Why We Must Sleep

"If sleep does not serve an absolutely vital function, then it is the biggest mistake the evolutionary process has ever made," Allan Rechtschaffen of the University of Chicago wrote in 1971 in a still widely quoted essay. "How could sleep have remained virtually unchanged as a monstrously useless, maladaptive vestige throughout the whole of mammalian evolution," he asked, "while selection has during the same period of time been able to achieve all kinds of delicate, finely-tuned adjustments in the shape of fingers and toes?"[26]

Some theorists suggest that enforcing rest alone may be the main purpose of sleep, but Rechtschaffen contends it must do something more than that. Heart rate and breathing slow down only a little. The energy savings you get from sleeping instead of simply resting quietly are modest. For a two-hundred-pound man, Rechtschaffen noted, a night's sleep offers the caloric savings of not drinking a cup of milk.

He and his colleagues have studied sleep deprivation in rats for the past two decades. In their studies, the rats may eat and drink as desired, and can move about freely in their cages. Two identical rats live in side-by-side twin cages with a common floor that is a motorized disk suspended over a shallow tray of water.

Both rats are monitored continuously. When Rat 1 falls asleep, the disk starts to rotate slowly. If the rat stayed asleep, it would bump into the dividing wall and be nudged into the water. Although in no danger of drowning, rats, by their nature, resist getting wet. By walking in the direction opposite that in which the disk is rotating, Rat 1 avoids being doused. Rat 2 also must walk whenever the disk is moving. Rat 1 gets almost no sleep, but Rat 2 can sleep whenever its partner is awake.

The rats deprived entirely of sleep eat more than usual, but they keep losing weight. They develop sores on their bodies and tails. Despite their increased activity, their body temperature falls, and they experience excessive heat loss. After about two to three weeks, they die. Their partners may develop some of the same symptoms but recover fully when allowed to sleep undisturbed. Rats deprived only of REM sleep suffer the same ill effects as those deprived totally of sleep but live about three weeks longer.

Animal rights activists have lambasted these studies, claiming they are cruel. The Chicago researchers maintain that their procedure is physically gentle, and that the animals are well cared for. The only thing the animals lack is sleep. Whether the rats feel stressed, and whether that affects their response is, of course, impossible to know. In this book, we've reported many benefits to humans made possible by animal research. Despite increasing sophistication of cell and tissue cultures, statistical studies, and computer modeling, researchers say, efforts to understand how the brain works require the study of sleeping and waking in animals, including humans.

Why the rats die is still not clear. The researchers suspect that the extreme loss of body temperature that develops may be an important key to why sleep is necessary. The normal downturn in temperature in sleep helps animals conserve energy. It reduces the need for food. Animals that stayed awake constantly would need to eat more. They would have to expend energy to find food. That would be a problem for some, including humans, who cannot see in the dark. To have all species on earth awake all the time would create an environmentalist's nightmare. Competition for food would dominate daily life.

Sleep and eating may be related in other ways. Americans not only sleep too little today, they also eat too much. One in three Americans is now obese, defined by federal guidelines as being 20 percent above their ideal weight.

When people are tired, Donald Bliwise notes, they eat more, and they eat more often.[27] Consumer magazines over the years have run articles on the theme "lose weight while you sleep." That is pure fantasy. It's intriguing to think, though, that a steady diet of good sleep may be a good aid to weight control.

Sleep probably has not one, but many functions. "Sleep has survived ubiquitously throughout all of mammalian evolution," Rechtschaffen observed. "Sleep persists in predators and prey; in carnivores and vegetarians; on the land and in the water; . . . in the smartest and the dumbest of all mammalian species. These facts suggest a primary, essential, functional core to sleep," he adds. "Sleep is a biological necessity in its own right."[28]

Bottom line: we sleep because we have to.

Timewise Tips for Good Sleep

Regularize your schedule. Get up about the same time every day regardless of how much sleep you got. This is the single most effective way to keep body rhythms in tune. A consistent bedtime helps, too, although it is less crucial. If you are like most American adults, you need to go to bed earlier than you do now. Try going to bed fifteen minutes earlier than usual for a week, and see if you feel more alert in the daytime. If you do, continue this process until you feel fully alert in the day, fall asleep fast, sleep soundly at night, and awaken spontaneously in the morning.

Program yourself mentally for sleep with daily rituals. Walk the dog, watch the news, have a snack. Include tactics you can "take along" on trips.

Keep your bedroom dark, or wear eyeshades. Darkness tells the brain it is time to sleep. Open shades or curtains as soon as you get up in the morning, since sunlight provides an alerting signal. If you have a secluded bedroom, leave windows uncovered, and let sunlight awaken you gradually.

Keep your bedroom quiet. This sends another sleep signal to the brain.

Keep your bedroom cool. This will promote the decline in body temperature critical to restful sleep. Caution: cold feet may slow rather than speed this process, by turning up your internal thermostat. If you do the obvious thing, and wear socks or use a hot-water bottle, you'll help blood vessels in the feet radiate body heat. In a study of various tactics to alter body temperature, Anna Wirz-Justice and her colleagues at the University of Basel, in Switzerland, found warm feet promote the rapid onset of sleep.[29] Being overly warm throughout the night may disrupt sleep, however, a good reason to turn the electric blanket down.

Go to bed only when sleepy. You're already halfway there.

Reserve bed and bedroom for sleep and sex. If you watch TV, snack, chat on the phone, and do paperwork in bed, you create cues for wakefulness, not sleep. Some people aren't bothered, but you may be.

If you can't fall asleep within thirty minutes, get out of bed. When the gate to sleep is closed, you can't force it open. You have to wait until it opens on its own. Be patient, but be ready. Don't start baking a cake.

If you nap, limit time lying down to thirty minutes in midafternoon. A regular nap at the sleepiest time of the waking day may help you sleep better at night by easing worries about not getting enough sleep. A twenty-minute nap is enough to boost alertness for several hours. If you're really sleep-deprived and need to catch up, set an alarm to awaken you after either ninety minutes or three hours, allowing you to enjoy one or two full sleep cycles. Caution: avoid naps if they make your nighttime sleep worse.

Take a hot bath ninety minutes before bedtime. Soaking in 105° F water for thirty minutes raised body temperature by nearly one degree in a group of women with insomnia, Cynthia Dorsey found in a study at McLean Hospital in Belmont, Massachusetts. On getting out of the tub, the women's temperature plummeted. They got more deep sleep afterward. The hot bath, or passive body heating, as Dorsey calls it, improved sleep as much as widely prescribed sleeping pills.[30]

Exercise regularly. Exercise can serve as a time cue to help foster sleep several hours later, particularly if you do it outside in daylight hours. Within a few hours of bedtime, it also may promote sleep by raising body temperature temporarily, much as a hot bath does. (See chapter 9: "Fitness by the Clock.") Daytime activity also complements nighttime rest; they are flip sides of a coin.

Avoid caffeine within five hours of bedtime. Even if it does not keep you from falling asleep, it's likely to make sleep more restless.

Don't drink alcohol or smoke near bedtime. A so-called nightcap may make you sleepy, but alcohol's rebound effect disturbs sleep. Nicotine is a stimulant that also interferes with sleep.

If you are a bedtime worrier, find thirty minutes earlier in the day to focus on problems. Write worries down, a tactic that often points to possible solutions. Or try Napoleon's trick: to combat bedtime worries, he allegedly envisioned a chest with many drawers. He mentally stuffed each problem in a drawer and shut it tight. When all were tucked away, he fell asleep.

Forget about counting sheep. It's too slow a method of distraction, according to Richard Bootzin of the University of Arizona. "A person can count sheep and still worry," he said, adding, "It's better to get out of bed, jot down some notes, and think about the problem in the morning, when problems seldom loom as large."

Use escapist fantasy. Robert Louis Stevenson said his father put himself to sleep every night of his life with stories of ships, roadside inns, robbers, old sailors, and commercial travelers before the era of steam. "He never finished one of these romances," Stevenson wrote. "The lucky man did not require to!"[31]

Learn relaxation techniques, such as muscle relaxation, meditation, or yoga, and use them regularly. These may help reduce stress both day and night.

If you awaken frequently in the night, turn your clock around so you can't see it. This may keep you from obsessing about how much sleep you have gotten so far, how long you've been awake, and how badly you may feel tomorrow if you don't get to sleep right away.

If you sleep poorly, use the sleep/wake diary on page 353 to help identify possible triggers. Note what helps and what harms your sleep. Sleep problems fall into four basic categories, covered by these complaints: "I can't sleep"; "I sleep too much"; "My bedpartner says strange things happen when I sleep"; "I can't sleep when I want." The first and last of these may reflect circadian rhythm sleep disorders. (See Sleep Disorders, page 339.)

If sleep problems persist, see your doctor. Medications you may be taking for other illnesses may be disturbing your sleep, or you may have a sleep disorder. If you snore loudly and are excessively sleepy in the daytime, for example, you may have sleep apnea. You may need a sleep specialist. Find accredited sleep centers near you at the American Academy of Sleep Medicine's Web site (www.aasmnet.org). Learn more about sleep at Web sites of the National Sleep Foundation (www.sleepfoundation.org) and the Sleep Research Society (www.sleephomepages.org). The American Sleep Apnea Association is at www.sleepapnea.org.

The Growing Years

Dramatic changes in body rhythms accompany the rapid physical and mental growth that takes place between infancy and adolescence. Changes in the amount and timing of sleep serve as signposts for this process.

Babies, though seemingly helpless, are not wholly passive recipients of cuddling and care. Within just a few days of their birth, they display an impressive ability to lock on to the world's schedule. At the entrance to adulthood, teenagers need as much sleep as they did when younger, but their biological clocks program them to go to sleep later. In this chapter, we explore these developmental landmarks and the years between.

BABIES

Even in the womb, babies display cyclic patterns of quiet and active sleep, responding to signals received from their mothers. On the day of their birth, they wake and sleep in a seemingly random fashion. By their second day of life, even if still in the hospital, they predictably sleep longer at night than in the day.[1]

Healthy full-term newborns may sleep as many as sixteen to eighteen hours a day, and may ask to be fed every two to three hours. New parents sometimes try to put their baby on what they view as a reasonable schedule. From the baby's point of view, that's not reasonable at all. The best solution, sleep specialists say, is a compromise, letting the baby call the shots while providing a stable, predictable home environment.

This means you feed your baby when it asks to be fed, and let the baby sleep undisturbed when it chooses to do so. At the same time, give the baby regular social cues. Talk and play with the baby in the daytime. Provide care but no entertainment at night. If family members get up and go to sleep at the same time each day, and share at least one meal, the baby soon will recognize familiar sounds and activities at certain times. You can build in other predictable events like bathtime or storytime. Additionally, you can provide strong light cues: open blinds or curtains in the morning and close them at night to teach the baby how the outside world organizes time. Breast feeding may provide another time cue, as melatonin from the mother helps synchronize rhythms in the baby.

These tactics will help your baby adopt your schedule with a minimum of conflict. A baby given this freedom, sleep specialists say, likely will eat and sleep better, and cry less than if you try to make the baby conform to your schedule from the start.

Cultural attitudes that shape parenting styles have a clear impact on twenty-four-hour rhythms. One study compared American and Dutch parents, finding that Americans touched and talked to babies more in the daytime and took them out more, while Dutch parents gave babies more waking time alone to foster their independence. The American babies spent more time in a state of active alertness both day and night. By six months of age, the American babies slept or rested quietly eight to nine hours at night; the Dutch babies, ten hours.[2]

Kate McGraw, a young mother and sleep researcher, studied the maturation of circadian rhythms in her own son, Tyler, starting when he was five hours old, and continuing throughout his first six months. Her intensive study provides an impressive demonstration of how quickly babies can adopt the world's schedule.

Either McGraw or her husband Dan observed the baby at all times, swapping shifts, and curtailing their own sleep for the duration of the study. They recorded when Tyler went to sleep and awakened, and when he started and stopped eating. McGraw breastfed Tyler throughout the study and added solid foods at the appropriate age. The couple also took hourly temperature readings, using a heat-sensitive ear thermometer that did not bother the baby in any way. In addition, they collected daylong samples of Tyler's saliva once a week to monitor his melatonin secretion, and they logged outings and visits to see if these events had an impact on his behavior.

Tyler slept in his own bed, in their bedroom, where he received natural light exposure through two unshaded windows. No artificial lights were used in the bedroom before sunrise or after sunset, except for a low-level nightlight to aid observations. For the length of the study, both parents and their two other children, aged seven and ten, regularly got up at 5:30 A.M., went to bed at 8:00 P.M. (except for the parent on caregiver duty), and they ate meals at the same times each day. The family agreed to this routine to make the baby's schedule changes easy to see in a statistical way.

By the end of his first week of life, Tyler's body temperature predictably dipped to its lowest point at night. In the second week, he reliably slept longer and more solidly at night. In the second month, he started to stay awake for 90 to 120 minutes at a time twice a day, in the morning and the early evening. In the intervening daytime hours, he stayed awake or napped for shorter intervals. His melatonin levels began to rise at night at six weeks of age, more evidence that he could tell night from day. By the end of the second month, he slept from sunset to sunrise with only a few brief awakenings.

For the first fourteen weeks, Tyler went to sleep at sunset. He then adopted the family's schedule and went to sleep later. When daylight saving time ended and family members stayed awake an additional hour, Tyler did, too, a social animal at a very early age.[3]

McGraw's study is the first to document the impact of light and social cues on a baby's development. While we can't generalize from one baby to all babies, this study adds to evidence suggesting that light and social cues deserve much more attention than they currently get. A related study compared two premature nurseries in the same hospital, where babies needed intensive round-the-clock care. In one nursery, the staff followed the customary practice of leaving lights on all the time and made no special efforts to reduce noise. In the other, they dimmed the lights between 7 P.M. and 7 A.M., and kept noise down. The babies in the second room slept longer and gained more weight, and they developed faster than the others after going home.[4]

Debate continues on whether babies need total darkness at night for optimal eye growth. In 1999, researchers at the University of Pennsylvania Medical Center reported that children who slept with a night-light or a room light on at night before age two were three to five times more likely to develop nearsightedness than those who slept in the dark. In 2000, separate studies headed by researchers at Ohio State University and the New England College of Optometry in Boston, Massachusetts, disputed these findings. They said nearsighted parents more often had nearsighted children, regardless of lighting in the children's rooms at night. Nearsighted parents, not surprisingly, make greater use of night-lights. The original researchers stood by their findings. They also cited animal studies showing that light/dark cycle disruption hampers eye development. More research on this issue is needed, but the importance of light/dark cues for strong circadian rhythms is clear. If using a night-light in your child's sleeping room, put it in a far corner, out of your child's line of sight.[5]

Some babies sleep well in the early months and develop trouble sleeping at the end of the first year. Although parents often worry when this happens, such children may be flourishing, not troubled, Dilys Daws, a child psychotherapist at the Tavistock Clinic in London, suggests in *Through the Night: Helping Parents and Sleepless Infants*. These children may be "fascinated by their discoveries of all that the world has to offer and loath to shut this off and go to sleep," she says. The nightmares and fears of tigers behind the curtains that develop in the second year, she adds, "are also signs of maturing minds and creative imaginings."[6]

AGES ONE THROUGH SIX

At twelve to fifteen months, infants still sleep perhaps fifteen hours a day over-all, but they get nearly all of their sleep at night. Some have abandoned their morning nap. Between ages two and six, most children still take a two-hour afternoon nap.

The persistence of the midday nap and the consistency of its length, despite differences in children's home lives and daily activities, suggests naps are part of a natural human biological rhythm, according to Marc Weissbluth, who tracked naps in nearly 200 children in his pediatrics practice from infancy until their seventh birthdays. "Preservation of good daytime sleep has important health benefits," Weissbluth said. "Kids who nap well are less fussy and more adaptable. They also have fewer problems falling asleep and staying asleep at night."[7]

You can help reinforce daily rhythms in a young child by talking about night as sleep time, and day as wake time or playtime. You also can teach your child that the bed is the best place to sleep by establishing a tuck-in ritual. Don't let your child fall asleep in front of the television and then carry him or her to bed, psychologist Jodi Mindell advises in *Sleeping through the Night*. Read favorite stories at bedtime, she suggests. Children find the familiarity relax-ing. Save new stories for daytime hours.[8]

Problems with schedules are the prime focus of parents' complaints about a young child's sleep, according to Richard Ferber of the Children's Hospital in Boston and author of *Solve Your Child's Sleep Problems*.[9] Often the child sleeps well, but goes to bed later or gets up earlier than the parent wishes. Sometimes parents themselves unwittingly contribute to schedule problems.

On the "too late" side of the spectrum, one mother put her toddler to bed at 8:30 P.M. The child couldn't fall asleep, and ended up watching television with her parents until 11 P.M. Then, because she'd been up late, her mother let her sleep until 9 A.M. "If the parents were to wake her consistently at 7 A.M.," Ferber said, "she'd go to sleep earlier, too."

While some children can't fall asleep, others won't go to bed. Their protests cause nightly struggles. Limit-setting, which may include restricting television viewing or too active play near bedtime, may remedy some situa-tions. Even young children may experience the delayed sleep phase syn-drome (see DSPS, page 342). Often these children are hard to awaken in the morning, too. Treatment in young children usually is easier than in adults, Ferber said, because children don't pay attention to clocks. One tactic is to let these children go to bed when ready, and, after a few days without bedtime battles, gradually awaken them earlier and put them to bed earlier until a bet-ter schedule is achieved.

Children, like adults, experience a forbidden zone for sleep in the middle of the evening, and some display a big surge in energy at this time. Ordinary sleep-inducing activities such as drinking warm milk or listening to quiet music or stories won't calm these children down. Parents may need both to wake them earlier in the morning and to shorten their afternoon nap.

The child who awakens "too early" may be going to bed too early. But simply keeping a child up later may not itself be enough. Parents may encourage early awakenings by feeding a child soon after he or she awakens. "A child who is fed at 5 A.M. today," Ferber said, "will be hungry at 5 A.M. tomorrow. Better to hold off breakfast until 6 A.M."

Parents also may have unrealistic ideas about when a child of a certain age should go to bed, or about how much sleep children need. Children as well as adults vary considerably in this respect: some are short sleepers, some long sleepers; some are larks, and others owls. Children allowed to stay up late and sleep late on weekends may have trouble readjusting to their weekday schedule, just as adults do. "To fix a child's sleep problem," Ferber asserted, "you have to start with an appropriate and consistent schedule."[10]

AGES SEVEN THROUGH TWELVE

Preteen children get gold medals for both their waking and sleeping skills: they typically are fully alert in the daytime, and fall asleep fast and sleep soundly at night.

With increasing independence, children often test the limits of parental authority regarding bedtime. Requests to watch a particular television show are a favored delaying tactic. Well-meaning parents might think that TV viewing may help a child go to sleep, but several studies suggest that, in the long run, it is more likely to sabotage sleep.

One study found one-fourth of nearly 500 kindergarten through fourth-graders in three middle-class suburban public schools had a TV set in their bedroom. These children proved more likely to have sleep disturbances than classmates who did not have a TV in their bedroom, did not use TV to aid in falling asleep, or watched less TV in general. Their sleep problems included bedtime resistance, trouble falling asleep, anxiety around sleep, and not getting enough sleep. Teacher evaluations suggested these children were sleepier in class than those without a bedroom TV.

Sleep problems developed even though nearly all the parents of these children said they kept their children from watching violent shows and limited their hours for TV viewing, according to Judith Owens and her colleagues at the Hasbro Children's Hospital and Brown University School of Medicine. These children watched TV about two hours a day on average, less, the researchers said, than generally is reported for American children the same ages.[11]

Curiously, neither television nor school, despite their heavy presence in children's waking lives, figure prominently in their dreams. True dreaming starts between ages seven and nine, according to David Foulkes, a longtime investigator of children's dreams at Georgia Mental Health Institute in Atlanta. Dreaming, he suggests, offers a window for viewing the growth of self-awareness over the life cycle. The so-called dreams that younger children sometimes relate probably arise in waking states, Foulkes writes in *Children's Dreaming and the Development of Consciousness.*[12] A child awakens alone in the dark, for example. This frightening experience may turn into a report of a "scary" dream.

When awakened in the sleep laboratory in rapid eye movement sleep, the state in which most dreaming occurs, children under age five typically say they were not dreaming at all. Dreams in five- and six-year-olds may concern simple events. Not until around age seven do children start showing up as active participants in their own dreams. Play is the central theme, generally involving positive relations with people or objects.

Around ages eleven to thirteen, dream content starts to reflect the traits and personal style of the dreamer. Assertive children dream of an active self, competitive children of self-initiated aggression, and those who display hostility, of anger. Dreams at this age are as long as adult dreams collected in the laboratory. Older teenagers become increasingly able to stand back, to observe themselves as actors doing things in their dreams. This constitutes evidence, Foulkes suggests, of further mental maturation.

AGES THIRTEEN TO NINETEEN

Parents know it. Teachers know it. Teenagers are zombies in the morning. Adolescents' proclivity to stay up late goes beyond the "nobody can make me go to bed before I'm ready" rebellion that's part of growing up. It's fueled by more than the lure of late-night television, the Internet, and social activities. Dramatic changes that occur in the body at puberty reset the biological clock, making it hard for teenagers to fall asleep before 11 P.M. Indeed, the average high school student goes to bed at midnight. Yet teenagers need nine hours and fifteen minutes of sleep on average, as much as younger children do.

They seldom get it, because high schools in the United States and around the world typically start between 7:00 A.M. and 7:50 A.M., about an hour earlier than middle and elementary schools. Classes begin before teenagers' biological wake-up time. In the 1990s this practice prompted growing nationwide concern. Researchers showed that sleep deprivation interferes with adolescents' learning, dulls moods, increases the likelihood of car crashes, and contributes to drug use. Starting high schools closer to 9 A.M.—an idea that still raises many eyebrows—is gaining momentum.

Some school systems in the United States and other countries already have done it. Mounting evidence that later start times boost both students' grades and moods may be among the most notable benefits of applying chrono-biology research to everyday health and well-being. Congresswoman Zoe Lofgren, a Democrat from California and the mother of two teenagers, pro-posed a Zzzzz's to A's Act to Congress in 1998 to encourage secondary schools to open after 9 A.M. The bill would provide school districts a federal grant of up to $25,000 to help cover administrative and operating costs involved in changing start times.

The decision to make a change is a multifaceted one. It affects opening and dismissal times not only of high schools but also of middle and elemen-tary grades, since school buses in most communities make all three rounds. It also affects schedules of teachers, parents, after-school sports, and fast-food restaurants and other retailers that depend on student workers.

Michael Scanlan is principal of the LaSalle Academy, a private Catholic high school in Providence, Rhode Island. His 1,200 students are expected to be in school by 8:10 A.M. Many arrive bleary-eyed. From the younger to the older teen years, from grades nine through twelve, Scanlan said, attendance falls steadily and tardiness rises. Insufficient sleep, he believes, undermines both classroom performance and relationships at home.

Teenagers Lead Busy Lives

Many work at paid jobs, some an astounding thirty hours in a typical school week, as much time as most students spend in class. (Forty percent of high school students nationwide work twenty or more hours a week at a paid job.) Some families need the income their teenagers bring in, but for many teenagers, cars are the prime impetus for paid work. After money for gas and car insurance, new clothes, movies, music, and other entertainment also serve as motivators. Some students participate in sports that require after-school practice five days a week, along with evening and weekend games. Others vol-unteer at hospitals or nursing homes. Some help care for younger siblings. Some are in clubs that meet at 7:30 A.M., before classes start. And some face an hour-long commute.

Ninety-five percent of LaSalle's students go to college, so getting good grades prompts considerable anxiety. But given all the other demands on their time, students may not start homework until 8 or 9 P.M. Some report they stay up late because they compete with sisters or brothers for time on the family computer. Their parents, at their age, Scanlan said, typically went to bed when their parents told them to. Today's parents often go to sleep before their children do.

LaSalle students in all grade levels are taking part in an ongoing study to chart changes in sleep and circadian rhythms throughout puberty. Randomly selected student volunteers in the Sleep for Science Project wear wrist activity monitors that record their sleep/wake patterns for two weeks, while they follow their usual schedules. They also keep daily diaries to report their bedtimes, wake-up times, and other daily activities. They then come to a white clapboard colonial-style house with a sun and moon flag at the door on the grounds of the nearby E. P. Bradley Hospital. Here, in the Brown University Sleep Laboratory, scientists monitor and record their sleep at night and in daytime naps, measure levels of various hormones, and assess performance of math, reasoning, and other skills over the course of the day.

Mary Carskadon directs this research. A pioneer investigator of adolescent sleep patterns, Carskadon started a summer sleep camp at Stanford University in Palo Alto, California, in 1976. Boys and girls enrolled at ages ten, eleven, or twelve and came to the campus each of the next five or six years for a seventy-two-hour study. They were asked to keep regular hours and sleep ten hours each night for the week before their visit, so that they would be well-rested when studies began. Carskadon then recorded their sleep for three consecutive nights from 10 P.M. to 8 A.M.

At the time, it was widely believed that people need less sleep as they grow older. Carskadon and her colleagues expected to find that older teenagers slept less than younger ones. "We were surprised to find that was not true," Carskadon recalled. All of the children, at all ages and developmental stages, when given the opportunity to sleep as long as they wished at night, slept about nine and one-quarter hours. Thus this appears to be the amount teenagers need.[13]

"Teenagers find the idea of getting this much sleep incomprehensible," she observed. "But they also tell you they are sleepy all the time. We ask them to go to school to learn," she said, "yet we make them go to school when they feel their worst. We are giving them the wrong message."

More Sleep Brings Better Grades

Carskadon and Amy Wolfson of the College of the Holy Cross, Worcester, Massachusetts, surveyed more than 3,100 students attending four Providence-area public high schools where classes started between 7:10 and 7:30 A.M. As adolescence progressed, the students still got up about the same time, but they went to sleep increasingly later. The nineteen-year-olds slept forty to fifty minutes less than the thirteen-year-olds. On average, all students slept less than seven and one-half hours on school nights.

About one-quarter said they usually slept six and one-half hours or less. Only 15 percent reported sleeping eight and one-half hours or more. On weekends, students typically went to bed about two hours later than they did on school days. They got up three and one-half hours later. The top students, the ones earning mainly A's and B's, went to bed earlier on both weeknights and weekends than those who received C's, D's, and F's. The high achievers slept about twenty-five minutes longer on school nights than did the low achievers.[14]

Although some educators and parents insist that teenagers simply need to manage their time better so that they can go to bed at a "reasonable" hour, Carskadon's work shows that even if teenagers were to go to bed early, they probably could not fall asleep. Secretion of melatonin, which indicates readiness for sleep, starts about 9:30 P.M. in younger teens, but not until 10:30 P.M. in older teens. A teenager who goes to sleep at 10:30 P.M. ideally would still be sleeping at 7:30 A.M., not already in school or on the way there, and certainly not driving. Teenagers are still sleepy at 8:30 A.M., Carskadon found, as much as are persons with serious medical sleep disorders.[15]

Sleep loss takes a toll on emotions, perhaps prompting some of the quick-silver changes seen in adolescence, according to Ronald Dahl, a psychiatrist who treats adolescents at the University of Pittsburgh Medical Center. "If faced with a frustrating task," Dahl noted, "a sleep-deprived teenager is more likely to become angry or aggressive." In a humorous situation, the same person might act silly. In Dahl's research, sleep-deprived teenagers asked to perform tedious computer tasks often reported increased irritability, impatience, and low tolerance for frustration. It's easy to see how sleep deprivation might lead to arguments with parents or siblings or teachers, and risky behavior behind the wheel. "The potentially fragile underpinnings of adolescent social competence, controlling thoughts and feelings at the same time," Dahl said, "may be most sensitive to the effects of inadequate sleep."[16]

Minnesota Starts Classes Later, Launches Study

The state of Minnesota has been in the vanguard of moving school start times back. The state's physicians, responding to concerns by sleep researchers, lobbied for later hours. In the 1997–98 academic year, Minneapolis became the first major metropolitan school district in the United States to embark upon a systemwide change. With 50,000 students, it is the state's largest school district. The city's seven high schools changed their start time from 7:15 A.M. to 8:40 A.M. The seven middle schools, which formerly had opened at 7:40 A.M., opened two hours later. Seventy-one elementary schools started at either 7:40 A.M., 8:40 A.M. or 9:40 A.M. The spread-out times accommodate school buses, which 90 percent of the students ride.

Putting themselves under a microscope, area school superintendents asked educational researchers at the University of Minnesota to study the process. Nearly six out of ten teachers said that more high school students were more alert in the first two classes of the day when school opened later, and that fewer students slept at their desks. Students also reported feeling more rested and alert on the late schedule, even though they were going to bed at the same time. They typically slept eight hours a night, one hour more than students in comparable schools in another upper midwestern city that did not change its school start times.[17]

Changing to a later start time caused the most difficulty for middle-schoolers, children aged ten to twelve. Teachers felt the 9:40 A.M. opening did not provide enough prime time in the morning. Teachers in elementary schools that opened at 9:40 A.M. complained that some students watched television for several hours before classes started. They had "eyes glazed over," one teacher said. Worse, the morning programming often included cartoons with violent themes that teachers said often were replayed in the classroom. The 8:40 A.M. openings were the most popular. Teachers pronounced students alert and ready to learn.

Changing school start times clearly altered family life. Affluent parents often were able to shift their own work schedules to take their children to school, while parents with limited resources faced the stress of having to cobble together solutions—arranging, for example, for a grandparent to take children to school or pick them up. Older students, whose classes now ended after 3 P.M., were no longer available to baby-sit their younger siblings in the early afternoon. Students who worked at paid jobs now had less down time between school and work, as many jobs started at 4 P.M. Some had to work later and got stuck with the least desirable tasks such as cleanup duties. Conflicts over access to the bathroom in the morning in some homes, when all family members felt rushed, sometimes set a negative tone for the day.[18]

Grades and scores on standardized tests provide an important measure of the experiment's success. "There is a clear trend line of improvement in academic achievement," Kyla Wahlstrom of the University of Minnesota reports. The Minneapolis suburb of Edina started high school classes an hour later beginning in the 1996–97 school year. Before the change, the top 10 percent of its senior class earned math and verbal scholastic aptitude test (SAT) scores between 580 and 720 (out of a possible 800). In the three years following the change, SAT scores ranged from 600 to 760. "This increase is remarkable," Wahlstrom said, "because these bright students already were doing well."

In the districtwide program, the three years of SAT data the researchers need to make valid comparisons will become available in June 2000, when high schoolers who participated in the program since its inception graduate. Grades clearly are up, Wahlstrom said, by about one-third point on average. Students who formerly maintained a C average now earn a C-plus, and B-minus students get B's. Students in both urban and suburban schools with later start times report significantly fewer feelings of depression and inadequacy than their counterparts in schools that start earlier, a change that cuts across all socioeconomic lines.

Success in making teenagers more alert and ready to learn, Carskadon stresses, requires much more than simply starting school later. Students need to learn about sleep and the effects of sleep loss in their biology, health, and driver's education classes. Parents and teachers need this information, too, and need to use it in planning school events. Many schools now make proms all-night events, for example, aiming to curtail drinking. Yet they still permit sleepy teenagers to drive themselves home in the morning.

Leaving home for college pushes bedtime even later. Orientation weeks at many campuses include midnight movies, tours, and pizza parties. College students go to bed and get up three hours later on average than high school students, Carskadon and her colleagues found in a four-year study of students at Brown University. Psychosocial pressures drive this change, the researchers concluded, not biological ones. "Until sleep gets more respect," Carskadon laments, "it's swimming upstream to try to maintain good sleep habits in college. But," she contends, "sleep is not optional."[19]

Timewise Tips for Teenagers

Aim to get nine hours and fifteen minutes of sleep each night. You probably won't . . . but keep this goal in mind. Getting enough sleep will help you feel better and think faster, and may boost your grades.

Try to stick to a regular bedtime on school nights.

Allow fifteen to thirty minutes before bedtime to wind down. Pack up your schoolbooks. Listen to relaxing music, read, talk to a friend on the phone. Don't jump onto the Internet; it's too energizing.

Exercise regularly, in late afternoon if possible.

Use caffeine judiciously. Don't drink caffeinated coffee or colas after 4 P.M.

Make school your first priority, even if you work at a paid job on school days. A little money in your pocket is nice now, but better grades mean a lot more money later on. Keep work hours to the minimum you can handle without letting grades slip.

If you nap when you come home from school, set an alarm so you won't sleep more than twenty minutes. A brief nap is enough to perk you up. Longer naps may make you groggy.

If you stay up late on Friday and Saturday nights, try not to sleep more than three hours later the next morning. If you're still sleepy that day, take a brief afternoon nap.

Timewise Tips for Parents

Encourage regular bedtimes. Your teenagers may resist rules, but your reminders may help.

Encourage your children to get enough sleep to feel alert in the daytime. If they skimp on school nights, don't hassle them about sleeping late on weekends.

Encourage your child to eat a healthy breakfast (fruit and yogurt on the run are better than chips and a can of cola).

Try to stick to a regular family dinnertime. Meals serve as another time cue that helps anchor your child's day.

Discourage bedtime TV viewing on school nights. This will be easier to do if you refuse to let children have a TV in their bedroom.

Monitor your children's schedules. Encourage them to view school as their main priority, and not to go overboard on extracurricular activities, whether school-related or a paid or volunteer job.

Watch for signs of extreme sleepiness: do you have to drag your child out of bed on school mornings? Is he or she more moody or cranky on school days than on weekends, after getting more sleep? Does your child fall asleep while watching TV, riding in your car, or at other quiet times? Have grades been slipping? Your child's doctor may have helpful advice.

Work within your local Parent-Teacher Association to ensure optimal schedules for learning.

Fitness by the Clock

Exercise at 4:30 P.M.
Everyday (New Years 2002
resolution)

Cyclic ups and downs in body rhythms govern sports performance. How strong you are, how fast, how accurate, how flexible, how quick-witted, how focused, and how able you are to keep going are among the numerous factors that vary over the day, some modestly and others markedly.

Exercising at the times your body is most suited for it has many pluses: you'll perform better, be less likely to get hurt, and probably enjoy it more. You may stick with it longer and see improvement sooner. Exercise at a regular time of day has another payoff: it helps keep the biological clock running on time and serves as a cue that helps keep mealtimes, sleep, and other body rhythms in line.[1]

The flip side is that not heeding these rhythms may throw performance off, increase the odds of injury, and make exercise feel more like work than fun. Exercising at the wrong time of day, round-the-clock studies suggest, may be the equivalent of working out after drinking the legal limit of alcohol or making do with only three hours' sleep.[2]

Most adults have only a little flexibility in choosing the time to exercise: before or after work, in the morning, or in the evening. If you're lucky, you may have access to a track or a room with exercise equipment at your workplace, giving you the option of using midday breaks. You probably can manage a walk or some stretching at lunchtime. Family and work obligations often hamper the best of intentions: you may have to get the kids to school, face a long commute to work in the morning, and prepare a meal and supervise homework at night. It's often hard to keep a regular schedule on trips. Urban design rarely promotes fitness. You might walk to a corner grocery for a few items, but not to a supermarket miles away for a week's groceries. Few cities provide convenient walking and jogging trails.

As a general rule, physical performance is best, and the risk of injuries least, in late afternoon and early evening. More than 60 percent of a group of elite athletes claimed to be at their peak in the afternoon, most often between

3 P.M. and 6 P.M. Stanford University researchers found. Roger Smith and his colleagues asked U.S. Olympic athletes and division I National Collegiate Athletic Association athletes when they felt they performed best. The ten men and eighteen women included runners, swimmers, basketball players, and participants in other sports. Slightly more than 20 percent said they were in top form between 9 A.M. and noon, and less than 20 percent chose 6 P.M. to 9 P.M. None claimed to fare their best before 9 A.M. or after 9 P.M.[3]

Major sporting events are held in late afternoon and early evening because that's when most people can attend them. This nonbiologic factor obscures recognition that these also are biologically the best times for sports. As an aside, it's worth noting that spectator interest also reflects biological rhythms, including those of attention, alertness, and mood. Fans are more content to sit and watch in the afternoon and evening than in the morning.

Media Coverage Sets Competition Times

Scheduling of events once depended on available daylight, also the key time cue for biological rhythms, but no longer. It's probably been years since you've heard, "Game called on account of darkness" for any event beyond a Little League contest. Broadcast media now control scheduling for major sporting events. To capture the largest television audience, Olympic events must compete with each other for the much desired 9 P.M. air time. Advertisers don't want to lose viewers to channel surfing so organizers try to avoid holding two major events at the same time.

Athletes' biological rhythms don't figure in such scheduling. Athletes' preferences carry no weight in scheduling either, according to John Lucas of Pennsylvania State University, an Olympics historian, unless the time of the event presents a demonstrable threat to health. Such concerns prompted a change in the men's marathon at the 1996 Olympics in Atlanta. This event, hugely popular with spectators, originally was scheduled to start at 6 P.M. Given Atlanta's hot, humid evenings, runners and coaches worried about the potential of heat injuries. The event's start time was switched to 7:05 A.M. Body temperature, as we'll discuss, has a potent influence on athletic performance.

Olympic athletes usually know the approximate time that they will compete months, even years, in advance. Indeed, athletes who compete internationally expect to have their events at about the same time from contest to contest and can tailor their training to some degree to this time. Some events, such as track, however, last just a few seconds. Others, such as javelin throwing, require participants to be on the field of play for several hours. Thus, some athletes may be more in sync with their body clocks than others at the actual moment of competition.

What Times Are Best for Sports Performance?

Real competitions provide clues to best and worst times of day, but they are biased by scheduling issues. To assess performance across the day, scientists ask people to perform the same task, running or cycling, for example, at different times. Boredom, fatigue, even what the subjects had for breakfast or lunch, may influence these results, so scientists often study single components of sports performance that they can isolate and measure, from sweat rate to elbow flexion. Their presumption, still unproved, is that such measures hold implications for actual sports competition. Here are important times for some key rhythms, geared to diurnal schedules:

6 A.M.–9 A.M.

Body temperature, lowest when you sleep, starts to rise. Low body temperature is the down time for many functions critical to physical performance, including flexibility, strength, and reaction time. This means you need to warm up more slowly in the morning and spend more time at it. If you exercise outdoors early in the day, particularly when it's cold outside, you run a higher risk of hypothermia. This is a good reason to dress in layers you can peel off as you warm up.

Joints are stiffest and muscles tightest just after you get up in the morning, a function not only of low nighttime body temperature but also of the relative inaction of sleep and daily lows in natural anti-inflammatory hormones. Once you start moving around, this stiffness diminishes. You still need to take it easy when stretching in the morning. Joint flexibility ranges by about 20 percent across the day, a meaningful difference.

Low body temperature makes mornings good for sports that require endurance and less than maximal output, like long-distance running. The generally cooler temperature outdoors in the morning offers further advantages to marathoners, diminishing their odds of suffering heat exhaustion. Heart strain is lower when outside temperature is cooler: cooling the body takes less effort then. The women's marathon at the 2000 Olympics in Sydney is scheduled for 9 A.M., September 24, and the men's is scheduled for 4 P.M., October 1. The daytime temperature in Sydney for the Olympics is expected to be in the sixties (Fahrenheit).

Low overall physical arousal benefits hand steadiness, which peaks in the morning. This skill is critical for archers and sharpshooters, who often like to fire in the lull between heartbeats. Many prefer to compete in the morning, when the heart rate is lower. They also require enormous grip strength, a skill that peaks in late afternoon or early evening. Archers face a dilemma shared by many athletes: their sport demands abilities that peak at different times of day. Peak performance thus sometimes involves a trade-off.

Accuracy and speed do not run in tandem. Accuracy, the skill you need to slam-dunk a basketball, as one example, is higher when temperature is low and falls as temperature rises. But reaction time and speed of performance, the skills you need to race across the court to the hoop, improve as temperature climbs.

If exercise feels like a lot of work, you may be less apt to do it. Round-the-clock studies show that people find the same exercise more formidable in the morning than in the evening. People who exercise in the morning work harder at the end of their workout, while those who exercise in the evening work harder at the beginning, according to Thomas Reilly and his colleagues at the Centre for Sport and Exercise Sciences at John Moores University in Liverpool.[4]

Whether you are a lark or an owl (see chapter 5: "Are you a Lark, an Owl, or a Hummingbird?") may influence your sports performance and preferences, too. Larks usually feel more energetic earlier, because body temperature rises earlier in the day in larks than it does in owls. Workplace studies show that larks perform a given industrial task better in the morning, and owls do so in the evening. Exercise studies don't show such distinct differences. In one, larks and owls pedaled a stationary cycle. Researchers found the two groups were similar in their exercise heart rate, perception of exertion, and in the amount of oxygen they consumed, all indicators of how hard they worked.

It's not clear whether larks or owls are attracted to sports they can do at times they favor, or whether the pros just become used to the time of day that their events take place. One study compared golfers, who competed in daylight hours, with water-polo players, who competed mainly in the evening. The golfers proved more larkish. In another study, cycling time-trialists who race early in the morning got higher lark scores. Most of us become more larkish as we grow older. After about age fifty, we may enjoy walking, jogging, or playing tennis in the morning more than we did when we were younger, assuming, that is, we don't suffer from arthritis, breathing problems, or other illnesses that interfere with these pursuits.

6 A.M.–9 A.M.

Eat a healthy breakfast. This is particularly important for gymnasts, jockeys, boxers, wrestlers, and others concerned about maintaining a specific weight. The body is more likely to burn food consumed in the morning immediately, and to store food eaten in the evening.

11 A.M.

The ability to withstand vague muscle aches that occur in association with extreme exertion peaks around this time. The type of muscle soreness that comes on two to three days after vigorous exercise is least severe in those who exercise in the evening.[5] Persons with rheumatoid arthritis and osteoarthritis find that inflammation and pain predictably vary over the day, making exercise easier at some times than others. (See Timewise Tips If You Have a Chronic Illness, page 104.)

2 P.M.–3 P.M.

This is the time of the post-lunch dip. Persons who exercise strenuously in the early morning may feel particularly sleepy now, and those embarking on strenuous exercise at this time move more slowly and display less stamina. Still, exercise benefits alertness later on. A few minutes of moderate exercise, such as a brisk walk around the block, can perk up an office worker bogged down by midafternoon lethargy.

2 P.M.–7 P.M.

As an indicator of muscle strength, hand-grip strength is easy to measure. It reliably peaks between these hours, with a difference from high to low over the day of about 6 percent. A golfer might hold the club a little more securely in a late-day match than first thing in the morning.

3 P.M.–5 P.M.

Airways are most open; breathing is easiest. Exercise takes less effort.

5 P.M.–9 P.M.

The strength of muscles in the back, legs, arms, and elsewhere varies substantially over the day. In one study, nine of sixteen swimmers, six of six runners, three of three shot putters, and a rowing crew performed better in the evening than in the morning.[6] Another study found that persons who trained only in the evening improved 20 percent more in muscle strength than persons who trained only in the morning.[7] Eye-hand coordination is best in these hours, too, especially important if you're playing racquet sports, shooting hoops, or throwing a Frisbee.

6 P.M.–8 P.M.

Body temperature is at its daily high in most people, although it may be highest earlier in larks, and later in owls. Muscles are most flexible and reflexes fastest. This is the best time for sports that demand both speed and all-out power, such as sprinting, speed-racing, and swimming. It's also the best time for sports that require exact timing and precise muscle control, such as gymnastics and figure skating. Expect your peak all-around athletic performance in a time window about three hours before and after your body temperature is at its daily high.

Pain tolerance is greatest when you are at or near your daily temperature high. Who can forget eighteen-year-old gymnast Kerri Strug's valiant performance at the 1996 Olympics? She injured her ankle on her first vault. Shaking the pain away, she sprinted down the runway, completed her gold medal–winning second vault, then turned to face the judges hopping on one foot. Grimacing in pain, she then sank to the floor. This superb athlete performs well at all hours, but time was also on her side that day. Her injury occurred at 4 P.M., July 23.[8]

A positive mood typically is highest in the evening. While every athlete needs high motivation, an upbeat mood may make that fire burn hotter. Good vibes are crucial for team sports, helping players work better together when the other team scores, officials rule against them, or the game is down to the wire.

Many sports require split-second decision making (pass or shoot?), recall of coaching advice, and rapid calculation. Different mental skills peak at different times of day, short-term memory in the morning, for example, and long-term memory in the afternoon. Variations also reflect situational demands. A coach's instructions probably can be remembered equally well, whenever given, assuming players pay attention in the first place.

Time-estimation ability varies with body temperature. This skill is critical in many sports: think of diving, gymnastics, precision skating, track. We tend to overestimate real time intervals slightly when our temperature is high. This is why persons in bed with a fever, such as children at home and patients in hospitals, think mothers and nurses take too long to respond to their calls. We underestimate time slightly when temperature is low. In late afternoon or early evening, you might perceive thirty seconds in real time as being a few seconds longer. In the morning, that same thirty seconds might seem a few seconds shorter. This ability, in theory, might cause an athlete to feel that time is passing more rapidly than it actually is late in the day, and to step up the pace. In the morning, the athlete might think time is passing more slowly, and cut back.

Menstrual Cycle May Alter Sports Performance

Women have won Olympic gold medals and set world records at all stages of the menstrual cycle. Medal winners are elite athletes, of course, trained to focus single-mindedly on sports performance. Other women may react more strongly to cyclic ups and downs in hormone levels that affect many bodily functions, as well as the psyche.

Body temperature in women is a little higher in the week before menstruation starts. Many women complain of bloating, breast tenderness, and sleep disruption then, all symptoms that may bother even the most ardent exerciser. Negative moods are highest at this time. Positive moods are highest from the end of menstruation through ovulation. Moods influence motivation to work hard, even to work out at all. (See Premenstrual Syndrome, page 324.)

Strenuous athletic training may disrupt the menstrual cycle, even causing periods to stop. Gymnasts, dancers, runners, and others who strive to keep their weight down and maintain low levels of body fat prove most vulnerable. One study found that 20 percent of female athletes, but only 5 percent of women in general, stopped menstruating because of their exercise regimen. An astonishing 50 percent of female runners covering eighty or more miles a week report that they do not menstruate. Running puts enormous repetitive stress on bones, stealing estrogen from reproductive-system activities to keep bones strong. Swimmers and cyclists, who do not have to support their body weight while exercising, have far less trouble with their periods than do runners.[9] The situation usually can be reversed by cutting back on training and adding some body fat, a trade-off not all women athletes are willing to make at certain ages and stages of their career.

Days 10–14 of the menstrual cycle may be a vulnerable time for a common type of knee injury, damage to the anterior cruciate ligament (ACL), according to researchers at the University of Michigan and the Cincinnati Sports Medicine Clinic. The ACL runs through the center of the knee joint and controls the pivoting motion of the knee. When stretched too far, the ACL may tear, an injury that typically occurs when an athlete plants her leg hard, then twists her body, a common move in such sports as basketball, soccer, and volleyball. Women are two to eight times more likely than men to suffer ACL tears, injuries that often require surgery and a year of rehabilitation. In studying forty young women with such injuries, orthopedic surgeon Edward Wojtys found that a disproportionately high number occurred mid-cycle. Levels of estrogen and another hormone called *relaxin* are highest mid-cycle, when ovulation occurs. How estrogen and relaxin contribute to knee injuries remains uncertain, but the link raises the questions of whether the cycle can be manipulated, and whether susceptibility to injury can be diminished by training women to use their leg muscles differently.

Home Field Advantage Includes "Home Time" Advantage

Researchers at the Stanford University School of Medicine studied twenty-five years of National Football League Monday Night Football (MNF) games, focusing on games in which West Coast teams played East Coast teams. Regardless of which coast the games were played on, the games always started at 9 P.M. eastern standard time to facilitate television coverage.

When the West Coast teams played MNF, they therefore started playing at the equivalent of 6 P.M. on their body clocks, when athletic performance is near its daily peak. By contrast, when the East Coast teams played MNF at home, they not only started at 9 P.M., but often played until midnight. This means they competed nearer to the daily lows for athletic performance.

Roger Smith and his colleagues studied the sixty-three MNF games between teams from both coasts that took place between 1970 and 1994. The West Coast teams won more often and by more points per game than the East Coast teams. Overall, West Coast teams won 63.5 percent of these games, while East Coast teams won only 36.5 percent. West Coast teams won by an average of 14.7 points per game, while East Coast teams won by an average of 9 points.

West Coast teams won 59.3 percent of all their home games but 71 percent of home MNF games. East Coast teams won 56.5 percent of all their home games but only 43.8 percent of home MNF games.

To reduce variables in their study, the researchers compared their results to the Las Vegas point spread. Las Vegas odds makers, aiming to ensure that equal amounts of money are bet on both teams, calculate team records, injury reports, winning streaks, and other factors, and then add points to the weaker team. They do not incorporate circadian factors, or at least have not stated publicly that they do. Simply selecting a West Coast team, Smith's group found, successfully predicted the winner against the Las Vegas point spread 67.9 percent of the time. The circadian bonus enhances the home field advantage for West Coast teams but nullifies it for East Coast teams.

Both East and West Coast football teams, the researchers say, now factor the adverse impact of jet lag and sleep deprivation on performance into their travel plans. West Coast teams usually travel to the East Coast two days before game time, and most East Coast teams travel to the West Coast one day before game time. East Coast teams might do even better, the researchers suggest, if they were able to alter their daily performance rhythms to mirror those of their West Coast competitors before MNF games on either coast.[10] Both teams now may be more evenly matched, biologically speaking. Beginning with the Fall 1998 season, MNF moved its game start time to 8 P.M.

In another study, researchers analyzed the nearly 8,500 regular-season games played in the National Basketball Association (NBA) in the eight seasons between 1987 and 1995. The majority of games involved no travel or travel within the same time zone. Home teams won 64 percent of their games by an average of 4.6 points. When coast-to-coast travel did occur, teams coming from the West Coast won more often. Most NBA games are night games, possibly giving the West Coast team a body-clock advantage, according to researchers Kyle Steenland of the National Institute for Occupational Safety and Health in Cincinnati and James Deddens of the University of Cincinnati.[11]

Baseball teams, however, win more games when they travel from the East Coast to the West Coast than the reverse, according to a study by Lawrence

Recht of the University of Massachusetts Medical School and his colleagues. Baseball teams play both day and night games, and travel more than football players overall, so time of day may be less critical than ease of adjustment to a new time zone. Westward travel generally is easier on the body than eastward travel. Still, both East and West Coast Major League teams won more games when they played at home.[12]

Even if you're not a professional athlete, it helps to be mindful of the home-time advantage when you travel. If your trip is short, calculate the time zone difference, and try to exercise at your usual home time if you can.

Jet Lag Undermines Sports Performance

U.S. Olympic gold medal–winning diver Greg Louganis struck his head on the springboard in preliminary trials for the 1980 Olympics in Moscow. Jet lag, he said, upset his coordination. World champion figure skater Debi Thomas fell in the first fifteen seconds of her routine at the 1988 Winter Olympics in Calgary, Alberta. She had to compete at 11 P.M., an hour she ordinarily would have been sleeping.

Jet lag symptoms are performance killers: trouble sleeping and concentrating, irritability, poor mood, altered estimation of time and distance, gastrointestinal upsets. These symptoms are worse in the first two to three days after crossing multiple time zones. The general rule is that adjustment takes about a day for each time zone crossed. Two or three weeks, however, may be needed to realign all rhythms completely.

Even north-south travel within the same time zone may leave an athlete fatigued. Stress, sleeping in a strange bed, competing in a new environment, eating unaccustomed foods, and other aspects of being on the road also may have a negative impact on athletic performance. On the other hand, the excitement of the trip may stimulate stellar effort. Moreover, people differ in how much jet lag bothers them, and individuals vary from trip to trip. Further, well-conditioned persons appear to adapt to schedule changes faster than those who are less physically fit.

Traveling athletes may perform better in their events if they anticipate competition times when training. West Coast runners who plan to participate in the Boston marathon, for example, probably will do better in that race if they synchronize their training time to the marathon's noontime start, 9 A.M. in their home time, and sleep on home time even after arriving in Boston. An East Coast race that started at 9 A.M. would pose more difficulty for a West Coast entrant. A runner would have to get up before 5 A.M. home time to warm up properly before hitting the streets at 6 A.M. Since it's primarily sunlight that keeps body clocks in line, light early in the day would advance the body clock somewhat, helping the West Coast runner adapt better to East Coast time. It might be impossible to shift fully before a trip, since that would require shifting not only sleep and training times, but also meals, work, and social cues that help regulate body time.

The U.S. Olympics Committee now encourages teams to do pregame training in the same region in which they will compete, a costly enterprise. Many teams arrive two to four weeks in advance. For the 2000 Olympics, some teams are considering breaking their journey into two stages, stopping for a few days at a halfway point. This strategy likely would reduce travel fatigue and minimize the stress of having to adjust to multiple time zone changes all at once.

You can take steps to prevent or reduce jet lag even before you leave home. (See chapter 12: "Getting the Jump on Jet Lag.")

Does Exercise Help or Harm Sleep?

Most people believe exercise promotes good sleep. In part, that's because we often confuse fatigue and sleepiness, which are not the same. If you take a ten-mile hike, you may be weary. But if you had enough sleep the night before, you probably won't be any sleepier than usual. Scientists have devoted considerable effort to try to determine the connection, if any, between exercise and sleep.

An important study reviewed every research report on exercise and sleep published in English between 1965 and 1995: thirty-eight studies in all. All of the reports focused on how the same persons slept on nights they did or did not exercise. Most of the more than 400 subjects were college students, healthy, young, good sleepers. Some were physically fit, some not.

Shawn Youngstedt of the University of California, San Diego, and his colleagues used a technique known as meta-analysis to compare results of all these studies. The most notable finding was that people slept about ten minutes more after they exercised than when they did not. The longer people exercised, the longer they slept, though the difference was in minutes, not hours. People did not fall asleep faster after exercising, but they did not take any longer to fall asleep either.

Exercise produced small changes in sleep states: about four minutes more on average of the deepest stages of sleep, thought to be the most restful, and about seven minutes less of rapid eye movement, or REM sleep, the time most vivid dreams occur. Exercise also delayed the start of dreaming by about thirteen minutes. The impact on dreaming sleep, though small, is interesting: antidepressant treatments have similar effects. This finding may account for exercise's well-known benefits on mood.

The impact of exercise on sleep may be tied to body temperature. People warm up while exercising and cool down when they stop. Sleep studies show that people who go to sleep when their temperature is dropping get more of the deeper stages of sleep, thought the most restful, than they would if they went to sleep when their temperature was rising. They also sleep longer. Other research shows that heating people up—asking them to sit in a hot tub or sauna for thirty minutes before going to sleep—increases deep sleep.

One theory is that exercise first artificially increases body temperature and then precipitates a faster decline in temperature than otherwise would occur, promoting more tranquil sleep. Athletes typically have a larger range between their daily high and low in body temperature than sedentary persons. It's a significant difference: about 50 percent. The low point of their temperature cycle is lower, by about 1° Fahrenheit.

Don't worry about trouble sleeping the night before a big event. A sleeping pill should not be necessary, and, indeed, may have unwanted next-day carryover. A little lost sleep probably won't harm performance. Your restlessness probably reflects some anxiety, actually a positive indicator that you are mentally energized and motivated to perform well. Good sleep in the days and weeks prior to the event is more important. Missing a whole night's sleep might harm your concentration the next day, but that's unlikely if you incorporate sleep fitness into your training regimen. Getting enough sleep, and getting it at regular hours, ideally at night, programs your body to sleep well even when you are under stress.

Getting enough sleep takes good planning. Don't skimp on sleep to exercise. Getting up early to work out may seem like a smart move, but to do it you must battle your body's natural predilection to stay up late. You also must resist the insistent allure of nighttime television, the Internet, and other entertainment to get to bed early: a tough task.

Too much exercise may make it harder to fall asleep. The weekend athlete who feels worn-out after an unaccustomed bout of exercise may think, "I'll sleep well tonight." The opposite may be true, as muscle aches and pains can sabotage sleep. A neighborhood jogger who wants to try a marathon needs to add miles slowly. Doing that is unlikely to disrupt sleep, and, as the research cited here suggests, may even improve it.

Is It Okay to Exercise near Bedtime?

This question is much debated. Many popular sleep books warn that exercise close to bedtime proves stimulating and disrupts sleep. Many also assert that exercise far from bedtime probably won't help sleep. The common advice to exercise four to eight hours before bedtime comes largely from studies showing that exercisers who did that fell asleep about eight minutes faster than when they did not exercise.

But some people report they find end-of-the-day exercise relaxing, a good way to get rid of tension and promote fatigue to help them drift off easily. Youngstedt and his colleagues studied sixteen highly fit male cyclists who rode bikes vigorously in the laboratory for three hours in daylight-equivalent artificial light, and went to bed thirty minutes after they finished. Despite this intense, prolonged exercise, the cyclists slept as well as usual.[13]

Toshinori Kobayashi and his colleagues at Ashikaga Institute of Technology assessed the effects of vigorous exercise at different times of day on sleep in ten college students who did not exercise regularly. All fell asleep faster and rated sleep better after exercising from 10:30 P.M. to 11:30 P.M. than they did after morning or early-evening exercise.[14]

Bottom line: with respect to sleep, exercise whenever you want.

Exercise May Help Troubled Sleepers Most

In the same way that even sleeping pills don't make good sleep better, exercise may not make much of a difference in the sleep of persons who already sleep well. But it may benefit those who need help most: insomniacs of all ages, shift workers, and travelers.

Thirty middle-aged adults with long-standing insomnia participated in a study at Stanford University School of Medicine. Each tried three different treatments for four weeks, in random order. In one month, they focused only on strategies of sleep hygiene, such as regularizing their schedule and skipping daytime naps. In the other months, they not only tried sleep hygiene but also one of two therapies: either forty-five minutes' exposure each morning to daylight-intensity artificial light, or a brisk walk for forty-five minutes each evening. The light treatment worked best, Christian Guilleminault and his colleagues found, enabling subjects to sleep fifty-four minutes longer each night on average. When they exercised, they slept seventeen minutes longer. Sleep hygiene alone had little effect. While the timing of the light or exercise may have influenced the results, both measures clearly provided benefits.[15]

In another Stanford study, forty-three older adults with moderate sleep problems enrolled in a four-month exercise program. They walked briskly or performed low-impact aerobic exercises for thirty to forty minutes four times a week before their evening meal. A comparison group of poor sleepers continued their usual sedentary lifestyle. By the study's end, the exercise group slept nearly an hour longer each night on average, fell asleep faster, napped less, and reported better overall quality of their nighttime sleep, while the nonexercisers continued to sleep poorly. Moderate exercise may have something positive to offer older adults with trouble sleeping, Abby King and her colleagues suggest.[16]

Older persons often suffer from sleep problems tied to the biological clock, including falling asleep too early, waking frequently, and waking too early. If this is an issue for you, evening exercise may help you stay up later.

Shift workers and jet travelers both suffer from out-of-kilter clocks. After changing to a new work schedule or crossing many time zones, they have trouble sleeping at hours they previously were awake, and trouble staying awake at hours they'd previously been sleeping in. Exercise and exposure to appropriately timed light together may speed up adaptation of the body clock to a new schedule faster than either would alone. It's not clear yet how much exercise is necessary to shift rhythms and which times work best.[17]

Timewise Tips If You Have a Chronic Illness

Whatever your illness, exercise can improve your flexibility and range of motion, strengthen your heart, boost your stamina, and perhaps even increase your longevity. It benefits mood, too.

Review your medications with your doctor. Some medications may interfere with how well or how safely you can exercise. Antianxiety drugs, antidepressants, antihistamines, and painkillers, for example, may cause drowsiness, interfere with coordination, and slow reaction times. The dosage of diabetes medications needs to be adjusted to accommodate the extra energy that exercise requires. Ideally, you will be able to tune into your body rhythms, and both exercise and take medications at the time of day when they will give you the most benefit and cause the fewest problems. Achieving this ideal may take some experimentation.

If you have heart disease, and are just beginning a cardiovascular conditioning program, work out in the late afternoon. The strain on the heart is less at this time than in the morning. Start slowly and cool down gradually, to allow your heart rate to return safely to a resting rate. Once exercise is routine for you, time of day is less important. A major study found that even persons who had had heart attacks, heart surgery, or other cardiac conditions and who worked out regularly had no added risk of suffering a heart attack when they exercised in the morning. (See page 280.)

If you have asthma, emphysema, or another lung disease, exercise in the afternoon, when airways are most open and breathing is easiest. This advice also applies to persons with transient upper-respiratory-tract infections. Exercise indoors on days when air quality is poor, since smog in urban areas tends to be most dense in midafternoon. (See page 214.)

If you have rheumatoid arthritis (RA), exercise in the late afternoon or early evening, when joints are most flexible. While everyone's joints are stiffer just after arising, the problem is more pronounced in those with RA. Swelling also is more severe in the morning. Fortunately, one of the body's natural inflammation fighters, cortisol, surges into the bloodstream around the time of awakening, easing RA symptoms as the day wears on. (See page 210.)

If you have osteoarthiritis (OA), exercise in the morning before pain becomes troublesome. OA is a wear-and-tear disorder that generally makes fatigue and pain worst late in the day. (See page 207.)

If you have restless legs syndrome (RLS), exercise late in the day when symptoms are worst. Creeping, crawling, prickling sensations mainly in the legs, but sometimes also the arms, characterize this disorder. RLS hinders sustained sitting and sleeping and prompts sufferers to keep moving to gain relief. (See page 330.)

What's the Best Time for Gym Class?

Costly athletic facilities such as ice rinks and swimming pools are scarce. To make them available to large numbers of youngsters, more and more schools now offer before-school sports. Do such schedules threaten children's safety? How does early-morning exercise affect classroom performance?

French researchers explored some of these questions in a study of 130 boys and girls, aged six to eleven. The children took gym for thirty to forty minutes 4.5 days each week, starting at 9 A.M. one semester, and at 2 P.M. the next semester.

The researchers gave the youngsters a variety of tests to assess classroom performance at 9 A.M., 11 A.M., 2 P.M., and 3 P.M. The results bring good news to educators who devise class schedules: gym time had little impact on most children's test results, Georges Huguet of the Pitié Salpêtrière and his colleagues found. Some children were more affected than others, an important reminder that everyone's inner clock is unique.[18]

For adolescents, before-school athletics may worsen an already-existing sleep debt. At a time when a growing number of high schools are opening later with the aim of improving students' sleep, before-school athletics seemingly are counterproductive. (See chapter 8: "The Growing Years.")

Timewise Tips

Exercise whenever it's convenient. If you can't fit exercise comfortably into your calendar, you may not exercise at all. If you are now a couch potato, exercise in the afternoon until you get in shape.

Exercise outdoors in the daytime when feasible to boost your daily exposure to bright light, keeping body rhythms in sync.

Exercise at optimal times on the body clock, according to your sport and your own "feeling best" times.

If you are an elite athlete, training and performing at optimal times on your biological clock may bring extra inches or seconds, even fractions of inches or seconds: the winning advantage.

Study. Visit the American Heart Association's fitness Web site, www. justmove.org.

Time to Eat

Soup for breakfast? Salad as a bedtime snack? Body rhythms make these odd choices for most people. Our inner clocks prompt us to seek energy foods in the morning, and sweets late at night. Body rhythms contribute to the famous female craving for chocolate just before menstruation. They cause most of us to gain a few pounds in fall and winter, but they also make spring and summer the easiest time to lose weight. *When* we eat proves a potent determinant of *what* and *how much* we eat, as well as how our bodies handle food.

WHEN WE EAT

Three Meals a Day by Nature's Design

Newborn babies cry for food about every ninety minutes. From their second to third month of life, most "ask" to be fed only four to five times a day. From their fourth to sixth months, they usually choose, or perhaps simply choose to go along with, the adult three-meals-a-day pattern.

The three-meal habit persists even in time-isolation lab studies, where participants follow the dictates of inner clocks and eat whenever they like. Nearly all subjects in such studies eat within an hour or so of awakening from their main daily sleep episode. Most then consume another two meals in the remainder of their waking day, at intervals roughly comparable to those in ordinary life.[1]

Most people in such studies live on internal days lasting a little over twenty-four hours. You might think they would eat more often, or more food than they normally do, but they do not. In these studies, people occasionally live on days that last as long as forty-eight hours, sleeping for perhaps eighteen hours straight. Yet they treat their long time awake as if it were a normal length day. They still eat only three meals, and they maintain their normal weight. The body adapts to different energy requirements. Understanding how this process works might yield better ways to help starving people, as well as those who eat too much.

In everyday life, as in the lab, hunger peaks three times a day. When healthy, normal weight adults rated how hungry they were every thirty minutes, their hunger jumped between 7 A.M. and 8 A.M., at noon, and between 7 P.M. and 8 P.M. It was most intense at noon.[2]

Regular Mealtimes Increase with Age

Most adults under age fifty eat breakfast about the same time on weekdays, and about an hour later on weekends and days off. Even with a late start on weekends, most eat lunch and dinner around the usual times. In midlife, people rarely sleep late on weekends and have meals about the same times every day.

University of Pittsburgh researchers asked more than two hundred healthy men and women aged twenty to ninety to keep track of daily behavior for two weeks. Participants recorded both when and with whom they ate, worked, did household chores, exercised, watched TV, slept, and engaged in other habitual activities, such as walking the dog or phoning relatives.

Behavioral rhythms interact with biological ones, Timothy Monk and his colleagues found. Behavioral rhythms make life more efficient: you don't have to decide anew each day when to eat or watch the news. You can tell family members, "Let's meet for lunch," and expect they know when to show up.

In the Pittsburgh studies, fifty-year-olds tackled the most activities each day, while seventy- to ninety-year-olds had the most consistent schedules from day to day. Still, there were many individual differences. A few twenty-somethings followed more regular schedules than most eighty-year-olds.[3]

Older persons who eat most meals with a spouse or other frequent companions generally have better balanced diets than those who usually eat alone. Widows and widowers who live alone sometimes report they "forget" to eat or have lost their appetite. Regular mealtimes may help people weather the grief of bereavement by giving the day more structure. People who eat regularly also usually have more regular sleep habits. They report more volunteer and social activities that get them outdoors in the daytime, so they get more exposure to daylight, further protection against depression. They're also more likely to take medications at regular times, and to have better functioning digestive systems.

People go to sleep and get up earlier as they get older, and they eat earlier, too, one reason restaurants in retirement communities attract large crowds with "early bird specials." Throughout life, larks eat earlier than owls. Recall that larks' favorite meal is breakfast, while owls prefer dinner. Larks spend more time on breakfast, and they eat more then, too. One in three owls reports being too rushed in the morning to have breakfast. (See chapter 5: "Are You a Lark, an Owl, or a Hummingbird?")

Fasting in Ramadan Alters Many Daily Rhythms

Muslims observing the monthlong holiday of Ramadan eat and drink only between sunset and dawn at the latitude in which they are living. The holiday follows a lunar calendar, shifting twelve days later each year. It is thus observed in all seasons, with great variations in the duration of daily fasting. Since people continue to work or attend school, the late meals often shorten the time available for sleep.

Mealtimes in Ramadan

♦ Selmaoui Brahim, a biochemist whose studies brought him from Morocco to the Hospital Pitié-Salpêtrière in Paris, France, describes the holiday schedule he follows in both locales:

"The first meal begins about ninety minutes after sunset, following prayers. It includes a sweetened milk drink, dates and other fruits, a type of crepe filled with honey, and vegetable soup. This meal is eaten slowly and enjoyed as a feast.

"Around 11 P.M., sometimes later, depending on the time of year, lunch is served. This meal might include meat, chicken, or fish, with vegetables. There will be many fruits for dessert.

"People then might take a walk or socialize for an hour or two. It would be hard to go to sleep immediately. In the summer, they might get only four hours of sleep. They get up before dawn for a breakfast of bread, yogurt, and fruit. If dawn comes very early, some skip breakfast in favor of a little more sleep."

Ramadan interests nutrition researchers because of the day-night reversals in eating patterns. Their studies may benefit night workers and jet travelers in any culture. One study found women who prepared food for their families in the daytime reported feeling hungry the first few days, but not later on. By not tasting food while they cooked, they may have learned to tune out appetite cues.[4] People often eat more food and more varied food in Ramadan, but few gain weight. Nor do most lose weight, despite remaining active in the daytime. Some report they drink fewer caffeine-containing beverages and smoke less.[5] The atypical mealtime schedule shifts the peak times of certain digestive and energy rhythms, but it does not alter most other body cycles.[6] Persons with chronic health problems, such as high blood pressure and diabetes, appear to manage well.[7]

Regular Meals May Keep Other Rhythms in Line

Jet-lagged travelers who eat at odd times on their body clocks often suffer from diarrhea or constipation for a few days until they adapt to the new time zone. (See chapter 12: "Getting the Jump on Jet Lag.")

Rotating shift workers develop gastrointestinal upsets more often than workers with regular hours. They experience diarrhea, constipation, heartburn, and peptic ulcers at more than twice the rates that day workers do. Since hunger and other digestive rhythms slow down at night, even in people who stay awake, night workers often pass up their usual normal-size meals. They snack frequently, often on high-fat, high-carb items such as potato chips and candy bars.[8] The brain may interpret being awake at the "wrong" time as a crisis calling for quick sources of energy, a high-stress situation that is hard on the body. (See chapter 13: "Clockwatching at Work.")

Persons with winter depression, or seasonal affective disorder, develop food cravings, particularly for carbohydrates, as day length dwindles in the fall. They eat more and gain weight. Their appetite returns to normal when days grow longer in the spring. Some must wear clothing several sizes larger in winter than in summer. (See under Mood Disorders, page 297.)

Persons with the eating disorder *bulimia* often consume vast quantities of food hurriedly, usually in the evening, when the body doesn't expect food and processes it slowly. Meal timing is only one of many biological rhythms that are out of sync in people who are depressed. (See under Mood Disorders, page 301.)

Some people even arise from their beds to gorge while sleepwalking. People with this rare *night-eating syndrome* often consume unpalatable items, such as raw bacon or cat food. Most have little or no memory of their behavior in the morning. They recognize the problem only because they leave the kitchen in great disarray and discover food remains in their beds or on their nightclothes. Most of the nineteen adults with this disorder described in one study ate every night, and often more than once a night.

When monitored in the sleep laboratory, most had a curious mix of rapidly cycling sleep and waking brain activity for sustained periods, according to Carlos Schenck and his colleagues at the Minnesota Regional Sleep Disorders Center in Minneapolis. That's why they were able to walk and eat in their sleep without being aware of it at the time. Most of these people had cut back on daytime food consumption to try to lose weight but ended up obtaining a hefty part of their daily intake at night. With medication to curtail sleepwalking and a balanced daytime diet, most got better.[9]

Many women report *menstrually related food cravings.* The hormone progesterone, highest in the days just before menstruation, may prompt food cravings and overeating. Seven in ten women crave chocolate, nutritionist Debra Waterhouse writes in her book, *Why Women Need Chocolate*. Premenstrual food cravings, usually for foods high in sugar, fat, or both, represent the body's effort to self-medicate, she contends. Enjoy them, she advocates, but in moderation.[10]

News reports on the alleged benefits of chocolate have an annual rhythm of their own, typically appearing in February, right before Valentine's Day. Chocolate may boost your sense of well-being, have a mild energizing effect, and supply some of the needed mineral magnesium, which also plays a role in stabilizing mood, some studies suggest. Chocolate may even promote longevity, according to a review of candy-eating in nearly 8,000 men, some as old as ninety-five, all participants in the ongoing Harvard University alumni health study. Men who ate one to three chocolate bars a month outlived non-chocolate eaters by almost a year.[11]

WHAT WE EAT

Body rhythms call for different mixes across the day of the three essential *macronutrients*: carbohydrates, proteins, and fats. These are the foods we need for energy and growth. The body's innate demands promote daytime activity and nighttime rest. The U.S. Department of Agriculture (USDA) recommends a diet of about 60 percent carbohydrate, 10 percent protein, and 30 percent fat, adding up to an average of 2,000 calories a day. The USDA Food Guide Pyramid translates these percentages into servings of specific kinds of food. The same foods may vary in their effects at different times of day.

Breakfast: Energy

CEREAL w/MILK, WHOLE WHEAT TOAST &
YOGURT OR EGG

In the morning, after fasting overnight, we need energy. Any type of food will lessen fatigue, while skipping breakfast will leave you as sluggish as you were on awakening. Pass up the simple carbohydrates in doughnuts and sweet rolls. Combine complex carbohydrates in whole wheat bread, cereal, and fruit, with protein in the form of milk or yogurt. A protein-rich meal supplies a bigger energy boost than a protein-poor, carbohydrate-rich one, according to Bonnie Spring of the Chicago Medical School.[12] To some teenage girls, breakfast is a stick of gum and a diet soda, not a good way to start the day. Educational research shows that children who eat a nutritionally balanced breakfast earn better grades, have fewer behavioral problems, and have higher attendance rates than those who don't consume an adequate morning meal. Adults who eat breakfast avoid midmorning irritability and lethargy.

Lunch: Sustained Alertness

TUNA, CHICKEN, FISH, TURKEY

A lunch with a high protein-to-carbohydrate ratio may sustain or boost alertness, some research suggests, while one higher in carbohydrates may foster fatigue at this time of day. Proteins are thought to trigger a rise in dopamine, a brain chemical associated with mental energy, and carbohydrates to increase serotonin, a brain chemical involved in sleepiness. To minimize the misnamed post-lunch dip—a normal midday decline in alertness—eat a small, high-protein meal, under 300 calories. Be aware that you're likely to eat more if you eat with other people than if you eat alone. Broiled fish, chicken with skin removed, tuna and cottage cheese, or beans and rice are good choices for your true "power lunch." Fresh or dried fruit can satisfy a noontime craving for something sweet. To enhance afternoon mental performance, avoid carbs such as pasta, potatoes, and sugary desserts for lunch. (See chapter 6: "Your Mind at Work.") Caution: if you have Parkinson's disease, protein may keep your prescribed medication from doing its job. Doctors often advise restricting consumption of protein foods to the time of day when difficulty moving poses the least inconvenience, usually in the evening. If you have any chronic illness, ask your doctor for specific nutrition guidelines.

Dinner: Relaxation

PASTA OR 4oz OF MEAT, FISH, CHICKEN, TURKEY
POTATOES

By the evening meal, your body anticipates sleep and wants a little fat to keep you going through the night. Four-ounce portions of meat, fish, chicken, or pasta with a sauce that includes unsaturated oil provide all you need. A meal high in protein will leave you with a greater feeling of fullness than one of equal calories that is high in carbohydrates. But a high-carbohydrate main course, such as pasta, may induce a calm mental state and promote enjoyment of an evening at leisure. Cravings for sweets are most common in late afternoon and early evening. The brownies you passed up at lunch will be harder to resist at dinner. Your stomach empties 50 percent more slowly after dinner than after breakfast, and your body processes food more slowly, too.[13] This works to your advantage, keeping you from waking up at night with hunger pangs. Moreover, the body stores carbohydrates in liver and muscle tissues at night more extensively than in the day. In the morning, it converts these stored carbohydrates to sugar to use as an energy source.

Bedtime Snack

Since carbohydrates foster sleepiness, they're a good choice for bedtime snacks. Examples include fruit or fruit juice and cookies, or cereal. A light snack is sufficient. Too much food at bedtime will interfere with sleep.

Some people swear by warm milk or cocoa at bedtime. Cocoa contains almost no caffeine. Even though milk contains the chemical building blocks for tryptophan, a brain substance that enhances sleep, a single cup contains too little to benefit sleep. Milk's alleged soothing benefits may be simply an enduring carryover of happy childhood bedtime memories.

For persons with diabetes, bedtime snacks serve an important purpose, helping to keep blood sugar from becoming too low overnight. If you have diabetes, you've probably heard of newcomers to the food market dubbed *nutriceuticals,* or medical foods. These provide the appropriate sources of sugar in a calorie-controlled package, in short, as a cookie or a candy bar. The advantage here is in the convenience, not the contents. Any measured carbohydrate snack is suitable. Other nutriceutical snacks offer alleged benefits to persons with angina, high blood pressure, and other illnesses. Discuss these with your doctor before using them.

HOW MUCH WE EAT

For most adults, breakfast is the smallest meal, and lunch and dinner are progressively larger. After 5 P.M., it takes more food to make us feel satiated, or satisfied, than it did earlier in the day.[14] This is a key reason we eat more in the evening. We also discern tastes better in the evening and enjoy food more. When food choices are limited or bland, boredom sets in. That's one reason the grapefruit diet and other one-food plans succeed, at least for a while: people soon lose interest in eating.

Like animals that hibernate, we eat more in the winter than at other times of the year, and more of certain types of food in one season than another. Humans and other animals typically eat more fat in the summer, more carbohydrates in the fall, and more proteins in the winter.[15] In spring and summer, the body uses carbohydrates as its main source of fuel, and it stores fat. In fall and winter, fat serves as our prime fuel source. Adults typically consume 6 to 7 percent more calories in the winter than at other times of year.[16] This pattern probably helped our ancestors survive the winter when food was scarce, but it makes maintaining weight harder when food is plentiful year-round.

Alcoholic beverages may comprise 10 percent or more of the calories of the typical American's diet. One drink contains roughly 100 calories. Moderate drinking confers some health benefits, as it lowers your risk of heart attacks and strokes. Health authorities define moderate drinking as one or two drinks a day for men, and one drink a day for women and anyone over age sixty-five.

Americans Eat Too Much and Exercise Too Little

Obesity is a major public health problem in the United States today. It is a key contributor to heart disease, high blood pressure, type-II diabetes, sleep apnea, and other ailments and reduces life expectancy by four years.

This country has the world's fattest population. Half of all adult Americans, 97 million people, are overweight. One in five of them is obese, as defined by federal guidelines based on the Body Mass Index, or BMI, plus waist size, an indicator of abdominal fat.

How Do You Shape Up?

♦ BMI is a mathematical formula that takes height and weight into account. Discover your BMI online by typing "body mass index" at any search engine, or by going to www.shapeup.org. To calculate your BMI yourself, you need a chart that converts inches into meters and pounds into kilograms. Divide your body weight in kilograms by your height in meters squared. (BMI = kg/m^2).

Here's what the results mean:

Normal weight = BMI of 19 to 24.9
Overweight = BMI of 25 to 29.9
Obese = BMI of 30 or more

If you are 5'6" and weigh 155 pounds, your BMI = 25. The BMI numbers apply to both men and women. Excess fat on your abdomen adds to your health risks. If you have a BMI of 25 or more and are male, your waist should measure less than 40 inches, and if you are female, less than 35 inches.

American adults now consume 500 more calories every day on average than their grandparents did in the 1930s. Portion-size inflation is rampant, and most people eat what they are served. The USDA says a standard serving size of cooked meat, poultry, or fish is two to three ounces. Many cookbooks call for twice that, and many restaurants offer substantially more. The USDA specifies three cups of popcorn and twelve ounces of soda as standard. Yet most movie theaters serve popcorn in sixteen-cup containers and offer forty-four-ounce soft drinks.[17]

To maintain normal body weight, your daily energy expenditure must equal your daily energy consumption. We're much less active than our grandparents were at our age. Today, only one in four high schools requires students to attend daily gym class. Only one in ten American adults exercises regularly. We drive rather than walk, and we watch a lot of television. Those who watch TV for three or more hours a day are four times more likely to be obese than those who watch for an hour or less a day.[18] A study at Stanford University showed that cutting back on TV viewing kept elementary school children from gaining weight. The researchers did not promote other activities as substitutes; the youngsters became more active on their own.[19]

Research on daily rhythms of the so-called satiety hormone leptin, discovered in 1994 at Rockefeller University, may produce a long-sought effective remedy for obesity. Made in the body's fat and muscle cells, leptin travels via the bloodstream to the brain. There, it targets the hypothalamus, home of the body's master clock, where it may help block appetite. Leptin levels are lowest around midday, and highest around midnight. Changing the timing of meals by several hours also changes the leptin rhythm. Animals given leptin eat less, lose weight, and are more active. While the relationship may not be this direct in humans, medications that include leptin or alter leptin sites in the brain now are under development at several pharmaceutical companies. Other recently discovered brain chemicals involved in controlling food intake also are an active focus of research.

Eat your biggest meal for breakfast
HOW OUR BODIES HANDLE FOOD

To Lose Weight, Eat Breakfast

The now-classic studies in weight control, conducted in the mid-1970s at the University of Minnesota, showed that people who ate only one 2,000-calorie meal a day for a week lost weight when they ate their meal in the morning. They gained weight when they ate the same meal in the evening.

In one study, the normal-weight volunteers ate their only meal for the day either at 7 A.M., within an hour of awakening from their night's sleep, or at 5:30 P.M., for one week. The meal's composition reflected a then-standard diet: 50 percent carbohydrate, 15 percent protein, and 35 percent fat. Those eating only breakfast lost just over 2 pounds on average in one week. Those on the dinner-only routine stayed the same or gained a little weight, Franz Halberg and his colleagues found.[20]

In another study, the same research group let normal-weight volunteers assemble their own meals from a selection of canned and frozen military rations. They still ate all their food either for breakfast at 8 A.M. for three weeks, or for dinner at 6:30 P.M. for another three weeks. The meals averaged about 2,000 calories overall, but most participants ate a slightly smaller breakfast and slightly larger dinner. On the breakfast schedule, they again lost weight. On the dinner schedule, they kept the same weight, or gained a little.[21]

Persons who picked their own foods lost around 1 pound per week on the breakfast-only schedule, only half as much as subjects who ate the higher-calorie meal the researchers provided in the earlier study. This suggests you may lose weight faster if you eat foods you *don't* like. The type of foods you choose also may account for this difference. Your body works harder at burning high-fiber foods such as vegetables, for instance, than those high in fat such as ice cream.[22]

The researchers also found that the different meal schedules shifted the timing of some body rhythms, including the release of growth hormone, insulin, and glucagon, involved in energy use and storage.[23] Discovering how to use meal times to shift rhythms would have practical implications for helping jet travelers and shift workers adjust faster.

A study of 350 French schoolchildren further shows how meal timing affects weight. Whether they were skinny, average weight, or fat, the seven- to twelve-year-olds all consumed about the same number of calories each day. The chubby children ate less for breakfast. Indeed, the smaller their breakfasts, the fatter they were.[24]

Overweight adults typically eat smaller breakfasts than persons who maintain normal weight. Obese adults in France generally eat their biggest meal for lunch, while those in the United States usually eat the most for dinner.[25] Obese people typically eat faster and take larger bites than those of normal weight.[26]

Snacking Does Not Spoil Your Appetite

Snacking is an easily overlooked source of added calories. Many people believe an afternoon snack will curb their appetite at dinner, but French researchers say that's not so. They invited young men to an eat-all-you-want lunch, and then left the men alone until they asked for dinner, roughly six hours later. In three later lunch sessions two weeks apart, the men were served exactly what they previously ate, plus a 250-calorie snack in either early, mid-, or late afternoon. The men still asked for dinner at the same time and ate just as much. The snack simply added to their total intake. Blood tests showed the snack caused only a brief jump in blood sugar, not enough to diminish their appetite for dinner.[27]

You can curb your appetite by slowly eating a small snack five to thirty minutes before dinner, however. Soup and high-fiber fruits and vegetables work better as "preloading" foods than less-filling cheese and crackers, Arthur Winter and Ruth Winter say in *Smart Food*.[28] To ensure that you get enough to eat, your brain waits to say "time to stop" until about twenty minutes after a stream of signals starts arriving from your stomach. You'll get the satiation message whether you eat a lot or a little—nice to know when you're dieting.

Even people who stick to a diet for most of the day often lose their resolve in the evening. Overweight persons report more intense feelings of hunger in the evening than those of normal weight. They also consume a larger proportion of their total daily calorie intake then. Food consumed at night prompts an increase in the unhealthy low-density type of cholesterol, and a decrease in the protective high-density type.[29]

HOW FOODS AFFECT MIND AND MOOD

Caffeine Is a Stimulant

You'll feel the alerting effects of caffeinated coffee, tea, or colas within fifteen to thirty minutes. Caffeine continues to be active for about three to five hours in most people, and for as many as ten hours in some. Its effects are modest when compared to those of other stimulant drugs. Caffeine stays in the body longer in women taking birth control pills, and in women in the luteal phase of their menstrual cycle, the time from ovulation until the start of menstruation. The more you consume, the more habituated to it you become, and the less you notice an impact.

While some people claim they can drink coffee at bedtime and still fall asleep quickly, caffeine near bedtime makes sleep lighter, causes more frequent awakenings, and shortens sleep time overall. Many sleep specialists advise not drinking caffeine within five hours of bedtime. Allow more time if you know you are unusually sensitive to it.

By the tenth century, monks drank coffee to help them stay awake for their nighttime vigils, just as shift workers do today, Mark Pendergrast reports in *Uncommon Grounds*.[30] Caffeine's effects on you may depend on both the tasks you are attempting, and your own individual sensitivity to it. Caffeine may help you type faster but won't necessarily make you more accurate. It may help you focus on a textbook but may not increase your comprehension. It may increase physical endurance if you exercise soon after consuming it, but it also increases your risk of dehydration when you sweat.

More people drink coffee at breakfast than at any other meal. Some claim it overcomes morning fogginess, but in fact, alertness rises on its own within an hour or two of awakening. To maximize caffeine's benefits for your alertness, use it sparingly, no more than a cup or two of coffee or tea, or two cans of cola a day. Don't consume it in the morning. Instead, use it shortly before your midafternoon slump, or at night, if you must stay awake. The bulk of research studies shows that for most people, the caffeine equivalent to that in a cup or two of coffee a day has no adverse impact on health.

If you frequently work at night, you need a fatigue management plan. Combining caffeine with a nap may help you perform better and stay more alert. Michael Bonnet of Wright State University School of Medicine found that doctors in training stayed sharper when they took a two-hour nap after 2 P.M. on the day before a night shift and then drank two cups of coffee at 1 A.M. Drinking two more cups at 7 A.M. helped them stay alert the following day.[31]

If you become sleepy while driving, pull over, drink a cup of coffee and then immediately take a fifteen-minute nap before the caffeine kicks in. This tactic suppresses sleepiness, Jim Horne of Loughborough University in Great Britain found, and reduces driver errors for as long as two hours.[32]

Caffeine-loaded "high energy" drinks, including caffeinated water, are now on the market. Such products include Jolt, Hype, Boost, Guts, and Zapped. Some health experts worry they further promote sleep deprivation. Caffeine also comes in many forms other than beverages. Two sticks of chewing gum with caffeine are the equivalent of a typical cup of brewed coffee. Chocolate contains caffeine, although the typical chocolate candy bar has only about 10 milligrams of caffeine, compared to about 130 milligrams in a cup of brewed coffee. Other foods, including coffee-flavored yogurt and ice cream, may contain as much caffeine as half a cup of coffee. It's also in medications designed to promote alertness, widely used by students at exam time, and in some pain relievers and cold remedies. Department of Defense researchers have devised a caffeine-supplemented food bar for use in field conditions where troops may not be able to brew the usual "cuppa Joe" (G.I. Joe's favorite drink).[33]

Contrary to popular belief, there is no biological mandate for the coffee break. This notion surfaced in the 1950s, soon after researchers discovered that sleep and dreaming occur in ninety-minute cycles through the night. Pioneer sleep researcher Nathaniel Kleitman postulated that a basic rest-activity cycle continued around the clock. "Brainstorms every ninety minutes," news stories of the day proclaimed. But studies of large numbers of people failed to prove this theory. Modern research in time isolation labs shows no ninety-minute cycle in hunger or other waking activity.

Alcohol Is a Depressant

While it slows down the central nervous system, it also may act as a stimulant, prompting boisterous behavior and talkativeness, for example.[34] It's a complicated drug, and its effects vary considerably over the day.

The same dose of alcohol is less intoxicating in the evening than in the morning. It is less intoxicating early in the evening, at 8 P.M., for instance, than later, near your usual bedtime, or in the hours you usually sleep. Since people often drink at late hours on weekends, they feel the buzz more strongly then, too. Alcohol also stays in the body longer in the evening, the time of day drinkers generally drink.[35] Weight, sex, and age alter alcohol's effects. If you are smaller, female, and older, you likely will be more sensitive to the same amount than someone who is larger, male, and younger. If you are sleep-deprived, alcohol will hit you harder. In an eight-hour sleeper who slept only five hours the previous night, one drink will act like two, according to studies by Timothy Roehrs of the Henry Ford Hospital in Detroit.[36]

Alcohol is not a good sleep aid. It may help you relax and fall asleep, but it makes sleep lighter and more fragile, particularly in the second half of the night. It also may cause intense dreams and morning headaches. It takes about an hour per drink for alcohol's effects to wear off in the evening. You'll sleep better if you stop drinking long enough before bedtime for your blood alcohol concentration to return to zero.

Sugar Has Short-Lived Effects

Simple sugars, in candy, cookies, and other baked goods, briefly boost blood sugar. You may feel a spurt in alertness for about twenty minutes. Then blood sugar will fall, and you may feel less alert than before you had your snack.

This message has not gotten through to teenagers or to school administrators. Vending machines dispensing candy and cola do a brisk business in high schools, particularly those that start as early as 7 A.M. Some crowded schools must schedule lunch periods as early as 10 A.M. This is too early to keep students primed for learning until the class day ends in the afternoon.

Is There a Best Time to Take Vitamins and Minerals?

The cells of your body need vitamins and minerals to do their work. You don't make these *micronutrients* in your body; you obtain them from the foods you eat. You can get all the micronutrients you need in a healthy diet. Still, 90 percent of adults don't eat the five servings a day of fruits and vegetables that the USDA recommends. Few adults consume the amount of calcium needed for strong bones. Hence, depending on your diet, you may need supplements.

There are thirteen vitamins. Four are stored in body fat (vitamins A, D, E, and K). Nine are not stored in substantial amounts. These include vitamin C, and eight B vitamins: thiamine (B_1), riboflavin (B_2), niacin, vitamin B_6, pantothenic acid, vitamin B_{12}, biotin, and folic acid (folate). You also need fifteen minerals, including calcium, iron, and selenium.

The food and nutrition board of the National Academy of Sciences established and continues to review guidelines for dietary reference intakes (DRIs) of micronutrients. DRIs include the familiar *recommended daily allowances*, or RDAs, listed on package labels. The way the body circulates, uses, and excretes vitamins and minerals varies over the day, but there are few studies of the optimal time to take these substances. It is known that they are absorbed better with food. "Take your daily multivitamin/mineral supplement with a meal," advises the *Tufts University Health & Nutrition Letter*. "A full stomach takes longer to empty, allowing more time for muscles there to agitate and break down the tablet at the same time that they shred food."[37]

Some vitamins and minerals interact with one another, or with other medications, decreasing their effectiveness. Calcium and iron, for example, if taken in separate pills, should be taken at separate meals. (The smaller amounts in a "multi" formulation are unlikely to cause problems.) If you take thyroid medication, you should not take either calcium or iron at the same time.

When it comes to micronutrients, more is not necessarily better. Too much boosts your risk of potentially dangerous side effects. Too much zinc, for example, can lower high-density lipoproteins, the "good" cholesterol. Too much vitamin B₆ may cause numbness in the legs and other neurological symptoms. Discuss food supplements with your doctor. If the doctor advises that you take them, ask for help in devising a schedule that integrates supplements with the other medications you use.

Timewise Tips

Eat a well-balanced breakfast. If you're always rushing in the morning, pack breakfast to go the night before. Suggestions: yogurt, a peanut butter, cheese, or turkey sandwich on whole-grain bread, a bagel with cream cheese, and fruit or fruit juice.

Don't skip lunch. Make it your largest meal. You'll burn more of the calories you consume at lunch than those you take in later in the day, and you'll be less likely to snack in the afternoon. Choose high-fiber, low-fat foods.

Pay more attention to your inner clock, and less to the one on the wall. Eat because you're hungry, not just because your watch says "It's mealtime."

Eat your evening meal at least four hours before bedtime. You'll improve digestion, burn more calories, and sleep better.

To help curb evening snacking, dim the lights in the kitchen after dinner. Darkness tells your body it's time to stop eating. Healthy snacks include veggies, fruit, or air-popped popcorn.

If you drink, avoid alcohol near bedtime to protect your sleep.

If dieting to lose weight, try "preloading" with soup, fruit, or vegetables before dinner, and immediately before leaving home for a cocktail party or restaurant meal. Consume most of the day's calories before midday, not in the evening.

If dieting, expect fastest results in the spring. Aim to lose one pound every week or two, a realistic goal for permanent weight loss. In the fall and winter, aim to prevent weight gain. This is a more achievable goal at this time of year than shedding pounds.

Weigh yourself in the morning, after emptying your bladder and bowels, when body weight is at its daily low.

Anytime Tips

Exercise regularly, ideally thirty minutes most days. Jump-start your day with morning exercise (assuming you have your doctor's okay), outdoor light exposure, and a good breakfast.

Keep a food diary if you are dieting, noting what and when you eat. A diary will show eating patterns, and help identify problem times or situations.

Practice portion-control. Put food on your plate in the kitchen. Don't bring serving bowls or platters to the table. Small plates can help foster the sense of eating large and satisfying portions. Eat slowly.

If you eat while watching TV, choose healthy snacks. This type of eating is driven more by habit than hunger. Try needlework or knitting to keep hands busy.

Study. For nutrition information, visit the Web sites of the American Medical Association (www.ama-assn.org/consumer.htm), the American Dietetic Association (www.eatright.org/), the National Institute of Diabetes and Digestive and Kidney Diseases (www.niddk.nih.gov), and the Tufts University Nutrition Navigator (http://navigator.tufts.edu).

For help with weight control, visit the Web sites of the National Obesity Foundation (www.obesity.org) and the National Initiative to Promote Healthy Weight and Physical Activity (www.shapeup.org).

Time for Sex

Tuning into body rhythms may help you enhance your performance and pleasure. It also may aid couples trying to conceive, women troubled by irregular menstrual cycles, premenstrual syndrome, or hot flashes and other menopausal symptoms, as well as men with diminished sexual interest and problems getting or keeping an erection.

SEXUALITY

Sexual desire, lust, love, call it what you will, is the stuff of magic and poetry. Understanding its biological substrate won't take that away. Both social and biological rhythms influence timing, frequency, and interest in sex.

Best Time of Day

Five healthy young Parisian men volunteered for the first systematic study of daily patterns in human sexual activity, conducted in the 1970s. The men recorded when they had intercourse or masturbated for fourteen months. Medical students or biochemists, they went to bed and got up at about the same time each day to keep their daily rhythms synchronized.

Three-quarters of their sexual experiences involved intercourse. As you might suspect, convenience played a bigger role than biology in its timing. The most popular time for sex was 11 P.M., with 8 A.M. in second place. The men had sex least often at their self-selected mealtimes and usual hours of sleep.[1] A 1997 survey of nearly four hundred men and women in Houston, Texas, shows the same pattern, with 10 P.M. the favored hour for intercourse, and mornings the runner-up.[2]

Most Popular Day of the Week

Saturday may be the most popular night for dates and parties, but Sunday is the preferred day for sex, at least for married couples. They make love nearly twice as often on Sunday as on any weekday. They also are more apt to make love more than once on Sunday. Overall, married couples have intercourse about 60 percent more often on weekends than weekdays. Two-thirds of weekday episodes of sexual intercourse occur between 10 P.M. and 1 A.M. On weekends, nearly 40 percent occur between 8 A.M. and 5 P.M. Newlyweds make love in the morning more often than do long-married couples.[3]

Preferred Time of Month

Among both married and single heterosexual couples, sex is most frequent on the eighth day of the woman's menstrual cycle, counting from the first day of menstruation. There is no medical reason to avoid intercourse during menstruation, although some religions prohibit it and some couples elect to abstain. The end of bleeding thus prompts a resurgence of sexual activity.

Sexual desire and fantasies in women peak about a week later, at mid-cycle, when they ovulate. A biological rhythm, the highest monthly secretion of estrogens, the prime female sexual hormones, fuels this interest. Women are about twice as likely to initiate sex at ovulation.[4] This is perfect timing, from an evolutionary perspective. Women seek sex most when they are most likely to conceive.[5] Women who take birth-control pills, which suppress ovulation, do not experience this mid-cycle peak of interest.

Women report they reach orgasm more often and that their orgasms are more intense both at ovulation and, again, just before menstruation.[6] Men married to women who are not taking birth-control pills initiate sex about 30 percent more often near the women's ovulation than at other times of the month. How can men tell the time is right? Scientists suspect the women emit certain odorless natural sex attractants, or *pheromones*, that send the male brain a powerful come-hither message.

Pheromones influence animal mating and other social behaviors, and recent studies suggest they affect human sexual behavior, too. Both sexes produce them. The mass market, as usual, has run ahead of science. A search on "pheromones" on the Internet yields numerous ads for love potions. One pitched to women claims it can distract a man watching football on TV.[7] Potent stuff, indeed!

Studies of lesbian couples further illuminate the biological rhythm in female sexual desire and responsiveness. Lesbian couples don't use birth control nor fear pregnancy. Like heterosexual women, as Natalie Angier notes in her book *Woman: An Intimate Geography*, they are more likely to initiate sex near ovulation, and report twice as many orgasms then than at other times of the month.[8]

Most Active Time of Year

Although popular culture links spring with romance, people have sex most often in the fall. This is true for the population as a whole, despite vacations, religious practices that either encourage or discourage sex, and similar events that may alter the frequency of sex for some individuals and groups.

In the Parisian study, for example, the men had intercourse more than twice as often on average in October as in February, their least active month. A biological rhythm, possibly tied to declining hours of daylight, may explain this pattern, Alain Reinberg of the Rothschild Foundation in Paris and Michel Lagoguey of the University of Paris suggest.[9] In late fall, men secrete more of the male sex hormone testosterone.[10]

Increased fall sexual activity has a predictable impact on the birth rate nine months later. As we noted in chapter 2, the birth rate in the United States and other countries of similar latitude invariably soars in late summer.

MENSTRUAL CYCLE

Every month, one of a woman's two ovaries usually produces one egg, sending it down one of her fallopian tubes to the uterus, which thickens in preparation for pregnancy. If pregnancy does not occur, the body sheds the built-up tissue and some blood through the vagina, and the process starts again.

Most girls in the United States today experience their first period around age twelve. They continue to menstruate until age fifty-one on average, with interruptions mainly for pregnancy and breast-feeding. Some illnesses, stressful events such as car crashes, and intense athletic training may halt periods temporarily, too.

When the ovaries stop producing eggs, bleeding ordinarily stops. At birth, a girl's ovaries contain an estimated two million eggs. This number dwindles to about 400,000 when menstruation starts, leaving only a few hundred unused eggs when it ends. In her lifetime, a woman ovulates about 400 times. Women using hormone replacement therapy in a manner that mimics normal monthly hormone production may continue to experience monthly periods, but they do not ovulate.

Our words "menstruation," "moon," and "month," all come from the Greek word for "measurer of time." A woman's menstrual cycle runs its course in about twenty-eight days, one lunar cycle. Periods usually start spontaneously in the week of the full moon in women not using birth-control pills or hormone replacement therapy, particularly those with ample exposure to natural daylight and dark cues. This natural rhythm is even more apparent in monkeys and apes that also menstruate. Scientists today are employing artificial moonlight to help women regularize erratic menstrual cycles.

Cycle length varies most at the start and end of the reproductive years. It is most consistent in women in their twenties and thirties, when fertility is highest. Cycles typically vary by a few days from month to month. One study found the longest cycles in January, averaging about twenty-nine days, and the shortest, in April, averaging about twenty-six days.[11]

Hormones produced in the brain by the hypothalamus regulate the menstrual cycle. The hypothalamus, remember, is also home to the body's master clock, the suprachiasmatic nucleus, or SCN. If you are female, events that upset your SCN, such as changing your hours of waking and sleep, jetting across many time zones, and working at odd hours, may upset your menstrual cycle, too. The hypothalamus also has a direct nerve-fiber connection to a special sensing organ in the nose, perhaps a fast track for pheromones.

The chief sexual hormones in women are estrogen—really *estrogens*, a family of related compounds—and progesterone, both made by the ovaries. In men, sexual hormones are called *androgens*. The chief one is testosterone, made mainly by the testes. The adrenal glands, located just above the kidneys, also produce testosterone in both men and women. Men make ten times as much; a very low level of testosterone in a man would be a very high level in a woman. Men make some estrogen, too, but women make ten times more. Starting at puberty, testosterone fosters bone growth and triggers the appearance of underarm and pubic hair. It also stimulates sexual desire in both men and women.

The Typical Menstrual Cycle Has Its Own Rhythms

The two halves of the menstrual cycle, before and after ovulation, resemble the rise and fall of a roller coaster when plotted on a graph. On the upside, eggs develop in special pockets, or follicles, of the ovaries, and estrogen levels rise. The first two weeks of your cycle is the *follicular* phase. Ovulation occurs at the top of the roller coaster. On the downside, assuming conception did not take place, estrogen levels fall. The empty egg follicle forms the *corpus luteum*, a factory that churns out progesterone for the rest of the cycle. This is the *luteal* phase.

Days 1–5:
Menstruation. The start of bleeding marks the first day of the cycle. On Day 1, estrogen and progesterone are at their monthly lows. This fact prompts the hypothalamus to send messenger hormones to tell follicles of one ovary, sometimes both, to prepare several eggs for release. The follicles produce a

highly active form of estrogen, estradiol, that alerts the uterus to build up tissue to prepare for the egg's arrival.

Many women report less interest in socializing when they have their periods. One researcher dubbed this experience "menstrual quietude."[12] "We all sometimes want to climb a tree and be left alone," psychologist Sharon Golub asserts in her book *Periods: From Menarche to Menopause.*[13]

Days 6–14:

Estradiol rises, and the walls of the uterus thicken. Eggs continue to mature. Progesterone levels stay low. Sexual desire and sexual activity rise. The number of days in the follicular phase (first two weeks) of the cycle often varies, making it hard to predict exactly when ovulation will take place.

This is the best time to have a mammogram *if you are in your forties.* You have this exam to see if breast-tissue abnormalities exist. Breast tissue is less dense in the first two weeks of the cycle in premenopausal women, making a mammogram easier to read. Women in their early forties are half as likely to get a false-positive result from a mammogram performed before ovulation than after it, Cornelia Baines of the University of Toronto found.[14]

Day 14:

When estradiol reaches a certain level, the hypothalamus produces a burst of another messenger hormone that triggers ovulation, sometimes experienced as a cramplike pain. The mature egg will tumble from the ovary down a fallopian tube, where fertilization will take place in the next twenty-four hours, if it is to occur at all.

Mid-cycle is the best time to have a Pap smear *to detect cervical cancer.* Cervical mucus is thinnest near ovulation, yielding the best sampling of cells, and increasing the odds of discovering cancer in its earliest, most treatable state. On the horizon: a home test for human papillomavirus, or HPV, which causes nearly all cases of cervical cancer. For this test, women collect their own cervical cell samples with a cotton swab. Columbia University researchers found the home HPV test as accurate as a Pap smear when women performed it themselves. When the HPV test was performed by medical professionals who could view the cervix and take a more complete sample, it proved even more reliable.[15] Attila Lörincz, scientific director of the Digene Corporation, which manufactures the HPV test, said the new test, unlike the Pap smear, does not require whole cells, and that most early studies suggest its accuracy is consistent across the month.[16] The new test is expected to serve as an adjunct for the Pap smear, not a replacement for it.

Estradiol levels are highest right after ovulation, indeed hundreds of times higher than on Day 1. Estradiol prompts high feelings of well-being and self-esteem, as well as peak interest in sex. It's also linked with heightened senses of vision and smell, enabling women to detect faint lights and certain odors best at this time of month. They also tolerate pain better. Testosterone levels in women also are at their monthly high, a further stimulus to sexual interest.[17]

Dream content changes with ovulation. Beforehand, dreams are more pleasant and more active. You might dream of finding a treasure. Afterward, if conception did not occur, particularly as menstruation nears, dreams contain more anxiety, passivity, and fears of injury. You might dream of being in a car crash. Dreams with explicit sexual content occur most often during menstruation itself.[18]

Days 15–22:

The ruptured follicle will form the *corpus luteum* and make progesterone. The unused egg-containing follicles will shut down. The luteal phase runs a relatively fixed fourteen days. Progesterone transforms the lining of the uterus into spongy tissue, rich in blood vessels, to provide a home for a fertilized egg. The release of progesterone prompts a rise of about 1° F in body temperature across the day. This rise does not signal the start of fertility. Rather, it indicates that ovulation took place. Two days in a row of elevated temperature suggests your fertile time for the month likely is over. On Day 22, progesterone is at its monthly peak, twenty-five times higher than it was on Day 1.

The second half of your cycle may be the best time to have surgery if you develop breast cancer. Studies of more than 5,000 women suggest surgery early in the luteal phase reduces odds of the cancer's recurrence and improves survival. (See page 233.)

Days 23–27:

If fertilization occurred, the egg is now implanted in your uterus, and both progesterone and estrogen remain high. If conception did not take place, levels of both hormones will fall, and the thickened lining of the uterus will break down. The unfertilized egg will break up and pass from your body unnoticed.

Some women report another peak in sexual interest and pleasure as menstruation approaches, often linked to the monthly high in pelvic congestion. At the same time, about three in four women report fluid retention, weight gain of two or three pounds, bloating, breast tenderness, poor sleep, irritability, blue moods, and other symptoms in the four or five days before their periods start, and for the first day or two of menstruation.[19] This constellation of physical and emotional symptoms commonly is called premenstrual syndrome, or PMS. (See Premenstrual Syndrome, page 324.)

Women with many chronic medical illnesses experience flare-ups at this time of month, too. Asthma, constipation, depression, diabetes, digestive disorders, fibromyalgia, heart palpitations, hot flashes, migraine headaches,

MENSTRUAL CYCLE CLOCK

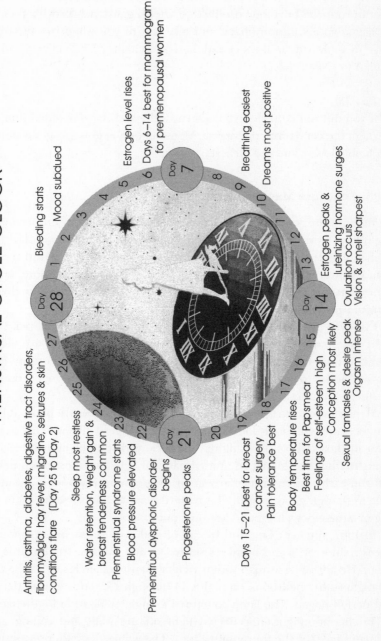

Arthritis, asthma, diabetes, digestive tract disorders, fibromyalgia, hay fever, migraine, seizures & skin conditions flare (Day 25 to Day 2)

Sleep most restless

Water retention, weight gain & breast tenderness common

Premenstrual syndrome starts

Blood pressure elevated

Premenstrual dysphoric disorder begins

Progesterone peaks

Days 15–21 best for breast cancer surgery

Pain tolerance best

Body temperature rises

Best time for Pap smear

Feelings of self-esteem high

Conception most likely

Sexual fantasies & desire peak

Orgasm intense

Bleeding starts

Mood subdued

Estrogen level rises

Days 6–14 best for mammogram for premenopausal women

Breathing easiest

Dreams most positive

Estrogen peaks & luteinizing hormone surges

Ovulation occurs

Vision & smell sharpest

multiple sclerosis, rheumatoid arthritis, and acne and other skin disorders are among those that worsen premenstrually. Abrupt changes in levels of circulating hormones may trigger these flare-ups, according to Allison Case and Robert Reid of Queen's University in Kingston, Ontario. Treatments that alter or suppress hormone production, they suggest, may provide relief. Their advice: keep a symptom diary, and take it with you when you see your doctor.[20] (See individual illnesses and diaries in chapter 15: "Sickness and Health from A to [Nearly] Z.")

Day 28:
If you did not conceive, your uterus will expel the unneeded lining tissue through the cervix into the vagina. Menstruation begins, progesterone falls to negligible levels, and the cycle starts over.

Light Exposure May Regularize Cycles

Light exposure, crucial for strong daily rhythms, also may ensure menstrual regularity. A cycle that consistently averages about twenty-eight days boosts a woman's odds of conceiving. About one in twenty-five women in the United States, however, has a cycle that averages thirty-five days or more, and often varies considerably. These women have higher rates of infertility than those with shorter and more regular cycles.

Evidence that fertility rates are lower in areas where people spend most of their time indoors suggests light's importance.[21] People who are blind have lower fertility rates than those who are normally sighted. Fertility rates are higher closer to the equator, where daylight hours are longer, than in far northern latitudes.

Menstruation starts earlier than average in girls who are blind at birth, or who become blind early in life. It also starts sooner in girls who live at sea level than in those who live at higher altitudes, with higher light intensity. First menstruation also shows an annual pattern. It begins most often in the late fall and early winter, particularly in girls who live in rural settings, suggesting a tie to changing day length. This pattern persists, but is less robust in girls living in large cities who spend less time outdoors.[22]

In 1967, physicist Edmond Dewan of Bedford, Massachusetts, noting that menstruation in some monkeys started in full moons, tried a little experiment. He advised a woman with irregular menstrual cycles to leave a lamp on all night in her bedroom, on nights 14 through 17, starting from the day her last period began. The lamp contained a single 100-watt bulb, the equivalent of bright moonlight. It reflected light off the walls and ceiling onto the woman's face for the four-month study. The woman's cycles previously varied from three to nine weeks, but they soon settled into a regular twenty-nine-day rhythm.[23]

Dewan's theories on light's possible benefits were popularized in a book, *Lunaception*,[24] but drew skepticism in scientific circles. Researchers took his findings more seriously, however, after studies in the 1980s showed that daylight-intensity light can shift rhythms in humans just as it does in other animals. In 1990 May Lin and her colleagues at the University of California at San Diego (UCSD) repeated and expanded Dewan's experiment. In their study, seven women with long or irregular menstrual cycles put a lamp with a bare 100-watt bulb three feet from the head of their bed, turned it on to read in bed for 30 minutes before they went to sleep, and left it on all night on Days 13 to 17. Nine other volunteers used a lamp containing a dim red photographic darkroom bulb, equivalent to pale moonlight. The red light was not bright enough to read by.

The women who used the 100-watt bulb developed shorter and more consistent menstrual cycles, which fell from about forty-six days to thirty-three days. When they stopped using the light, their cycles got longer. Cycle length did not change in the women who got the dim red light treatment.[25]

In subsequent UCSD studies, Katharine Rex and her colleagues experimented with different light intensities and ways to deliver the light, as well as different days for the treatment and different durations of light exposure. Some studies used electronic light masks, which do not disturb bedpartners. Most of these studies showed that even pale light on Days 13 through 17 could help women with irregular cycles, and did not shorten cycles in women who already had normal-length cycles.[26] "This apparently powerful—yet simple and seemingly safe—methodology," said Daniel Kripke, who directs chronobiology research at UCSD, "should lead to exciting progress in our understanding of human reproductive endocrinology."[27]

How could light have such a dramatic impact on the length of a woman's cycle? One theory is that women with irregular cycles may have an abnormality in their secretion of the hormone melatonin, thought to be important for reproduction. The light may somehow restore their melatonin rhythm to normal.

Timewise Tip for Women with Irregular Periods

Use a lamp with a bare 100-watt lightbulb. Place it about a yard from your head. Turn it on at bedtime on Days 13 through 17, and leave it on all night.

Why Close Friends Often Menstruate at the Same Time

In 1971 a student at Wellesley College persuaded 135 women in her dormitory to keep track of the start of their periods over the school year. Martha McClintock, now a psychology professor at the University of Chicago, found that periods in roommates and close friends moved closer together as the months passed. The amount of time the women spent in each other's company appeared to be the key determinant of this menstrual synchrony.[28]

Other researchers explored this phenomenon in other settings. One study focused on twenty-seven Bedouin families. The Bedouin women lived in close proximity for many years, in a highly sexually segregated society, and in comparable surroundings. Few used birth-control pills. These conditions were optimally conducive to menstrual synchrony, according to Aron Weller and Leonard Weller and their colleagues at Bar-Ilan University in Israel.[29] In another study, the Israeli researchers found that sisters living in the same house had their periods at about the same time, whether or not they shared a bedroom.

The same researchers also looked at fifty-one pairs of working women who had shared a relatively small office for at least a year, and worked there full-time, seeing few other people in the workday. Here, close friends tended to get their periods within three to four days of each other, while coworkers who were not close friends got theirs about eight to nine days apart.[30]

The Israeli studies suggest that close, but not too close, relationships promote menstrual synchrony. Mothers, daughters, sisters, and good friends have such ties. Roommates and workplace acquaintances, even though they spend a lot of time together, may not.[31] Women in very intense and intimate relationships, such as lesbian couples, also do not cycle together.[32]

McClintock continues her research in the field. In 1998 she and her colleagues provided strong evidence that pheromones may underlie menstrual synchrony. They took odorless underarm secretions from some women and wiped them under the noses of others. The recipients shortened or lengthened their cycles to mesh with those of the donors at the time the secretions were taken. The changes much exceeded normal cycle variation, shortening by up to fourteen days, and lengthening by up to twelve days.[33] This work raises the possibility that scientists may be able to devise pheromone-based drugs to help infertile women regularize their menstrual cycles, or to help others prevent pregnancies.

McClintock thinks menstrual synchrony is merely one example of social regulation of ovulation throughout the lifespan.[34] In rats, she notes, such synchrony has a practical purpose. If many females are in heat at the same time, males other than the dominant male have more opportunities to mate, thus increasing diversity in the gene pool. Females who give birth around the same time share the care of all the infants, promoting their survival.

Even in humans, menstrual synchrony may reinforce bonding in women in the same family, as well as among friends. Young girls who are best friends often start menstruating at about the same time. As young adults, good friends have babies at about the same time. As older women, they go through menopause together. Men sometimes are surprised to learn that women discuss "female" matters in great detail with each other. The shared biological rhythms create an added social glue.

PREGNANCY

Fertilization of an egg occurs in a narrow time window, roughly the twenty-four hours right after ovulation. Sperm, however, may survive in a woman's body for three to five days. *The right time to conceive thus runs from the five days just before ovulation through the day of ovulation.*[35] Intercourse even one day after ovulation is unlikely to result in pregnancy. If you are trying to avoid pregnancy, you still need to take precautions, because it's hard to tell on your own when ovulation occurs.

Almost no one has perfectly regular cycles. The wobble in the system generally occurs in the first half of the month, that is, before ovulation. This is the reason the rhythm method of birth control has a higher failure rate than birth-control pills or barrier methods of contraception. It predicts the date of ovulation from general biological rhythm principles that may not apply to a specific woman.

Some women feel a cramping pain when they ovulate. Some study their cervical mucus, which becomes watery, rather than sticky, just before ovulation. Some take their temperature, watching for the rise of about 1° F that indicates ovulation has occurred. Taking your temperature first thing in the morning, as doctors often advise women to do, is subject to error because people often awaken from REM sleep, a time when temperature normally fluctuates. Also, the rise in temperature may occur over several days.[36]

Timewise Tip If You Want to Get Pregnant

To determine your date of ovulation reliably, use a home urine test kit that measures monthly shifts in hormone levels. Pharmacies offer a wide selection. A computerized device, the ClearPlan Easy Fertility Monitor (Unipath Diagnostics, $200) uses urine test strips to determine the amount of estrogen, which rises steadily in the first half of the cycle, and of luteinizing hormone, which the pituitary gland produces about sixteen to thirty-two hours before ovulation. If you perform urine tests as specified, this device will show your fertility status each day of your cycle. It also stores test results in its memory, increasing its ability to predict your five most fertile days each cycle after several months of use.

Can You Choose to Have a Boy or Girl?

Does the time you have intercourse determine your baby's sex? Women at several medical centers participated in a study to answer this question. The women charted their monthly cycles, recording signs of ovulation, including cervical mucus changes, and changes in body temperature. They also recorded when they had intercourse. After nearly one thousand women became pregnant, Ronald Gray of Johns Hopkins University and his colleagues calculated the probable day of insemination relative to the day of ovulation. When the babies were born, the researchers studied the records to see if timing had any influence on a baby's sex. They came up empty-handed. As long as there are grandmothers, there may never be a "last word" on this topic, but this research suggests that timing insemination in the hope of determining a baby's sex is as reliable as, say, a toss of the dice.

Pondering the baby's sex before it is born preoccupies expectant parents. Biological rhythms may offer useful clues. Several studies show mothers-to-be with severe morning sickness early in pregnancy have girls more often than boys. High levels of a hormone that appears late in pregnancy when the baby is a girl are implicated in morning sickness. Of more than one million babies born in Sweden in the eight years of one study, 49 percent were girls, a normal distribution. Of nearly 6,000 women who had such severe nausea and vomiting in their first trimester that they had to be hospitalized, 56 percent later had girls. Johan Askling and his colleagues at Karolinska Institute, Stockholm, theorize that the women who became ill early on produced too much of the "girl" hormone, too early in pregnancy.[37]

A mother's dreams about her baby's sex turns out to be a pretty good predictor, too, accurate 71 percent of the time in women with more than a high school education, Johns Hopkins University researcher Janet DiPietro and her colleagues found. Presumably, the women picked up some subtle biological clue, but what that was, and how they did it, remains unclear.[38]

Pregnancy Disrupts Sleep

About eight out of ten women report their sleep is more disrupted in pregnancy than at other times, particularly after the baby starts moving around.

Months 1 to 3 (First trimester):
Many women report they are much sleepier than usual and need more sleep now than either before pregnancy or in its later months. The rapid rise in progesterone following conception may be the trigger.

Months 4 to 6 (Second trimester):

Sleepiness usually fades, even though progesterone stays high throughout pregnancy.

Months 7 to 9 (Third trimester):

Pressure on the bladder from the baby often prompts several trips to the bathroom at night. Difficulty finding a comfortable position, leg cramps, and heartburn are other common complaints.[39]

After the baby is born:

Sleep disturbance is greatest in the first month, particularly for first-time mothers.[40] The new mother will face sleep deprivation and fatigue until her baby sleeps through the night. Her sleep then will improve, but it is an enduring fact of life that even women whose children consistently sleep through the night sleep less soundly than women without children.[41] Most women encounter a brief bout of new-baby blues, and a few develop a severe postpartum depression. (See under Mood Disorders, page 305).

Timewise Tips to Improve Sleep If You Are Pregnant

Sleep on your left side to provide best blood flow to your baby, and to your uterus and kidneys. Use pillows or rolled-up blankets to help you maintain this position.

Avoid consuming fluids near bedtime.

Nap in the daytime both to boost energy and make up for lost sleep at night.

See Timewise Tips for Good Sleep, page 77.

Nighttime Is Prime Time for Births

Tales of racing the stork to the hospital at 3 A.M. are part of many families' lore. These always sound like great and exotic adventures. They are, in fact, the norm. Humans and other day-active species give birth most often at night, and night-active species do so in the daytime. Birth in the body's natural rest period increases the likelihood that mother and baby will be in a safe space at a vulnerable time.

Spontaneous labor in humans starts around midnight more than twice as often as around noon, its least frequent start time, a study of labor in more than 200,000 women shows. Records collected on more than two million natural births in the 1970s showed 20 percent more babies were born between 2 A.M. and 6 A.M. than between 2 P.M. and 6 P.M.[42] Later studies support this nighttime peak. This is true for all babies, not just first babies.

Even in the modern world, nighttime labor and delivery may offer some advantages. Women whose contractions spontaneously start after dark spend about two hours less in labor on average than those whose labor started after dawn. Women whose labor starts at night experience less bleeding and fewer complications associated with childbirth than those whose labor starts in the daytime. Babies born at night are in better shape right after birth than those born in the daytime.

Medically stimulated or induced labor, more common in recent years, somewhat obscures circadian patterns of labor and birth. Physicians typically perform such procedures in the daytime. One-third of births in the United States in 1997 were stimulated or induced, or both, the National Center for Health Statistics reports. This practice also alters the weekly distribution. More babies are born on Tuesday than on any other day. Sunday and Saturday are the least common days. In 1997 births in the United States were 27 percent less likely to occur on Sunday than on Tuesday.[43]

While mothers-to-be often wonder if it would be safer to let nature take its course, obstetric interventions in the daytime in modern maternity facilities pose no added risk for mother or child. There are clear benefits for medically complicated pregnancies, as more staff members are on hand in the daytime. One possible downside of nighttime deliveries is that fatigue and human errors are higher on the night shift. (See chapter 13: "Clockwatching at Work.")

It is a myth that babies are born most often under a full moon. People simply are more likely to remember a full moon at a baby's birth, according to astronomer Daniel Caton of Appalachian State University. Caton's team debunked this folk belief by using a computer to correlate records of 50 million live births in the United States with dates and states of the moon.[44]

PERIMENOPAUSE AND MENOPAUSE

The stereotypical view of the so-called change of life as a time of angst is fading. Menopause is a natural event, not a disorder. Most women feel happier and more fulfilled after menopause than they did earlier in life, the North American Menopause Society reports. More than half of 752 women responding to this professional society's 1998 survey said relationships with spouses or partners improved, and their sexual relationship stayed the same after menopause. The rest were about equally divided between those who said their sex life got better and those who said it deteriorated.[45]

Women today have fewer complaints about menopause than their mothers did, possibly a reflection of better ways to remedy the consequences of midlife hormonal shifts, derived from new insight into the underlying biological rhythms.

If you are a woman in your thirties, your hormone levels already are starting to fall. In your mid-forties, you might go for a month or two without a period, and then have two within a single month. Your flow might be lighter or heavier than usual. The years just before your last period and the year after it are now called *perimenopause.* The end of menstruation, *menopause,* occurs at age fifty-one on average.

What Causes Hot Flashes?

The falling levels of estrogen send confusing messages to the hypothalamus, which regulates body temperature. Sudden rises in temperature trigger hot flashes, the most common complaint of perimenopause, and one that 75 percent of women experience. Hot flashes—some women jokingly call them "power surges"—involve a sudden rush of warmth over the face, chest, back, shoulders, and upper arms. A woman may visibly redden, and feel heart palpitations and anxiety. These sensations may last from a few seconds to a half hour or longer. As body temperature readjusts, she may perspire, and then she may feel cold. If sleeping, she may awaken frequently from severe hot flashes, known as night sweats, that force a change of nightgown and sheets.

Hot flashes follow a daily pattern, peaking in most women in late evening, when body temperature is still near its daily peak. They peak in some women in the morning, close to the time body temperature is lowest.[46] Hot flashes continue for six months to five years on average, although some women experience them into their seventies.

They are the prime cause of sleep disruption in women over age fifty, Suzanne Woodward of Wayne State University School of Medicine reports. Her studies show that hot flashes in sleep occur about once an hour. Most prompt an arousal of three minutes or longer. Independently of their hot flashes, women who have them still awaken briefly every eight minutes on average. The sleep process dramatically blunts memory for awakenings, Woodward said, and in the morning women seldom realize how poorly they slept.[47]

Instead, they often focus on the daytime consequences of poor sleep, which include fatigue, lethargy, mood swings, depression, and irritability. Many women and their doctors, Woodward said, dismiss such symptoms as "just menopause." This is a mistake, she suggested, because treatment can reduce or eliminate hot flashes, aid sleep, relieve other symptoms, and improve a woman's quality of life. Treatment also helps keep frequent awakenings from becoming a bad habit that continues after hot flashes subside.

Drop in Estrogen Affects Many Bodily Functions

Beyond hot flashes, falling levels of estrogen may cause vaginal dryness, leading to pain during intercourse, vaginal itching at other times, and increased frequency of urinary tract infections. These difficulties may reduce a woman's interest in sex. Falling levels of testosterone that also start well before menopause may further undermine sexual desire and decrease genital sensitivity. Declining hormones also affect memory and cognition, as well as the health of the heart and bones.

"Menopause is a state of hormone deficiency that should be treated," declares the American Association of Clinical Endocrinologists (AACE), a physicians' group. Some doctors, and some women, however, contend it is a natural life process, better left alone. In its guidelines for doctors, the AACE suggests that all women should consider hormone replacement therapy (HRT) not simply to replace missing hormones but also as preventive medicine.[48] HRT may consist of estrogen alone, or estrogen and progestin, a form of progesterone; both forms of therapy reduce hot flashes. Testosterone may be included, particularly for women who report a decrease in their sexual desire, sensitivity to sexual stimulation, and capacity for orgasm.

Studies suggest that women using HRT are one-third to one-half less likely to die of heart disease than women not using it, an important benefit since heart disease is the leading cause of death in American women.[49] Because of estrogen's bone-strengthening effects, HRT users have fewer fractures from osteoporosis and less tooth loss. They may have a lower risk of Alzheimer's disease, colon cancer, diabetes, and osteoarthritis. While women using estrogen alone have a higher risk of uterine cancer, taking estrogen with progestin cancels this particular risk. This two-hormone combination has become the standard therapy for women with an intact uterus.

But HRT users may be more likely to develop breast cancer than nonusers. The estrogen-progestin regimen may elevate a woman's risk of breast cancer more than estrogen alone does, a National Cancer Institute study of more than 46,000 women at twenty-nine screening centers throughout the United States suggests. Catherine Schairer and her colleagues found the increased risk occurred largely in current users and in women who had used HRT in the previous four years.[50] Their findings also suggest the risk of developing breast cancer increases with longer use of HRT, a fact that complicates the decision-making process, since it is not until ten years or more after menopause that risks of hip fractures and heart attacks surge. HRT also may increase a woman's risk of stroke, fibroid tumors, and gallstones. All these findings are prompting doctors to review current dosing regimens and to consider alternative strategies. Every woman needs to assess carefully with her own doctor the benefits and drawbacks of HRT in her particular situation.

An exhibit traveling to science centers across the United States through 2004 gives women the opportunity to literally weigh the pros and cons of hormone replacement therapy for themselves. Seated at a scale, you will be able to balance metal weights labeled "may decrease my risk for heart disease," for example, against "may be linked to the development of breast cancer," according to their importance to you. The $3.2 million exhibit, "The Changing Face of Women's Health," is the collaborative effort of nine major U.S. science centers and the U.S. Centers for Disease Control and Prevention.

Because of the health concerns and questions, and perhaps also because the cost of treatment serves as a barrier for some women, fewer than 30 percent of the 35 million postmenopausal women in the United States currently use HRT. Some uncertainties may be resolved by the ongoing Women's Health Initiative study of HRT in 27,000 women nationwide. Results should be available starting in 2005.

Timewise Tips for Menopausal Women

Use the menstrual cycle diary (page 329) to log hot flashes and other symptoms. Try to identify events that triggered them, such as drinking coffee, or eating hot or spicy foods.

To minimize hot flashes:

- Keep your home and bedroom cool, especially when preparing for bed.
- Use a fan even in winter.
- Do not take warm baths.
- Wear cotton nightclothes, and use cotton sheets.
- Keep a thermos of ice water at your bedside and drink from it if you awaken with a hot flash.
- If sharing an electric blanket, use one with dual controls.
- Learn to breathe from your abdomen, not your chest. Slow breathing reduces frequency and intensity of hot flashes.

Talk to your doctor about HRT. Estrogen and other hormones come in a variety of forms, including pills, skin patches, injections, creams, and a ring that is inserted in the vagina. Estrogen patches, as one example, are applied once or twice a week, on the same days of the week, and worn continuously. No specific time of day is advised. The medication is released at a constant rate. You may need to use HRT for a month or two before its benefits with regard to hot flashes stabilize.

To mimic normal monthly rhythms and prevent endometrial cancer, a woman who still has her uterus must also take progestin. For women who cannot use conventional HRT or choose not to, a new family of drugs known as selective estrogen receptor modulators, or SERMs, may provide some of estrogen's benefits while avoiding some of its side effects. The first of these drugs, raloxifene (Evista), was approved by the FDA in 1998 to prevent and treat osteoporosis.

Some women prefer natural estrogens in foods or supplements derived from foods. Black kohosh and genistein and other soy-based products may reduce hot flashes. Their benefits for reducing heart disease and osteoporosis are not proven. There are no published studies on their effects when taken at different times of day.

Testosterone use still is controversial, both because testosterone may have unwanted side effects in women, such as growth of facial hair, and because research findings regarding its benefits, particularly in older women, have been contradictory. Tablets containing low doses of testosterone are available. A small testosterone patch designed for women is undergoing study. "Testosterone is not an aphrodisiac," notes psychiatrist Susan Rako. It usually takes several weeks to show benefits, she reports in her book *The Hormone of Desire*.[51] There are no published studies of testosterone's effects in women when taken at different times of day.

If you are using HRT, schedule your annual mammogram in the part of the month when you are not taking progestin. In general, women who have gone through menopause have less dense breast tissue than younger women. About 25 percent of those using hormone replacement therapy, however, show increased breast density in the ten days of the month that they take progestin.[52] Seek your doctor's advice on stopping hormone therapy briefly before your mammogram. Some studies suggest this tactic also may lower the likelihood of a false-positive result.[53]

Practice good health habits to reduce postmenopausal illnesses: exercise regularly, consume adequate calcium, don't smoke, maintain a healthy weight, cut fat in your diet to reduce heart disease and breast cancer risk, and get an annual mammogram and Pap smear.

Study. Visit the Web sites of the North American Menopause Society (www.menopause.org) and the American Association of Clinical Endocrinologists (www.aace.com).

HORMONE RHYTHMS IN MEN

Testosterone is both predictable and quirky. While men secrete it in daily and annual patterns, it also serves as a barometer of their moods and mind-set. Testosterone surges in men who win football, soccer, and tennis games, as well as champion chess matches. It plunges in losers. It even goes up and down in male fans who watch their teams win or lose, a biological show of team spirit.[54]

Testosterone is higher in actors and lawyers than in ministers, higher in single men than those who are married, higher in *Animal House*-type college fraternities than in quieter groups.[55] It rises in anticipation of sex, falls if the situation disappoints. "If there was ever a hormone designed to blow hot-blow cold, it seems to be testosterone," Deborah Blum writes in *Sex on the Brain: The Biological Differences between Men and Women*.[56]

Testosterone levels prove higher on average in sleep than in wakefulness, as Israeli researchers discovered when they took blood samples hourly across the twenty-four-hour day.[57] It's been known since the 1980s that testosterone secretion follows a rhythmic pattern, tied to the different states of sleep. Testosterone levels rise shortly before the start of each REM period, and dip after it.[58] Hormone levels are highest in the morning hours, at the end of a night's sleep. In the waking day, morning testosterone levels may be 35 percent higher than those in the midafternoon and evening. Levels of this hormone typically are lowest between 7 P.M. and 10 P.M.

Men produce more and faster sperm in the afternoon, however. Italian scientists compared seminal fluid collected around 7 A.M. or 5 P.M. The fifty-four volunteers provided the semen samples on separate occasions after abstaining from intercourse for several days. Having lots of speedy sperm boosts the odds that one of them will reach the egg in the few days each month when conception is possible. *For couples trying to conceive, the late afternoon thus may be the best time for intercourse,* Angelo Cagnacci and his colleagues at the University of Modena suggest.[59]

Sperm counts also vary over the year, providing a marker of annual rhythms in sexual activity: the more active a man is, the lower the number of sperm released in each ejaculation. Several studies show sperm counts are lowest in the summer and fall, the peak season of conception, and highest in the spring.[60] Heat is known to harm sperm; changes in daylength also may be a factor.

MALE MIDLIFE CHANGES

Men do not go through andropause the way women go through menopause. The production of androgens, the male sexual hormones, does not cease, as women's periods do. But both sexes share certain midlife changes.

Hormone levels start falling in both sexes in the thirties. In men, the principal hormone, testosterone, declines about 1 percent to 2 percent a year between ages forty and seventy. Also starting around age forty, the range of daily ups and downs in testosterone secretion gradually flattens. Men in their seventies typically produce 40 percent less of the hormone than they did in their forties, although they still may be capable of fathering a child.

The rate of testosterone's decline varies from man to man. Smoking more than ten cigarettes a day makes it fall sooner. Diseases such as mumps and injury to the testicles and some medications curb testosterone, too. If testosterone levels fall too low, men may even get hot flashes like those women experience at menopause. They also may develop enlarged breasts. Low levels of testosterone, however, do not make a man's voice change.[61]

Low levels of testosterone may blunt a man's interest in sex and cause difficulty getting or keeping an erection and infertility. They also may decrease his bone and muscle mass, strength, and stamina and prompt weight gain. On the mental and emotional sides, low levels of the hormone may induce irritability and depression and diminish the ability to concentrate. These problems typically surface when men are in their fifties and sixties.

All this makes andropause sound suspiciously like menopause, although you almost never hear doctors attributing such symptoms to, say, "the empty car syndrome." Some male physicians maintain that the emotional side of andropause is fictional. A French medical-journal article suggested the term "andropause" was slander.[62] A German medical report asked, "Do we need the concept of male climacteric?"[63]

What Treatment Is Available?

Hormone replacement therapy with testosterone, HRT for men, may preserve bone or prompt building of new bone, increase muscle mass, improve mood, boost interest in sex, and increase a man's erectile ability. Whether HRT will improve or worsen a man's risk of heart disease isn't yet known.

HRT is not for every man. It may increase the risk of prostate cancer, and certainly should not be used by a man who already has this illness. It may worsen the sleep-related breathing disorder, sleep apnea, and cause acne, hair loss, and other problems.

Testosterone for use as HRT comes in pills, patches, injections, or implantable formulations. The patches, developed in the 1990s, are popular because they are user friendly. They provide maximum concentrations of the hormone in the blood in early morning hours and minimum concentrations in the evening, simulating the normal daily pattern of testosterone release in healthy young men. A man using a *Testoderm* patch, as one example, would apply it to his scrotum on awakening in the morning.[64] Testosterone penetrates skin in this area at least five times more readily than skin elsewhere on the body. Other patches are available for men who prefer to wear them in a different location.

Erectile Dysfunction Now out of the Closet

Erectile Dysfunction, or ED, trouble getting and keeping an erection, once wrongly termed "impotence," moved from the bedroom to the living room as a topic of discussion with the introduction of sildenafil (Viagra) in the United States in 1998. One-time presidential contender Robert Dole testified to the efficacy of the "little blue pills."

While ED may affect men of any age, it becomes more frequent with aging. More than half of the forty- to seventy-year-old men in the Massachusetts Male Aging Study reported on a questionnaire that they had minimal, moderate, or complete ED.[65] Findings from this study suggest that more than 152 million men worldwide experienced ED in 1995. Because the population is rapidly aging, projections for 2025 show a prevalence of approximately 322 million men with ED, an increase of nearly 170 million.

A 1976 study documenting daily biological rhythms in erections prompted the now routine use of the sleep laboratory to help identify likely causes of ED. Researchers at the Baylor College of Medicine found that healthy males of all ages, from infants to those in their eighties, normally had erections in REM sleep.[66] Ismet Karacan and his colleagues monitored erections in the sleep lab by attaching a strain gauge to the penis. They reported that healthy men in their twenties average four erections a night lasting a total of 191 minutes, roughly one-third of their time asleep. Healthy seventy-year-olds have three erections a night, lasting ninety-six minutes, one-fifth of their sleep time. Little boys experience regular sleep-related erections, SREs, even though they make only small amounts of testosterone in their adrenal glands. That suggests that SREs, along with rapid eye movements and other aspects of REM sleep, may have a functional value, notes Max Hirshkowitz of Baylor.[67] These activities may provide a self-test, the body's way of making sure all systems are "go."

Men who lack normal SREs often have a physical illness such as diabetes or high blood pressure. These illnesses may interfere with the nerves controlling blood flow to the penis, or to the blood vessels whose engorgement sustains erections. Some medications used to treat these and other illnesses also may cause ED, and adjusting the dose may improve the ED. Testosterone deficiency may cause ED, and testosterone replacement may correct it. Smoking and alcohol abuse also contribute to ED. By contrast, ED in men with normal SREs is more likely to have psychological roots such as anxiety, depression, or anger, for which counseling may be useful. SRE tests help doctors to focus quickly on appropriate treatment.

Whatever the cause, sex therapists say, psychological or relationship issues often coexist. Viagra, and other medications for ED, are unlikely to solve such problems by themselves.[68] Taking advantage of biological rhythms in sexual responsiveness, however, may help a couple proceed with more confidence. The last hours of sleep are most dense with REM sleep. Erections at this time are strongest, too, the reason that men often awaken with one. For men with ED, sex thus may be easiest in the morning.

Timewise Tips for Men with Erectile Dysfuntion

See your doctor if you have ED. If the cause is not readily apparent, your doctor may suggest a sleep-lab study.

Make a morning "date" with your partner. Try setting your alarm clock for an hour or so before your usual wake-up time to exploit your sleep-related erection.

If using Viagra, which takes about an hour to work, leave the pill and water on your nightstand. Set an alarm clock ninety minutes before your usual wake-up time, take the pill, set the alarm to go off an hour later, and go back to sleep. Caution: don't use Viagra or other drugs for ED if you are taking nitrate drugs, such as nitroglycerin; if you have high blood pressure; or if you have had a heart attack or stroke. Sudden deaths have been reported in some Viagra users with underlying heart disease. The cause is still under investigation. For current information, see www.viagra.com. Also see "When Is Sex Safest?," page 281.

Consider couples' counseling. The nonsexual side of your relationship may be more important than you now suspect.

Study. Visit the Web sites of the American Medical Association (www.ama-assn.org/insight/spec_con/sexdysf/) and the American Society for Reproductive Medicine (www.asrm.org/patient/sexdys/html).

Getting the Jump on Jet Lag

Welcome to the Timeful Hotel. Our motto is: "You'll send jet lag packing." We're conveniently located at the airport to help you adjust body clocks painlessly before or after you cross multiple time zones. Tell the desk clerk where you're going, or where you've been, and what your flight times are. Frequent fliers: take a minute to update your computer file, reporting how long you normally sleep and when you typically eat and exercise. If you take medications at specific times, add that information, too.

Along with your room key, you'll get a schedule showing the best times to sleep and to be awake to speed adjustment to your chosen time zone. You'll gradually move your sleep and wake times earlier if flying east, or later if flying west. If you are on a brief visit and want to stay on home time, we'll show you the easiest way to do that, too. If our local time is the same as your home time, we'll give you fast steps to ease your return.

Our schedule also tells when to get bright light, when to be in dim light, and when to be in bed in the dark. Time goes fast in the Timeful Hotel's premier attractions, our three "beat the clock" wings: Day Land, where it's always day, all the time; Night Land, the reverse; and Local Locale, where there's no time like the present.

The Timeful Hotel, a fantasy conceived by chronobiologist Charmane Eastman,[1] doesn't exist—yet. It's a doable concept, though, probably no more costly to build and staff than the typical luxury resort and conference center. Astronauts already are using bright lights to switch their sleep, wake, and meal times to prepare for space flight. Some power plants and other industries now provide daylight-bright ceiling lights to help control-room workers stay wide awake on the night shift. Some hotels offer lighting devices in guest rooms, round-the-clock food service, and other programs to ease travel stress.

You don't have to wait for the Timeful Hotel to open to take advantage of the many new clock-resetting strategies. These tactics, based on biological rhythm research, can help you function more effectively whenever you travel.

Eastman and other researchers are scrambling to find even faster ways to take the "lag" out of jet lag.

Jet Lag Is a Modern Malady

We fly like eagles. But body clocks follow like turtles. Their slow pace of change works to our advantage when we stay put: it keeps us anchored on home time. We'd be mighty uncomfortable if the hands on our inner clocks spun to and fro every time we walked in or out of a dark movie theater or stayed up late.

Our ancestors did not suffer from ship lag, wagon lag, or even train lag. Early modes of transportation couldn't take them six hundred miles, the approximate distance of one time zone, in a single day. Shifts in body rhythms occurred outside their awareness.

Then planes came along. Suppose you fly tonight from New York to Paris, a trip six time zones eastward. You may stroll down the Champs Elysée tomorrow, but your body will act as though you still are walking on Fifth Avenue. If you take a ship from New York to France, a voyage of about six days, and keep your wake/sleep schedule in tune with the rising and setting of the sun, you will be on French time when you disembark. The "lag" in jet lag is the gap between the time on your body clock and the new local time.

Anyone who doubts that inner clocks exist, or thinks they don't matter, never had jet lag. For several days after you arrive in a new time zone, body temperature, normally lowest when you sleep, may be lowest when you are awake. Since alertness rhythms parallel those of body temperature, you probably will feel less sharp and focused than usual, and more fatigued overall. You may find it hard to fall asleep and stay asleep at night.

You may awaken more often to use the bathroom. Being out of sync may make you feel sluggish, light-headed, and weak. You may be more clumsy or forgetful. You may want supper when it is dinnertime in New York. That's midnight in Paris. The upset stomach that travelers often blame on unfamiliar foods may be the result of balky body clocks. On top of all this, you may have headaches, muscle aches, and general malaise.

These symptoms probably won't be severe enough to keep you confined to your hotel room. But they may hang on for several days. Jet lag complicates sensitive diplomatic missions, throws off athletes' and musicians' performances, fouls up business deals, and makes busloads of tourists snooze through the sights they came to see. It undermines skills needed for driving, adding to the potential hazards of having to navigate unfamiliar roads.

With the rise of multinational corporations, more and more people, many of them top decision-makers, spend so much time away from home that they develop a chronic jet lag syndrome. They are never home long enough to readapt before taking off again. Their complaints resemble those of persons who rotate job shifts around the clock. (See chapter 13: "Clockwatching at Work.")

One Traveler's Perspective

♦ To chronicle the transportation of freight around the world—tropical fish from Manila to Los Angeles, racehorses from Chicago to Tokyo, strawberries, gold, computers, pajamas, everything we eat and wear and use and amuse ourselves with—writer Barry Lopez made forty flights within a few months. He covered about 110,000 nautical miles, often riding in the cockpit with the pilots. "On the road, like the pilots, I endured the symptoms of a jagged, asynchronous life," he reported in *Harper's* magazine.

"No matter how exhilarating a trip might have been, I sensed on leaving the plane that a thrashing like the agitation of a washing machine had ended and that, slightly dazed, I was now drifting off my path, a yawing ship. My tissues felt leaden. Memory seemed a pea suspended in the empty hull of my body. I had the impression that my mind was searching for the matching ends of myriad broken connections and that it was vaguely panicked by the effort. The fabric of awareness felt discontinuous. Time shoaled, losing its familiar depth and resonance. I craved darkness and stillness."[2]

Pilots and road warriors suffer every bit as much as first-time travelers. Experienced travelers, however, usually devise personal strategies for coping through trial and error. A 1999 ad campaign for IBM's Lotus software assured ordinary mortals, "Superman can fly but still gets jet lag." The message, as articulated by Lotus's director of worldwide advertising in *The Wall Street Journal,* was "You can be in control of your life, your destiny, your business . . . You're empowered to go beyond the limitations you've had so far in your job."[3]

We may aspire to be superman or superwoman. But short of staying home, none of us can avoid jet lag entirely. Body clocks have a mind of their own. They hold us in their thrall. Alleged jet lag remedies abound: just surf the Internet! Slick ads tout diets, foods, pills, and special drinks, most with no more than testimonials to support them. Findings from biological-clock research, however, offer truly effective help.

Daytime Symptoms Bother Travelers Most

Some three hundred Norwegians, nearly all physicians who attended a medical meeting in New York City for five days, agreed to participate in a study conducted by Robert Spitzer of the New York State Psychiatric Institute and his colleagues.

The day they left for home and for the next five days, the volunteers answered questions about whether and how much they suffered from nine common jet lag symptoms and how much jet lag bothered them overall.

The researchers encouraged the volunteers to use a sleep mask when attempting to sleep on the plane and not to drink alcohol. Once home, they were to try to go to bed and get up at their normal time and not to take any medicine other than the capsules that were part of the study (more on these later).

After four days in New York, 85 percent of the 257 persons who finished the study reported having no or only "a little bit" of jet lag. On their first day home, after crossing six time zones, 63 percent said they had at least "moderate" jet lag. Daytime symptoms bothered this group of travelers much more than poor sleep did.

Most Annoying Jet Lag Symptoms

Symptom	Day 1 % of travelers	Day 6 % of travelers
Sleepiness during the day	72	4
Fatigue or tiring easily	69	1
Decreased daytime alertness	40	1
Trouble concentrating or thinking clearly	40	1
Lethargy or sluggish feeling	32	2
Light-headed, dizzy, or other uncomfortable sensations in the head	30	2
General feeling of weakness	29	2
Physical clumsiness	17	1
Trouble with memory	13	0

Adapted with permission from Spitzer, R.L., et al. Jet lag: clinical features, validation of a new syndrome-specific scale, and lack of response to melatonin in a randomized double-blind trial. *American Journal of Psychiatry.* 1999; 156: 1392–1396.

Travel Fatigue Makes Jet Lag Worse

Long plane trips themselves generate discomfort, even if you do not cross any time zones. Fortunately, symptoms of travel fatigue usually fade in a day or two. Moreover, you can minimize these problems by advance planning and in-flight tactics. (See Timewise Tips, page 160.)

Travel fatigue symptoms include dryness of the mouth, nasal passages, skin, and eyes. These are caused by reduced oxygen levels and drier-than-desert air in the aircraft cabin. If you drink beverages containing alcohol and caffeine, both diuretics, you'll add to your moisture loss. If you stick to water and fruit juices, you'll reduce it.

The cramped conditions of the typical coach seat leave many people with a backache and stiff muscles. If you sit for hours, fluids collect in lower limbs, making ankles and feet swell. Stand up and move around when you can. Avoid carbonated drinks, as they may produce intestinal gas and distend the abdomen while you are in flight. Vibration, noise, and air turbulence may trigger a headache, as may secondhand smoke. More and more international airlines now offer smoke-free flights, a boon not only to passengers but also to flight attendants who long campaigned for a smoking ban.

Even frequent fliers often tackle a monumental "to do" list in the days before travel. Feelings of anxiety, weariness, and irritability may not surface until you sit back on the plane and reflect on both the tasks you did and those you left undone. There always are last-minute chores. Few people sleep as well as usual the night before a big trip. Sleep loss itself undermines performance and well-being.

Culture Shock Doesn't Cause Jet Lag

Sleeping in a strange bed, eating strange foods, hearing a strange language, and other experiences that make travel different from life at home do not cause jet lag. You can use the excitement and pleasure of these experiences to distract you from the discomfort of having out-of-kilter body clocks.

In one laboratory study of jet lag, eight middle-aged men spent fifteen days alone in a time-isolation apartment, with no windows, clocks, or other indicators of time. Timothy Monk of the University of Pittsburgh and his colleagues told them when to go to bed, get up, and have meals. The scientists also monitored their sleep, recorded their body temperature continuously, and regularly assessed their performance on a variety of physical and mental tasks, as well as their moods.

One night—night as perceived by the subjects—the researchers secretly shortchanged them on sleep. Each volunteer went to bed as usual but was awakened six hours early. This is the equivalent of leaving New York in the evening and flying to Paris. After the meal and the movie, when cabin lights finally are dimmed, you might snatch an hour or two of sleep. You'll arrive in Paris with a sleep deficit of about six hours.

In this study, the subjects did not go anywhere. They did not know about the stolen sleep. They followed the same daytime routine and slept in the same bed at night. Yet their body clocks were as upset as those of any traveler. The disruption lasted as long as for someone crossing six time zones eastward, about a week.[4]

Flying East Is Harder than Flying West

When traveling east, you have to go to bed and get up earlier than usual. Eastward travel, in essence, shortens the day. When traveling west, you typically stay up later and sleep later. Westward travel thus lengthens the day. Because the body clock typically runs slightly longer than twenty-four hours, staying up later is easier than going to bed earlier.

Expect to be sleepier than usual in the morning after traveling east, and sleepier in the evening after traveling west. Conversely, you may be more alert than usual in the afternoon after heading east, and in the morning after a trip west. Savvy travelers use these facts to their advantage. A businessperson from the east coast of the United States who travels to London, traversing six time zones, for example, would want to avoid important meetings between 9 A.M. and 11 A.M., British time, a down time for the traveler. Between 2 P.M. and 4 P.M., however, when British associates are fighting their midday slump, the U.S. visitor would feel sharp and productive.

When you fly west, your body clock runs in the same direction as your plane. When you go east, some rhythms shift earlier, and others, later. After you fly eight time zones eastward, for example, some rhythms will move eight hours earlier, and others, sixteen hours later. The resulting jumbled state until you adjust induces the symptoms that make traveling eastward more troublesome than traveling westward.

Body clocks adjust faster after westward travel in most people. Two groups of German researchers, Jürgen Aschoff and his colleagues,[5] and Karl Klein and Hans Wegmann,[6] found body clocks shift by about ninety minutes a day on average after you fly west, and about sixty minutes a day after you fly east. Thus, if you cross about five time zones east, it takes about five days on average for clocks to realign themselves, while it takes about three days if you fly west. These findings prompted the easy-to-remember dictum that it takes roughly a day to adapt to each time zone crossed.

Regardless of direction, some rhythms shift faster than others. Within two or three days after you cross six time zones, you may fall asleep at your customary time, but wake up more frequently to go to the bathroom. Rhythms of the kidney adjust slowly. Most rhythms readjust fastest in the first few days after travel. It may take two or three weeks to realign all rhythms completely. If you keep on traveling across time zones, you'll continue to have some of your rhythms out of sync.

North-South Flights Don't Cause Jet Lag

North-south flights in the same time zone, even those lasting many hours, may cause travel fatigue but they don't cause jet lag. A trip from Canada to Mexico, however, especially in winter, may involve big differences in the times of dawn and dusk in the two locales. When traveling north to south, your sleep and mood may change, perhaps for the better. If you were to fly south to north, the opposite might be true.

Local culture may prompt changes in your schedule. Americans who go to

Spain, where the evening meal typically is served much later than in the United States, tend to eat later and stay up later while visiting. Americans thus may get over jet lag faster in Spain than in France, where the time zone is the same but the people generally dine earlier. Americans would have less of a gap between their bedtime at home and at the new local time in Spain than in France. Those who visit Scandinavia in the summer, when there is near-constant daylight, also may stay up later than usual. Winter visitors to far northern countries may go to bed earlier than usual.

Many people find homebound journeys less discomforting than outgoing ones, regardless of the direction of travel. Laboratory studies show the east/west differences in severity of jet lag persist, but psychological factors, such as a return to familiar surroundings, may make jet lag less noticeable.

If traveling around the world, expect less jet lag if you go west. One notable exception: if you have a depressive disorder, you may do better if you travel east. The sleep deprivation associated with eastward travel mimics manipulations of sleep sometimes used to treat depression. It may improve your mood rather than dampen it as more often happens in travelers who are not depressed. For persons with depression, westward travel often proves more problematic.

You don't have to leave home to suffer jet lag. Staying up three hours later than usual on Saturday night is the equivalent of flying from New York to San Francisco, or from Hong Kong to New Delhi. On Sunday night, in essence you attempt to make the return trip. You'll probably take longer than usual to fall asleep and find it hard to get up at your usual time Monday morning. Monday fogginess is so pervasive in our society that it's given rise to such maxims as "Don't buy a car built on a Monday" and complaints such as "Monday morning blahs." Classroom teachers know this phenomenon well, often reporting that they spend Monday mornings talking to the tops of their students' heads.

Daylight Saving Time (DST) also mimics jet travel. The spring change is akin to traveling east, and the fall change to traveling west. Springing forward is harder on the body than falling back. Although only a one-hour difference, the spring DST change packs a bigger wallop than a flight one zone eastward. Jet lag is negligible after a trip from, say, St. Louis to Orlando, because the sun rises and sets an hour later in Florida than it does in the Midwest. DST asks you simply to pretend sunrise and sunset occur an hour later. It expects you to heed the clock on the wall, a much weaker pacesetter than the sun. It takes about three or four days to adjust after the spring DST change, but only about a day to adjust in the fall.

Some sleep disorders also produce a syndrome akin to jet lag: they cause people to stay up later and sleep later than desired, or the reverse, to go to bed too early and wake up too early.

Why You Sleep Poorly

Sleeping and waking typically snap back fast, letting you fall asleep at your usual time within two or three days after crossing six time zones east or west. Body temperature, however, takes longer. In the five or so days that the temperature rhythm takes to regain its usual pattern, your temperature probably will be higher than usual while you sleep. This makes it more likely that you will toss and turn, and awaken more often than you ordinarily do.

Most flights heading from the United States to Europe depart at night. This custom has no apparent business rationale, and it adds to travelers' woes. Flights from the west coast to the east coast of the United States, and from Hawaii to the U.S. mainland, which occupy about as much time as some flights to Europe, often take place in the daytime. "Red-eye" flights are a notable exception, giving a passenger full days at either end, at the expense of a night's sleep. For an eastward flight from San Francisco to London, you might leave at 5 P.M., fly for ten hours, and arrive at 11 A.M. the next morning. If you stay up until your usual bedtime, 11 P.M., you will be attempting to go to sleep at 3 P.M. home time.

Flights heading west from the United States usually depart in the daytime. Leaving San Francisco at noon, you would fly for eleven hours and reach Tokyo at 4 P.M. This is a difference of seven time zones, so you arrive at 11 P.M. San Francisco time. If you stay up until your usual bedtime hour, 11 P.M. in Tokyo, you will be going to sleep at 6 A.M. home time.

In both of the above scenarios, if you adopt local time on arrival, you will have a long day. That first night, feeling quite sleepy, you probably will fall asleep fast and sleep reasonably well, even though it is the wrong time for sleep according to your body clock.

The second night you won't be as sleepy. Your misaligned temperature clock may make you sleep fitfully. By carrying the resulting sleepiness through the day, you'll sleep better the third night. By the fourth night, your sleep and temperature clocks will be nearly synchronized, and sleep should be close to normal. If you traveled east, it may take longer than usual to fall asleep for the first few days. If you traveled west, you may fall asleep easily but awaken too early.

Canadian Airlines announced a new transatlantic flight schedule in 1998: its Dayliner service is the first flight of the day from Canada to England. Its Starliner is the last flight from England to Canada. These schedules give Canadian travelers a few extra hours to work or enjoy the normal waking day in England.

You can get a head start on shifting sleep rhythms a few days before leaving home. Go to bed and get up earlier if heading east, and later if heading west. A change of just an hour or two shouldn't throw off your home schedule by much, but it can make a substantial difference on the road. Adaptation is fastest in the first few days.

When Can Sleeping Pills Help?

Taking a sleeping pill on the plane may help you catch some sleep you'd otherwise forfeit. It's wise to try the medication at home a few times, so you know how it affects you and how long it takes to wear off. You wouldn't want to be groggy when you land. Sleeping pills with a short duration of action are particularly useful in counteracting the difficulty of falling asleep that often follows eastward travel. These include zaleplon (Sonata) and zolpidem (Ambien). (See When Can Sleeping Pills Help?, page 349.)

A few travelers have reported transient memory loss after taking benzodiazepine sleeping pills, particularly triazolam (Halcion), which has a half-life of from 1.5 to 5.5 hours. These persons appeared to be their usual selves on and after the flight and even gave lectures or attended meetings soon after arrival that they later could not remember. This effect is unusual and appears to be aggravated by use of alcohol while taking these medications. Hence, it's wise to avoid this combination.

After arrival, sleeping pills generally do the most good on the night after a night with good sleep, that is, the second and fourth nights. While better sleep by itself will reduce some of the unpleasantness associated with jet lag, sleeping pills also may act as *chronobiotics*, medications that shift body clocks. They do this by inducing sleep at the time you desire.

To avoid shifting to the new time zone, try to schedule your sleep so that some hours coincide with time you would have been sleeping at home. This practice serves to anchor sleep and other body rhythms, as well. Eleven P.M. to 3 A.M. in Washington, D.C., is 5 A.M. to 9 A.M. in Amsterdam, for example, an appropriate time to sleep in both time zones. Avoid sleeping late in the morning. Get up at your usual hour. If sleepy, nap in the afternoon.

We All March to Different Drummers

Your symptoms may vary from one trip to the next, even if you cross the same number of time zones. You may have certain symptoms, while your companion on the same trip has different ones. You may suffer acutely, and your companion only mildly, or seemingly not at all.

Morning people, or larks, report less jet lag than evening types, or owls, when traveling east. Owls do better than larks when traveling west. That's because larks find it easier to go to bed and get up early, and owls find it easier to stay up late and get up late.

Members of tour groups suffer less jet lag than do solo travelers. Groups keep regular hours for meals and other activities, creating numerous time cues to hasten adaptation. They often spend considerable time outdoors, enlisting the environmental light and dark cycle to reset body clocks. One study of travelers who crossed six time zones found those who spent time outdoors every other day adapted 50 percent faster than those who stayed inside—an important message for business travelers and conference goers.

Summertime travelers can expect to adapt faster than those who travel in winter, *again a function of higher daylight exposure.* Winter sports enthusiasts would be an exception.

Extroverts adapt faster than introverts, probably because they interact more with others and benefit from group routines.

Persons who are overweight report less jet lag. They typically pay more attention to eating meals at regular times than persons of normal weight.

Younger travelers suffer less jet lag than middle-aged and older travelers. Margaret Moline and her colleagues recruited six men aged eighteen to twenty-five and eight men aged thirty-seven to fifty-two to spend two weeks in the chronobiology laboratory at the New York Hospital–Cornell Medical Center. For the first week, the volunteers followed their usual schedules. Then their sleep was cut short by six hours on one night to mimic a trip from New York to Frankfurt, six hours eastward. For the first four days after the shift, the older group awakened more frequently and got less sleep than the younger subjects. They also felt sleepier during the day and reported that it took more effort to do daily tasks. Body temperature rhythms in both groups, however, adjusted at the same rate.[7]

Persons who exercise regularly do better than those who are sedentary. Regular exercise serves as another time cue. The physically fit, as a group, also sleep better than those who are out of shape.

Military troops usually adapt faster than civilians. They travel in groups and spend more time outdoors. They also are young and in good health, traits associated with flexible rhythms and good sleep. Troops also travel for reasons that distract them from jet lag symptoms. Jet lag is a key concern for military forces, however, since troops who travel long distances may have to go into action immediately.

Bright Light May Speed Clock Resetting

Appropriately timed exposure to sunlight or artificial light of equal intensity may help you adapt more quickly to a new time zone. (See chapter 4: "How Your Body Clock Works.")

Light exposure soon after your body temperature is lowest—a time that shifts when you travel—speeds adjustment to travel in an easterly direction. It makes you more alert earlier in the day in your new time zone. It also starts hormone secretion earlier and makes body temperature rise sooner. Light exposure right before the temperature low point has the opposite effect. It speeds adjustment to westward travel, which requires later sleep and wake times.

In the laboratory, researchers can synchronize light exposure closely with body temperature readings, or with other markers of body rhythms, such as secretion of the hormone melatonin. They can control precisely the timing, dose, and intensity of the light.

In an early study of light for jet lag, Charles Czeisler and James Allen at Harvard University Medical School designed a light routine for Mike Long, a reporter for *National Geographic.* In 1986 Long flew to Boston from Tokyo after a month in the Far East. On the flight, he wore welder's goggles to shield his eyes from daylight. In Boston, he spent three days in the chronobiology laboratory at the Brigham and Women's Hospital, isolated from time cues and exposed to bright lights for several hours when his body temperature was lowest. His temperature rhythm shifted from Tokyo time to Boston time, a difference of eleven hours, in three days, roughly twice as fast as is usual. According to the researchers, the first two days' exposure jolted Long's clock and blunted its normal daily ups and downs. The third exposure restarted his clock at the desired time. "My jet lag," Long wrote in his article, "vanished in the lights."[8]

In everyday life, it's not possible to measure temperature and melatonin rhythms easily and precisely. Trying to target your lowest temperature closely is risky. Light at the wrong time may send your body clocks in the wrong direction, much as if you were to set out from Chicago for Rome but ended up in Honolulu.

Fortunately, even without knowing the exact low point on your body temperature clock, you can make use of general principles of light exposure. The easiest way to get bright light while traveling is to spend time outdoors in the morning if going east, and in late afternoon if going west. The easiest way to avoid light is to stay indoors, or, if you must go outside, to wear the darkest sunglasses you can find, ideally with top and side protection. Dark goggles, the type welders use, are highly effective in blocking light, but few tourists are brave enough to wear them on the street.

Planning your schedule carefully is not difficult. Suppose you fly from New York, where your temperature low occurs at 4 A.M., six time zones eastward to Paris. On arrival, your temperature low will occur at 10 A.M. Paris time. You'd thus want to avoid bright light before 10 A.M. the first day, but spend time outdoors in the late morning. This will tell your body clock to start the next day earlier. On your return trip, assuming you've stayed in Paris long enough to become acclimated, your 4 A.M. trough in Paris will occur at 10 P.M. New York time. Light in the late afternoon will push that time later.

One day of attention to light exposure is not enough. "Even if you follow instructions perfectly," Yale University light researcher Dan Oren cautions, "exposure to light at the wrong time on Day 2 can undo what you did the previous day." In *How to Beat Jet Lag*,[9] Oren and his colleagues provide a program of instructions to follow for several days after flights anywhere in the world.

They target their strategies to persons whose temperature minimum occurs before 5 A.M., who they believe represent the majority of the population. As the following excerpt from *How to Beat Jet Lag* illustrates, you need to pay attention to much more than getting and avoiding light at certain times. You also need to sleep and be active at the right times.

SIX TIME ZONES EAST JET LAG COPING GUIDE

For example:
From the U.S. East Coast to Western Europe

1. Board plane for take-off.

2. After 10 P.M. in your original time zone, being exposed to light will interfere with your effort to beat jet lag. Therefore, wherever you are at 10 P.M. in your original time zone, put on dark glasses. If you expect to be asleep at 10 P.M., put on a cloth eye mask before going to sleep. When you wake up, be sure to put on dark glasses when you take off your eye mask. Be careful as you walk with the glasses on. NOTE: Don't wear dark glasses if the light level is too low for them to be worn safely.

3. **First morning at destination:** After about eight hours, the plane has crossed six time zones and lands. Be sure to continue to wear dark glasses and be as inactive as possible until 10 A.M. in the time zone of your destination. Until 10 A.M., being exposed to light and being active will interfere with your effort to beat jet lag. Be careful as you walk with the glasses on.

4. At 10 A.M. in the time zone of your destination, remove dark glasses or eye mask. After 10 A.M., especially from 10 A.M. to 1 P.M., exposure to light and being active will help you beat jet lag. If possible, maximize your exposure to sunlight during these hours. NOTE: Do

not look directly at the sun or a halogen bulb. If you are flying during this period, try to sit next to a window. If you are on the ground, try to be out of doors as much as possible. If indoors, try to stay near a window or in a brightly illuminated room.

You are likely to be tired during the first day at your destination, but this will be due to lack of a full night's sleep rather than to jet lag. It's best not to nap during the day or evening, so that you can get a full night's sleep at the end of the day. If you wish to nap, do so between 2 and 8 P.M., and keep your nap as short as possible.

5. **First night at destination:** Try to go to bed between 9 P.M. and midnight, local time. Avoid the tendency to stay awake past midnight. After midnight, staying awake, being exposed to light, and being active will interfere with your effort to beat jet lag. Before going to bed, close the curtains, put on a cloth eye mask, and have your dark glasses available so that you can put them on in place of the mask when you get out of bed during the night or in the morning.

6. **Second morning at destination:** Sleeping or remaining inactive until 8 A.M. would be helpful. If you arise before 8 A.M., be sure that you replace your eye

mask with dark glasses. Avoiding early morning light by wearing either an eye mask or dark glasses until 8 A.M. will help you beat jet lag. Be careful as you walk with the glasses on. NOTE: Don't wear dark glasses if the light level is too low for them to be worn safely.

7. Be sure that you are awake and active after 8 A.M. Also, remove dark glasses at 8 A.M. Being awake, active, and exposed to bright light from 8 until 11 A.M. will help you beat jet lag. If possible, maximize your exposure to sunlight. NOTE: Do not look directly at the sun or a halogen bulb. Try to be out of doors as much as possible. If indoors,

try to stay near a window or in a brightly illuminated room.

8. **Second night at destination:** Try to go to bed before midnight, local time. After midnight, staying awake, being exposed to light, and being active will interfere with your effort to beat jet lag.

9. **Third morning at destination:** Arise at the time that will be customary during your stay at your destination. Avoid sleeping late. Being active and exposed to bright light in the morning will help you lock in to local time. NOTE: Do not look directly at the sun or a halogen bulb.

Adapted, with permission, from *How to Beat Jet Lag: A Practical Guide for Air Travelers,* by Dan Oren, Walter Reich, Norman Rosenthal, and Thomas Wehr. New York: Henry Holt. 1993:45–49.

Travelers have to put some effort into following such schedules. There may be obstacles: they may have to attend meetings indoors, or they may encounter a dark, rainy day. Devices that deliver measured doses of daylight-equivalent artificial light may be a practical aid.

Some travelers take along light visors, lightweight portable devices worn on the head like a baseball cap, with a battery-operated light attached below the brim. You also can use a light box, a bank of fluorescent lights mounted on a metal reflector. These come in tabletop units. Some have handles, and some are even small enough to fit in the overhead luggage bin. Some hotels provide them for guests.

In 1994 the Baltimore Symphony Orchestra traveled to Korea, Taiwan, and Japan, thirteen time zones eastward. They had to cope with a complete reversal of day and night, the hardest change for the body to manage. Chronobiologist Eastman offered suggestions on jet lag prevention before the monthlong tour. Taking into account midday rehearsal times and evening performances, she prescribed going outdoors in the afternoon, particularly between 4 P.M. and 6 P.M.

Symphony orchestra members, in essence, work on split shifts. Many habitually take a nap in late afternoon to promote high alertness at their evening performances. The question came up: What would enhance alertness more, sunlight exposure or a nap? The answer: do both. Eastman suggested taking a half-hour nap early in the afternoon, soon after lunch, a drowsy time of day, so as to permit outdoor activity in the late afternoon. Most orchestra members who relayed their experiences afterward and said they had made an effort to go outside reported that their jet lag was mild and not troublesome.

A fifty-nine-year-old musician said that he had not managed to get outside late in the day, and it took him ten days before he felt comfortable on the new time schedule.

The music critic for *The Baltimore Sun*, Stephen Wigler, who accompanied the orchestra, reported that three days after arriving, musicians still showed signs of jet lag. "At a rehearsal yesterday afternoon, the players seemed to drag themselves to the buses that took them to the hall. And at the evening concert, they seemed to be playing through the headaches, fatigue, scratchy throats and sleepiness that characterize jet lag," he said, although performing "like the professionals they are." Midway through the concert, he noted, the musicians apparently experienced a wake-up call, producing "a thrilling conclusion."[10] Wigler didn't mention that problems with bus schedules that day had pushed the rehearsal into the afternoon, robbing musicians of their nap time.

Three days later, the symphony's performance drove the audience "wild with enthusiasm," Wigler wrote, prompting the crowd to demand curtain call after curtain call, receiving three encores in exchange.[11] This stellar performance continued throughout the rest of the tour. Besides being attentive to getting enough sleep and going outside at the right time, the musicians traveled in a group, stayed in the same hotel, and ate meals together, all factors that ease jet lag.

Finding the very best schedules for light exposure to minimize jet lag is an area of active investigation. Questions remain about when light exposure most effectively alleviates jet lag, as well as how much light a person should get, for how long, and how often.[12] For the present, many travelers are willing to try a trial and error study on themselves. If you're among them, just keep the basic principle in mind: get light in the morning after traveling east, and light in the afternoon after traveling west.

Can Melatonin Prevent Jet Lag?

Suppose you could pop a pill today that would take your body clocks to London or Moscow or Tokyo as fast as the plane flies? You might even use such a drug at home to get ready to participate in a global teleconference.

The hormone melatonin might be used. (See Timewise Tips on Using Melatonin, page 351.) Taking it in capsule form at certain times may trick the brain into thinking that night starts earlier or ends later. This is the rationale for its use to prevent jet lag, since night occurs at a different time in the new time zone, with respect to when you sleep and stay awake at home.

Suppose you plan to fly from New York to London, five time zones east. Nine P.M. in London is 4 P.M. in New York. Thus, taking melatonin in midafternoon at home on the day you depart will tell your brain that night falls sooner. Caution: You might be sleepy that afternoon, a good reason not to attempt work that requires a high degree of concentration or to drive for the rest of the day. Suppose you plan to fly from Los Angeles to Sydney, six time zones west. Nine P.M. in Sydney is 3 A.M. in Los Angeles. Taking melatonin at 3 A.M. before you go would be impractical. But taking it once you've arrived, if you awaken in the middle of the night, will tell your brain that it's still night. This would not be a good strategy, however, if you must attend an early-morning meeting.

In both cases, taking melatonin at your new local bedtime after arriving will help lock sleep in the desired time slot in the new time zone. You'd take it thirty to sixty minutes before bedtime for about four days. For trips of less than five time zones westward, melatonin probably won't be useful. The sleep/wake cycle normally adapts to such trips in one to three days.

In a series of studies Josephine Arendt and her colleagues at the University of Surrey conducted over more than ten years, some five hundred travelers tried different doses and schedules of melatonin. More than a hundred persons in the same studies took only a placebo, a look-alike but inert substance. Results show that travelers who used melatonin typically suffered only about half as much jet lag as those using a placebo. Melatonin proved most effective in trips of more than eight time zones. Whether trips were eastward or westward made no difference.[13]

But not all studies of melatonin show benefits. The Norwegians returning home from New York in the study mentioned earlier, for instance, took different doses of melatonin, or a placebo, at different times, starting on the day of travel and continuing daily for the next five days. All took a bedtime and an evening capsule, although not all capsules, of course, contained melatonin.

Most of the travelers displayed jet lag symptoms. Almost all felt much better five days later. But those who took melatonin did no better than those who took only the placebo.[14] Why not?

Perhaps these physicians, who attended a medical meeting in New York City in the winter, spent little time outdoors while in the United States. They may have shifted only partially to New York time, making their return home much easier. Further, they complained most about daytime symptoms. As busy physicians just back from a trip, most likely facing a large stack of mail and phone messages, they may have focused more on symptoms that interfered with their work than on disturbed nights, the typical traveler's biggest complaint.

If you take melatonin at any time other than bedtime, avoid driving. Melatonin might make you sleepy when you don't want to be. If planning to take melatonin to prevent jet lag, try it at bedtime at home first, to be sure you have no ill effects, such as nausea, headache, or extremely vivid and disturbing dreams.

Despite all the hype about melatonin, much remains unknown. Studies suggest melatonin is less effective in shifting rhythms than is bright light. You don't have to make an either/or choice. You can get light at the proper time, and also use melatonin, if desired. Scientists are working actively to determine how much melatonin to take, when to take it, and for how long. As with any medicine, taking the lowest effective dose for the shortest possible time always is wise.

While clearly more study is needed, curbing jet lag at present is melatonin's best-tested and most successful application. It also may be one of the safest, as most research suggests taking low doses, less than 5 milligrams, for only a few days. For up-to-date information on melatonin, check the Web site of the Society for Light Treatment and Biological Rhythms, www.sltbr.org.

Does the Jet Lag Diet Work?

Fast answer: no. The so-called jet lag diet surfaced in the early 1980s, after U.S. soldiers being sent to Europe tried a diet that alternated feast and fast days for four days before their flight. The troops traveled together on planes where the light-dark schedule and mealtimes were immediately shifted to destination time. The soldiers reset their watches when they boarded. On arriving, they followed a sleep and activity schedule designed to help them adjust to the new time zone. All of these factors collectively may have made the trip easier.[15] Nonetheless, the diet alone received considerable coverage by news media and in popular books, and it still attracts some attention.

A laboratory study that simulated jet lag showed the diet offered no benefit. Fifteen young adults spent two weeks in the chronobiology laboratory at the New York Hospital–Cornell Medical Center, following their usual schedules. On the last four days of that week, seven consumed meals prepared according to the jet lag diet, while the others ate ordinary meals. Then their sleep was cut short by six hours on one night to mimic a flight from the United States to Europe. The volunteers stayed in the laboratory another week. After the simulated trip, Margaret Moline and her colleagues report, all slept equally poorly. Their body temperature, mood, and performance adjusted at comparable rates.[16]

Military nutritionists aiming to ease rapid deployment of troops across many time zones continue to explore the question of whether what or when you eat can speed rhythm shifts. Research from Cornell and elsewhere suggests that mealtimes are an important time cue, helping to keep a host of body rhythms in line. After crossing multiple time zones, it's useful to eat on local time, even if you are not particularly hungry. Both the meal and the social experience of eating at a conventional mealtime help reinforce adaptation. Eating lightly for the first couple of days may minimize gastrointestinal distress associated with having disrupted rhythms in digestive hormones.

A dietary substance that may help counter the fatigue and sleepiness that are prominent in jet lag is so widely used that most people don't even think of it as a drug: caffeine. In a study at the Walter Reed Army Institute of Research, Mary Kautz and her colleagues gave subjects caffeine equivalent to that found in about one, two, or four cups of brewed coffee after forty-eight hours without sleep. The four-cup dose, 600 milligrams of caffeine, improved cognitive performance, objective alertness, and self-ratings of mood over the next twelve hours as well as 20 milligrams of amphetamine did in a comparable previous study. The caffeine had fewer side effects than the amphetamine. The findings suggest that caffeine may help postpone sleep up to twelve hours.

A medication that first came on the market in the United States in 1998, modafinil (Provigil), aims to improve wakefulness in persons with the sleep disorder narcolepsy. It is currently under study to see if it also aids wakefulness in healthy persons. If that proves to be the case, it may function as a chronobiotic to shift performance rhythms in travelers.

Plan Your Visit to the Timeful Hotel

In chronobiologist Eastman's imaginary Timeful Hotel, sleeping rooms have special features, because all guests sleep at different times: some preparing to fly east, some to fly west, some coming from the east, and some coming from the west. Everyone's schedule changes by a few hours each day, as guests zip into their desired time zone. The sleeping rooms provide a comfy bed, choice of pillows ranging from soft to firm, and opaque drapes with magnetic closures to make the room totally dark when you sleep. You can turn on white noise: wind in the trees or waves lapping the shore. Electronic sensors notify housekeeping to straighten the room when you leave. Thick walls and insulated doors shield you from vacuuming and hallway chatter. Melatonin, if you want it, is in your mini-bar.

Room lighting will be programmed to help shift your schedule. A simulated natural sunrise will awaken you easily and gently. Ceiling lights will ramp up gradually to daylight levels. When your schedule says "night," the lights will dim, although you'll still have ordinary room lights akin to those in most hotels now. The television in your room will be programmed to show morning news or nightly news, according to the schedule you're on.

On leaving the tower that houses the sleeping rooms, you'll cross an indoor bridge, a physical and psychological transition to the appropriate wing. Day Land is bright twenty-four hours a day, with natural light when available, and daylight-equivalent artificial light at other times. You can go swimming, stroll in a garden, play tennis, ride a bike, and otherwise enjoy the day at any hour. In the morning—your morning, whenever that is—you'll find waffles, muffins, and other breakfast foods in a friendly coffee shop in the company of like-minded diners. You have a wide choice of lunch places, too. It always feels like daytime whenever you're here. The hotel staff is peppy and energetic, and your fellow guests also are wide awake, or trying to be.

Night Land, by contrast, is dim. You can have a leisurely dinner, see a movie or play, go to a disco, or drop in at a bar, where you can watch videos of baseball games and other night sports events on a big screen. A small diner, Mom's Kitchen, serves cocoa, cookies, and other bedtime snacks. The ambiance in Night Land will be familiar to persons who have been to gambling casinos in Las Vegas, Atlantic City, and elsewhere. There's one crucial difference: by eliminating windows and clocks, casinos aim to blur awareness of the passing of time. In the Timeful Hotel, all cues focus on acclimating you rapidly to day or night in your new time zone.

The Timeful Hotel's conference center is located in Night Land. Travelers spending most of their time in Day Land will not have schedules perturbed by attending meetings in rooms dimmed for talks and slide presentations. By contrast, Night Land visitors would topple their adjustment if they were to venture into the bright light of Day Land.

If you're staying in town, you'll visit both Day Land and Night Land to speed set your body clocks, and then visit Local Locale to enjoy its resort facilities. This area is open to the elements. You'll see normal dawn to dusk shifts in daylight, and the moon at night. If it's morning, the restaurants will hand you a breakfast menu. Expect soup, salads, and sandwiches midday. There are good places for dinner, and Mom's Kitchen has an outpost here, too. Clocks with the correct local hour are everywhere. Background noises reinforce the time: traffic sounds at rush hours, school bells, factory whistles.

Some contemporary hotels already offer some features of the Timeful Hotel. Indeed, jet lag prevention strategies are viewed as a good marketing ploy to attract frequent fliers. "Sleep-Tight" rooms available at some Hilton Hotels in the United States invite guests to use a light box to jump-start their day. Guests receive guidelines for timed light exposure and light avoidance to shift their rhythms, based on chronobiology studies. The rooms also contain a dawn-simulating alarm clock that turns on gradually, starting thirty minutes before a desired wake-up time. Black-out drapes, a white-noise machine, and a brochure, *Sleep and the Traveler,* are among other features. Hilton developed its travel program in conjunction with the National Sleep Foundation in Washington, D.C.

The Hotel Okura chain offers guests light boxes, a relaxation video, sessions with a personal coach at its health club, and a jet lag menu that includes a protein breakfast for "an energized morning," and a carbohydrate meal to promote evening relaxation. The Okura also provides guests with a copy of its *Jet Lag Survival Manual.* At the Ritz-Carlton Hotel in Kuala Lumpur, Malaysia, a "one-night stay" runs for twenty-four hours, starting whenever the guest arrives.

Timewise Tips

More than half of 1,100 business travelers in one survey admitted that they "did nothing" to fight jet lag. Not surprisingly, they also reported that they slept worse away from home. The rest tried a grab bag of tricks. Eating and sleeping at the new local time was the preferred tactic. Still, fewer than one-quarter of the respondents said they used this approach.

The consequences were clear: most of these travelers, who came from the United States, Germany, Japan, and the United Kingdom, said they felt sleepy in the morning. Some reported nodding off when bored. About half said they drank more coffee and alcohol and experienced more stress on the road than at home, according to this survey, conducted for the Hilton Hotels Corporation and the National Sleep Foundation in 1996. Some travelers complained of poor memory and not feeling as good as they liked. About one-third admitted driving while drowsy.[17]

You need not suffer such symptoms. Use the tips below to hasten adjustment. For trips lasting less than three days, try to remain on home time. Stay indoors and schedule activities as best you can by your home time clock.

Before you go:

Try to arrive early for important events. Athletes, musicians, and many business travelers routinely do this. Try to avoid scheduling important meetings immediately after arrival.

Arrive in the evening if you can, whichever direction you travel. You will be able to sleep off travel fatigue and wake up on local time.

Request a specific seat assignment. Being far from (or near) the bathroom, next to a window, in the back where there's more likely to be nearby empty seats on which to stretch out—all can add to your comfort.

Start adapting while still at home. A week or so before the trip, start going to bed and getting up earlier if flying east. Go to bed and get up later, if flying west. Changes of even an hour or two will give you a solid head start.

Shift mealtimes, exercise, medications, and other daily routines in the desired direction.

Try not to skimp on sleep before you go. How well-rested you are is a key determinant of how long it will take you to recover from jet lag.

Ask your doctor how to modify times for any medicines you regularly take. (Don't be surprised if he or she isn't sure. The information is out there, but many physicians haven't yet incorporated it into their practices.)

Don't take a sleeping pill on the plane, unless you also use the pills at home and know that you can awaken a few hours later without feeling groggy.

If planning to use melatonin, try it at home at your normal bedtime. See how you sleep and how you feel the next day. Take whatever you plan to use with you. It's not available in all countries.

Use travel guides, friends' advice, and Internet chat rooms to size up the airports you might use. Some have less traffic, a better layout, more efficient baggage service.

Consider breaking up a long flight with an overnight stopover. You will cross the same number of time zones but may feel less travel fatigue.

Have a decent meal before you get on the plane. Eat lightly until reaching your destination.

Bring along a small tape recorder and earphones to tune out the distractions around you.

Take gum to relieve pressure on ears when landing. Buy it before you leave home; many airports don't sell it. Earplugs designed to prevent build-up of pressure in ears are sold in many pharmacies; they'll also screen out sounds, and discourage talkative neighbors. Take a moisturizer to soothe dry skin, an eye mask to block light, an inflatable neck pillow, a toothbrush; in short, anything you need to improve your in-flight comfort.

Take a watch that shows two time zones if your trip will be short, and you wish to stay on home time. These are popular with pilots and widely available. Set the watch to show destination time when you board the plane.

On the plane:

Set your watch to show destination time when you board.

Grab a pillow and blanket.

If it is night at your destination, try to sleep. Using an eye mask will facilitate sleep. If it is day, try to stay awake, or nap only between the hours of 2 P.M. and 4 P.M. in the new time zone. Some airlines now offer first-class passengers fully reclining bed seats. Ear plugs will come in handy if those around you are snoring.

Stick to water and fruit juices. Drink enough to prevent dehydration on long flights. Flight attendants and pilots aim for at least eight ounces of water for every hour in the air. To reduce intestinal gas and trips to the bathroom, avoid carbonated drinks and caffeinated beverages. If you consume alcohol, remember that one drink in the sky has the impact of two on the ground.

Loosen or take off your shoes. Wear shoes with laces that can be easily adjusted if swelling occurs. Stand up every hour or two. Walk in the aisles if you can. Exercise in your chair: tense and relax muscles, stretch arms, roll shoulders, lift knees, and the like—all good tactics to reduce the risk of cramps or stiffness.

Eat lightly. Airline food is, well, airline food. It will be easier to sleep if you're not feeling stuffed.

After you get there:

Plan important activities in advance. When traveling east, schedule key events for the afternoon; when traveling west, arrange them for the morning. "Fortunately, few business trips demand high-level on-the-spot decisions," an attorney with a multinational firm maintains. "Most trips involve mainly passing papers around, and lots of talk, and they end with taking matters under advisement. Still," he adds, "no one wants to be caught napping."

Eat and exercise on local time. Both activities provide additional time cues to help you readjust faster.

Spend as much time outdoors as possible in the morning if heading east, and in late afternoon if going west. Exercising outdoors in daylight at the right time reinforces the appropriate time cues. At the local time for sleep, rest in the dark, even if you can't fall asleep.

If feeling sleep-deprived, nap in the afternoon. Even twenty minutes will boost alertness.

Familiarize yourself with meeting-room locations if your next-day's sessions will be held in the hotel where you are staying. Take note of fire exits, too. These tactics may ease some uncertainty and aid bedtime relaxation.

Set an alarm clock and request a wake-up call, even two wake-up calls. You'll worry less about not waking up at the right time.

Expect a little tossing and turning at night. Jet lag aside, sleeping in a strange bed almost always proves disruptive. Small stuff—a photo of your family on the nightstand, reading another chapter in a book you've been enjoying at bedtime at home, watching the late news—may help counter the strange bed/strange place effect.

Leave cookies or fruit on your bedside table to quell middle-of-the-night hunger pangs. Save the bedtime chocolates until the next day; they contain caffeine.

Drink caffeinated beverages only when feeling sleepiest to get the most benefit from caffeine's alerting effect. Avoid caffeine within five hours of bedtime.

Avoid alcohol near bedtime. It's a myth that it helps most people sleep. While it may make you feel drowsy, its effects wear off quickly, disrupting sleep.

After you return home:
Anticipate lowered performance the first few days.

Spend as much time outdoors in daylight as possible, in the morning if you came east, and in the late afternoon if you came west. Go to bed at your usual time and rest in the dark, even if you can't fall asleep. Get up at your usual time, too. If sleepy in the daytime, try to nap in midafternoon.

Drink caffeinated beverages only when feeling sleepiest to get the most benefit from caffeine's alerting effect.

Avoid alcohol near bedtime. As its effects wear off, sleep may be disrupted.

Summing Up

With advance planning and attention to how you organize your day in a new time zone, heeding both the "do" and "don't" tactics listed above, you can avoid many of the unpleasant consequences of jet lag. This is the practical payoff of hundreds of chronobiology studies.

Research that benefits travelers also aids persons who suffer chronically from jet lag without leaving home, the millions of persons worldwide who frequently change their hours for work and sleep, sometimes rotating around the clock. They drive trucks, pilot planes, deliver babies, tend the sick, bake bread, run power plants, trade on the stock market, report and produce news, and more. We'll look next at how they manage.

Clockwatching at Work

Jeff, Angie, Katie, and Dawn smile at readers from the front page of each issue of the PATT newsletter. In yearbook-style snapshots, a grinning Jeff wears his baseball hat backwards. Angie, a blonde, and Katie, a brunette, show off luxurious hair that cascades below their shoulders. Dawn smiles shyly.

The four teenagers could be anyone's children, anyone's brother, sister, niece, cousin. Members of PATT, Parents Against Tired Truckers, want everyone to think about that, and to remember why the organization was founded. They don't want other families to lose those they love the same way.

Jeffrey Izer, age seventeen, of Lisbon Falls, Maine, and the others were heading to a hayride on the evening of October 10, 1993, when the engine on Jeff's car overheated, and the car stalled. The teenagers pushed the Ford Escort station wagon into the breakdown lane of the Maine Turnpike, well off the road. They got back in and waited for help. The car's flashers and interior lights were on, witnesses told police.

The kids wrote "Help!" on the fogged windows. They joked with each other. They even said prayers. Suddenly, with no honking, no screeching of brakes, no warning of any kind, a tractor-trailer weighing 80,000 pounds slammed into the rear of the car and ran over it, instantly killing Jeff, along with Angie Dubuc, sixteen, Katie Leighton, fourteen, and Dawn Welding, fifteen. A fifth teenager, Linda Tardif, fifteen, though gravely injured, survived.[1] A newspaper photo shows the virtually unrecognizable car, a coffin of twisted metal.

A woman driving behind the truck told police she saw its right tires come up off the road "as if the tractor-trailer was going up and over something." The eighteen-wheeler tipped slightly to the left, then bounced down to the right, and swerved right, caroming off the turnpike and down an embankment. The woman did not see the truck's brakelights light up.[2]

The truck's driver, Robert Hornbarger, of Clearville, Pennsylvania, walked away with only minor injuries. There were no skid marks and no indication that Hornbarger took evasive action. He said he did not remember what happened. Although investigators concluded that he fell asleep at the wheel, a grand jury decided not to indict him for manslaughter. Hornbarger pleaded guilty only of falsifying his logbook by reporting rest breaks that he had not taken, a misdemeanor charge. He received the maximum penalty for this offense: four months in jail and a $1,000 fine.

The jury's decision galvanized the teenagers' parents. Jeff's mother, Daphne Izer, a school nurse, took the lead in 1994 in establishing PATT, an organization modeled on MADD, Mothers Against Drunk Drivers. By 1999 PATT had seven thousand names on its mailing list, from across the United States, as well as in Canada and as far away as Australia. PATT members work with sleep and safety experts to raise awareness of the consequences of drowsy driving and to advocate changes in truckers' work schedules. Some truckers have joined the group, too, recognizing that its battle "against tired truckers" focuses squarely on the poor schedules and working conditions that force them to put their own lives on the line.

Out-of-Date Schedules Foster Driver Fatigue

Regulations governing truckers' schedules in the United States date from 1938, when trucks were smaller and lighter, a far cry from today's behemoths that may weigh 200,000 pounds when fully loaded. Traffic back then also was far less dense. The rules permit truckers to drive for ten hours and go back on the road after only eight hours' rest. No distinction is made between day and night driving. In Canada truckers may drive for up to thirteen hours before taking a rest.

Drivers often attempt to live on eighteen-hour days. This schedule makes fatigue inescapable. Highway crashes, in trucks as well as autos, peak when daily alertness is lowest. Drivers are more than twenty times more likely to fall asleep at the wheel at 6 A.M., near the low point on the body clock, than at 10 A.M., when alertness is high. Drivers are three times more likely to fall asleep while driving at 4 P.M., the midday low in performance, than at 10 A.M.[3]

Safety experts no longer call crashes "accidents." "Continued use of the word 'accident' promotes the concept that these events are outside of human influence or control," the U.S. Department of Transportation proclaimed.[4] Fall-asleep crashes, safety experts say, are predictable and preventable. Changing the way we think and talk about crashes also may change the way we drive.

Under present laws, drivers get paid only when their wheels are turning. They earn no money while they load and unload their freight, or wait to load and unload it, tasks that often consume many hours. In our "just in time" economy, manufacturers and distributors both aim to minimize inventory. They see trucks as warehouses on wheels. The nation's three million long-haul truckers are expected to move merchandise fast, and they do an impressive job of it. By the end of the twentieth century, trucks commanded more than 80 percent of the nation's $531 billion freight bill.[5]

But there is a human toll. "Innocent people are being killed to get a load of widgets delivered," Izer declared in testimony before the Senate Commerce Committee in 1998. The driver's incentive should be "to be safe," she asserted, "instead of 'on time at any cost.' "[6] The U.S. Department of Labor says truck driving is the nation's most dangerous profession: about 800 drivers die on the job in this country every year. In each of these crashes, four other persons die, on average, along with the driver.

Safety experts regard fatigue as the most common cause of fatal highway crashes, more common even than alcohol. A study by the National Transportation Safety Board (NTSB) found fatigue the probable cause of 31 percent of crashes in which a driver of a heavy truck was killed, and alcohol and other drug use the probable cause of 29 percent.[7] Fatigue and alcohol use often occur together; sleepiness magnifies alcohol's effects. In a sleepy driver, one or two drinks may act like three or four in one who is well rested.

Poor Schedules Blamed for Major Industrial Catastrophes

The demands on truckers are not unique. In our increasingly twenty-four-hour society, more and more of us work at all hours of the day and night. This fact has important implications for workers' health and safety and for those of the rest of society as well. Unlike the machines we operate, we humans function much better in the daytime than at night.

A night worker, even one who has slept reasonably well the preceding day, is no more alert between 2 A.M. and 8 A.M. than a day worker who has had only four hours of sleep for two nights in a row, according to studies cited in *Wake-up America*, the National Commission on Sleep Disorders Research 1993 report to Congress.[8] The costs of mistakes by sleepy workers in the United States, including lost production, missed days from work, and medical costs, exceed an estimated $100 billion annually.

By the end of their first night on a night shift, about half of all shift workers have been awake for at least twenty-four hours. These workers are likely to perform tasks calling for attention, reasoning, decision making, and other mental skills at least as badly as someone with a blood alcohol concentration of 0.1 percent, the standard for being legally drunk in many states. Nicole Lamond and Drew Dawson of Queen Elizabeth Hospital in South Australia reached this conclusion after studying healthy young adults who went without sleep or consumed alcohol in a laboratory setting.[9] Their research suggests how sleep loss may have contributed to some of the twentieth century's most grievous industrial catastrophes. At the low point of the day, and after missing some sleep, people fail to see things they seldom overlook when fully alert.

- The crisis at the Three Mile Island nuclear power plant started between 4 and 6 A.M. on March 28, 1979. Workers did not notice that an important valve was stuck. A major loss of core coolant water occurred at the Pennsylvania plant before workers discovered the problem. It took feverish efforts to prevent a complete meltdown. The workers involved had rotated that very day from the day shift to the night shift. "Except for human failures," the President's Commission on the catastrophe concluded, "the major accident at Three Mile Island would have been a minor incident."[10]

- The *Exxon Valdez* ran aground at 12:04 A.M. on March 24, 1989, in well-charted waters off the coast of Alaska. There was no fog and no other traffic nearby. The spill of eleven million gallons of crude oil despoiled wildlife, ruined the area's fishing industry, and necessitated a $2 billion cleanup of 1,200 miles of pristine shoreline. A court assessed the Exxon Corporation $5 billion more in punitive damages. Many people still believe the captain, who had been drinking onshore the previous evening, caused the grounding. The captain was not even on the bridge at the time. He was off-duty, in his cabin. The third mate, the person in charge at the time, was qualified to take the ship to sea. Nonetheless, on the night before the accident, the third mate probably got only about four hours sleep, the NTSB concluded, less than he needed to maintain alertness. He had worked a physically demanding day, napping briefly between his afternoon shift and supper. In the twenty-four hours before the accident, it was estimated that he slept less than five hours.[11] Such schedules are common in shipping, where the usual work schedule, six hours on duty alternating with six hours off duty, prevents crews from sleeping more than five hours straight.

- The space shuttle *Challenger* exploded just after its noon liftoff on January 28, 1986, killing all seven aboard, including a teacher, Christa McAuliffe, who was to have taught the nation's schoolchildren lessons from space. The Presidential Commission that investigated the disaster concluded that the launch crew's excessive overtime, irregular working hours, insufficient sleep, and fatigue played a contributory role. Some key managers had less than two hours' sleep the night before the launch, and had been on duty since 1 A.M.[12]

- The meltdown and explosion of a reactor at the Chernobyl nuclear plant near Kiev in the Soviet Union on April 26, 1986, spewed radiation across Europe in history's worst nuclear power accident. More than 200 times more radiation was released at Chernobyl than in the bombings at Hiroshima and Nagasaki combined. Ukraine government sources reported in 1998 that 3,600 of the 800,000 "liquidators" who helped clean up contaminated areas without proper equipment or training have died from radiation exposure. Health groups put the death toll even higher. The number of persons in Ukraine and neighboring Belarus who developed thyroid cancer since the explosion has jumped by 7,900 percent.[13] Pripyat, the city built for the 40,000 Chernobyl employees and their family members, stands empty. It was evacuated two days after the catastrophe. Government sources publicly estimated the damage suffered by Ukraine at up to $130 billion. Soviet officials blamed the 1:23 A.M. event on both faulty equipment design and human errors. Engineers involved in the disaster had been at work for thirteen hours or more.[14]

- The chemical disaster in Bhopal, India, occurred at 12:40 A.M. on December 4, 1984, just after a shift change at the Union Carbide plant. Workers did not recognize that pressure in a pesticide chemical tank had increased fivefold between the last reading of the previous shift and the first reading of their shift. Water leaked into the tank through a faulty valve, mixed with the chemical, and created pressure strong enough to rupture the tank and release poisonous gas. The gas drifted in a low cloud over the nearby city, killing 6,000 people and injuring 30,000 more. Fifteen years later, ground water remained contaminated with toxic mercury, according to the environmental organization Greenpeace.[15]

One in Five Americans Works Evenings or Nights

Nearly one in five Americans with full-time jobs—those involving more than thirty-five hours a week—toils outside traditional daytime work hours, defined by the U.S. Bureau of Labor Statistics as roughly between 6 A.M. and 6 P.M. These 15.2 million Americans work evenings, nights, irregular schedules dictated by their employers, and rotating shifts, in which they switch from days to evenings to nights, typically on a weekly basis.[16]

Many who work odd hours don't fit the stereotypic image of a shift worker. They include actors and musicians who perform at night, morning television news anchors who rise at 3 A.M., computer wizards in Silicon Valley who work past midnight, physicians on call, diplomats negotiating treaties at all hours, stock brokers and business executives dealing with clients around the world. About 2 to 10 percent of workers in any type of job work outside traditional hours.[17] Any of us who sometimes stay up late or get up early, travel frequently, or miss a significant amount of sleep for any other reason, may experience acutely some of the problems shift workers suffer chronically. As the Internet matures, more and more homes will maintain a continuous connection, more akin to telephone service than the now more common "dial up and sign on" system. The opportunity to be online twenty-four hours a day, seven days a week, also means more and more of us can expect to work around the clock. "Round-the-clock markets," *Business Week* says, "make 'closing prices' an obsolete concept."[18]

Businesses around the world face new demands to provide goods and services at all hours. Companies that invest in costly equipment want to maximize its use. Some industrial processes require nonstop operations. The more shift workers there are, the more shift workers society needs. More families eat out, for example, and seek service from haircuts to doctor appointments outside the weekday daytime window.

Types of Schedules Vary Widely

In agricultural economies, people often work from dawn to dusk, roughly a twelve-hour day, with some times of the day and seasons of the year more hectic than others. At the start of the twentieth century, workers in iron foundries and steel mills also put in twelve-hour days, and switched between days and nights every two weeks. Every twenty-eighth day, they got one day off. Reformers persuaded Congress to pass the Adamson Act of 1916, making the eight-hour day the standard for calculating overtime. The forty-hour week came into being with the Fair Labor Standards Act of 1938.

Many round-the-clock companies in the United States still run on twenty-eight-day schedules, with workers spending seven eight-hour days on morning, evening, and night shifts, with either two or three days off in between shifts. The most common shift schedule in this country, however, probably is five days on a single shift, followed by two days off. Filling three shifts requires at least four crews, and sometimes five, depending on the need for varying numbers of workers on different shifts.

Twelve-hour shifts have come around again. A 1999 survey of five hundred companies with twenty-four-hour operations in the United States and Canada by *ShiftWork Alert*, an industry newsletter, found twelve-hour shifts slightly more prevalent than eight-hour shifts. The respondents included chemical, paper, consumer goods, and other manufacturers, as well as utilities, hospitals, hotels, retail outlets, and transportation companies.

On the most common twelve-hour schedule, workers work two days and get two days off, then work three days and get two days off, then two days again, with three days off, before the pattern repeats. Such schedules provide every other weekend off. In a typical twelve-hour schedule, workers alternate between working from 6 A.M. to 6 P.M., or the reverse. Workers like twelve-hour schedules because they get fourteen days off out of every twenty-eight. Employers like them, too, because they simplify scheduling and record keeping. But concerns persist about the impact of such long work periods on fatigue and safety. "Despite their apparent popularity," says British shift-work expert Simon Folkard, "prolonged shifts will almost certainly reduce safety levels, especially towards their end, and may well result in reduced efficiency."[19]

Not all workers do all of their work at once. School-bus drivers work early in the morning and late in the afternoon. Sailors traditionally work on four-hour "watch" schedules. Devising schedules for twenty-four-hour community services, such as police, firefighters, and power and gas workers, is tricky because the demand for such services is uneven. Even in hospitals, where patients are equally sick at all hours, staffing is higher in the daytime than at night. Remember the mythical Maytag repairman? There are plenty of jobs where workers put in time only on an "as needed" basis. Workers in the United States today follow more than a thousand different work schedules.

Why Shift Workers Rarely Adapt

You might think that adapting to a change in work hours would be the same as traveling across time zones, easier, perhaps, since you get to stay home. You'd be wrong on both counts. "Shift lag" lasts longer and often proves more severe than jet lag.

Schedules that rotate by eight hours each week often are likened to flying from San Francisco to London to Tokyo at weekly intervals, and then repeating the trip. Stressful as such trips might be, travelers get substantive help from changes in sunlight and darkness, and from sleeping, eating, and exercising at familiar times of day in the new time zone. In travelers, these time cues thus promote adjustment. In shift workers, the identical time cues discourage it, even actively fight it.

If you leave work at 7 A.M., you will be exposed to sunlight, which sends a potent "wake-up" message to your biological clock that fights your intention to go to sleep soon. Social cues also tell you it's morning. You will see children on their way to school, and merchants arranging their wares for the day ahead. Your day may be over, but for most of society the day is just beginning. If you go to sleep in the daytime and wake up to answer the phone or use the bathroom, you may be exposed to daylight cues that confuse your sleeping brain. Since your body is designed for daytime activity, it seldom lets you sleep as long in the daytime as at night.

Most body rhythms in persons who fly across eight time zones return to normal in about eight days. Shift workers who rotate eight hours seldom stay on the new schedule for eight full days. On days off, most stay up in the daytime and sleep at night, regardless of the hours they were working or soon will start. Thus any adjustment that gets started is soon reversed. Then they shift schedules again.

Numerous studies show that body clocks in shift workers rarely adapt fully, even after many days on a particular shift, and even after many years of shift work. Timothy Monk likens this experience to salmon attempting to swim upstream. It's hard to leap to the top of a waterfall, but easy to fall back down. Shift workers often live with chronic jet lag, a condition dubbed the "shiftwork maladaption syndrome." Although this condition sounds like a disease and causes plenty of misery, it is a perfectly normal response. Maladaption occurs only when you try to work and sleep at "wrong" times on the body clock, to live according to schedules that run counter to those for which your body was designed.

How Out-of-Kilter Clocks Harm Workers' Health

Banners hanging over streets and signs posted in Rouen, France, in May 1980, welcomed visitors to the Fifth International Symposium on Night and Shift Work. The painters who prepared these banners and billboards did not speak English. They simply copied information supplied by conference organizers. When writing "shift work," however, they left out the "f." Many who work off-beat hours think the painters got it right. Shift workers typically complain more vociferously about their jobs than day workers do.

Shift workers also may have higher rates of some illnesses. These may be the biological-clock equivalent of miner's lung or cancers in workers exposed to toxic chemicals, the long-term consequence of chronic misalignment of inner rhythms.

The existence of such problems, and their link to shift-work schedules, are just beginning to come to light. Some health disorders in shift workers develop slowly and only after many years of exposure. Some are written off as the result of smoking or lack of exercise, unhealthy behaviors that are more common in shift workers than in day workers. Other health problems have escaped attention because people who become ill while working on shifts switch to jobs that do not require schedule changes. Older workers often opt out of shift work or receive promotions to the day shift, the shift preferred by nine out of ten workers.[20]

Shift workers in general take fewer days off for illness than day workers, Italian shift-work expert Giovanni Costa reports. They may be able to take advantage of free time in the day to see the doctor. Or they may tolerate health problems better as part of the job and feel a bond of solidarity that makes them more reluctant to burden fellow shift workers by their absence.[21] Some persons who doubt their ability to cope with changing hours may never attempt shift work at all, which means that studies of shift workers may be looking at a population that overall is healthier than the population at large.

There have been virtually no studies attempting to correlate increased susceptibility to toxic chemicals used in a wide variety of industrial processes at different times of day, with the likelihood of problems on particular shifts. The traditional way to assess occupational risk assumes susceptibility is equal at all times of day, but chronobiology research clearly shows risks are higher at some times of day than at others.[22]

An estimated 15 percent to 30 percent of those who try shift work find they cannot tolerate it. About 10 percent of shift workers relish the variety of frequent schedule changes, especially the opportunity to have free time off at different times of the day, and, on some schedules, substantial blocks of time off between shift changes. The remainder tolerate shift work reasonably well. Even these workers may be at increased risk for some health problems.

Given the lack of attention to biological clocks in medical education, it is no surprise that many physicians fail to suspect a link between patients' illnesses and their work schedules. A dermatologist assessing a skin eruption would ask a patient about exposure to workplace chemicals. A physician treating a patient with troubled sleep, gastrointestinal upsets, or depression may ask about work and stress but may not think to ask specifically about work schedules.

Night work most often brings workers an additional $.26 to $.75 an hour. About 9 percent of shift workers earn a shift premium of $1.50 per hour or more, according to a survey conducted by *ShiftWork Alert*.[23]

Some parents prefer shift work because it provides more time overall when at least one parent can be with the children. "I get to tuck my son into bed before I go to work at night, and wake him up when I return," one night worker wrote to an online shift-work forum. "I can coach Little League, be the Cubmaster, and do a lot of things during the day with him, while other fathers languish on the job."

Some people like shift work because it permits them to care for an elderly or sick parent. Others like working in the evening or at night so that they can go to school in the daytime. Some are night owls who choose permanent night or evening work because they function best on such schedules.

Sleep and Digestive Problems Bother Shift Workers Most

"I don't get enough sleep."

Attempting sleep in the daytime, when alertness normally is highest, means that sleep and alertness spar. If you're sleepy, you will sleep, but alerting forces in the brain will keep you from sleeping as long as you would at night. Noise disturbs daytime sleep more than it does nighttime sleep, because daytime sleep is lighter. Night, day, and evening shifts affect sleep in different ways.

Night workers get two to four hours less sleep, on average, than they do when working in the day.[24] They get their fair share of the deepest stages of sleep, thought to be the most restful, but they miss some of the lighter stages, which ordinarily make up the bulk of sleep, and they miss some rapid eye movement, or REM, sleep, believed important in regulating mood. Many night workers elect to go to sleep within an hour or so of ending their shift, a pattern that contrasts with the day worker's habitual routine of work, leisure, and then sleep. Many night workers also take a nap shortly before going to work, a good strategy for compensating for their shortened main sleep episode.

Fatigue enters the picture, too. The night worker who sleeps from 8 A.M. to 1 P.M., and does not nap, will have been awake for eighteen hours at the end of the night shift. A day worker who gets up at 7 A.M. will have been awake for only ten hours when work is over at 5 P.M.

Day workers who must get up between 4 and 5 A.M. complain most about difficulty getting up when the alarm goes off, and about not feeling refreshed. Workers dislike this type of schedule the most, according to Torbjörn Åker-stedt of Karolinska Institute in Stockholm. Having to get up extremely early makes people feel sleepier through the rest of the day. Workers on this sched-ule also get two to four hours less sleep than they do on a more traditional schedule, with less lighter sleep and less REM sleep. Expecting to have trou-ble getting up in the morning itself sabotages sleep.

Afternoon and evening workers show more variation in the times they choose to sleep than workers on other shifts. Some go to bed well after mid-night and sleep until 8 or 9 A.M., or even later. Few take naps. The big com-plaint about the evening shift is not that it interferes with sleep but that it interferes with social and family life, removing the worker at the preferred time for leisure activities.

Persons working evening, night, or rotating shifts use alcohol as a sleep aid more often than day workers do, according to a 1996 survey of a representa-tive sample of more than 2,000 Detroit adults. Shift workers also use pre-scription sleep medications more often and for a longer time than day workers. In both instances, workers said their main problem was difficulty falling asleep.[25]

Female shift workers report sleeping less and having sleep interrupted more often than male shift workers. Married female night workers with chil-dren get the least sleep of all. Difficulty sleeping may persist, unfortunately, even after a night worker switches to a regular daytime schedule. Former night or rotating shift nurses assessed in the sleep laboratory, Marie Dumont of the University of Montreal found, got less of the deeper stages of sleep than nurses who had never worked nights.[26]

Morning newscasters, however glamorous they look on the air, readily admit to sleep deprivation. Some must get up at 3 A.M. to get to the studio to prepare for going on the air at 6 A.M. A 1998 survey found 142 morning news-casters in the top thirty-five U.S. television markets averaged only 5.7 hours of sleep each night. Nearly all reported high levels of daytime sleepiness related to their job schedules, particularly in the early afternoon. Some reported nodding off while waiting for traffic lights to change. To compensate for sleepiness, about half drank coffee, as many as twelve cups a day, and half took naps.[27]

Long commutes steal time from sleep, too. People who commute more than seventy-five minutes each way every day average forty minutes' less sleep on work days than those who travel less than forty-five minutes, a survey of riders on the Long Island Rail Road shows. The long commuters also reported more trouble staying awake in the daytime. Nearly 4,700 riders on the nation's largest commuter rail line responded to a survey by Joyce Walsleben of New York University and her colleagues.[28]

Persons who must sleep in the daytime must contend with the brightness of the room, and noise from traffic, children at play, the ringing phone, neighbors cutting grass, and other sources. Many shift workers have adopted elaborate strategies to circumvent these sleep disrupters, such as installing room-darkening and sound-baffling drapes, wearing eyeshades and earplugs, unplugging the phone, and even sleeping in a basement or attic.

"My stomach often is upset."

Gastrointestinal symptoms, such as diarrhea, constipation, and heartburn, are two to three times as common in shift workers as in permanent day workers. Some problems, commonly termed *Graveyard Gut*, are particularly troublesome on the first few days after a shift change. More serious ailments, such as peptic ulcers, also show increased frequency among shift workers. After five years on the job, shift workers show two to five times the incidence of peptic-ulcer disease as do day workers. Large companies that operate around the clock reportedly commonly spend hundreds of thousands of dollars in health care costs for stomach remedies for workers.[29]

These problems stem from both when and what shift workers eat. Digestion is a daytime function on the body clock. Like other body rhythms, digestive activities shift slowly and only partially to a nighttime work schedule. Irregular mealtimes disrupt the amount and pattern of secretion of hormones, acid, and enzymes necessary for the normal digestion of food. Eating in a hurried atmosphere, not uncommon when people eat at work, contributes further to indigestion. Both day workers and night workers who gulp a meal at their desks or workstations are at higher risk of such problems than they would be if they ate in a more leisurely manner. Changes in mealtimes also mean that acid may be present in the stomach at times when enzymes and other substances that protect the stomach lining are not. This situation may trigger stomach ulcers.

Soon after night work began in the nineteenth century in the mills of New England, horse-drawn lunch wagons started to ply their trade at night on nearby streets.[30] Night workers tend to snack more than day workers, often on fatty and hard-to-digest foods, such as potato chips, fried foods, and pizza. They munch more on candy bars, in hopes of boosting energy, although any beneficial effects from a candy bar on energy likely dissipate within twenty minutes. Night workers often have to make do with vending-machine food, with generally meager offerings of fruit, soup, and other healthy choices. Eating after work hours follows a different time pattern, too. "Eating a big breakfast when I get home from work, and then going to bed, seems to have resulted in weight gain," one worker wrote an online shift-work forum. "I used to be fit and trim," he said, "and now I'm starting to look like the Michelin man!"

A growing number of companies have installed refrigerators and microwaves at their work sites, enabling employees who bring food from home to store and prepare it themselves. Some even staff a nighttime cafeteria, which fosters socializing, an activity that in itself aids relaxation and improves digestion.

Shift workers drink more caffeinated and alcoholic beverages than people who work only during the daytime, both, perhaps, an attempt to help manage alertness and sleep. Some shift workers report their coffee intake in pots, not cups, or drink caffeinated sodas steadily throughout their shifts. In a survey of nearly 8,000 shift workers conducted between 1996 and 1998 by Circadian Technologies, Inc., a Boston-based shift-work consulting firm, at twenty sites in the United States and Canada, 15 percent of the workers said they typically drank ten or more cups or cans of caffeinated beverages a day. Thirty-five percent said they smoked, about twice the rate of the general population. Caffeine, alcohol, and smoking are all risk factors for digestive problems.

Many who take pain relievers for problems such as muscle soreness or backaches don't appreciate that such medications may cause or worsen stomach irritation. Medications such as aspirin and ibuprofen cause the fewest problems when taken at the start of the rest cycle, that is, at bedtime, rather than at the start of, or in the middle of, the work day.

"I'm worried about having a heart attack."

The risk is real. After working shifts for five or more years, both men and women have a 30 percent higher risk of having a heart attack than do comparable groups of day workers, Swedish researchers found. Anders Knutsson of Umeå University Hospital and his colleagues asked more than 2,000 persons with first-time heart attacks about their work histories, and compared them to an otherwise similar group of persons living in the same communities. Shift work proved to be the single common thread in those having heart attacks. Although more of the shift workers smoked, the researchers took that into account when making their calculations. They found that job strain, age, job educational level, and smoking did not alter their findings.[31]

Other studies also affirm that shift workers smoke more than day workers. Smoking alone doubles the risk of heart disease. It is an even greater risk factor than shift work alone.

Shift workers have higher cholesterol levels than day workers, and they also develop high blood pressure more often. Their blood pressure rhythms may change, too. Like hundreds of other bodily functions, blood pressure normally dips at night. In shift workers who slept in the daytime, blood pressure stayed closer to waking levels than it did in day workers, a Cornell Medical Center study showed. Joseph Schwartz and his colleagues monitored blood pressure in 100 female nurses working on a variety of schedules around the clock. Nurses who worked evenings and nights proved six times more likely to be nondippers than day workers and had higher average blood pressure overall. African-American nurses were seven times more likely than non–African Americans to be nondippers. African Americans, in general, suffer from high blood pressure at higher rates than other population groups. Failure of blood pressure to dip normally in sleep puts added stress on blood vessels and is linked with damage to the heart, brain, kidneys, and other organs.

The changes in mealtimes that occur with shift work also may increase the risk of developing heart disease. In a study at the University of Surrey, twelve healthy adults moved their schedule forward by nine hours. They ate the same test meal on either the day schedule or the night schedule. David Ribeiro and his colleagues then sampled their blood for the next nine hours. When the volunteers ate at night, their blood levels of a specific type of fat, triacyglycerol, or TAG, a known risk factor for heart disease, rose significantly higher than it did when they ate in the daytime. It took at least two days on the night schedule before their blood levels of TAG started to return to their pretest levels. The researchers currently are studying whether eating low-fat meals on the night shift helps blunt the nighttime rise.[32]

"I should have paid better attention."

In 1995 three newborn babies in an Annapolis, Maryland, hospital developed such severe trouble breathing that they had to be placed on respirators. All were found to have received narcotic drugs, most likely from syringes improperly filled in the hospital pharmacy. Fortunately, all three babies survived. The pharmacist implicated in the error, who had worked at the hospital for nine years, was fired. The blunder occurred at 3 A.M.

There's no doubt that mistakes are higher on the night shift. While few fortunately are headline-grabbing catastrophes, many harm the workers involved, or those in their care. Some also damage expensive equipment or slow down production.

Nighttime errors typically involve a failure to respond appropriately. People lapse into brief episodes of sleep, known as microsleeps, more often at night than in the daytime. Many of us commonly do this in the evening, while reading the newspaper, say, or watching television. Nighttime is the worst time for monotonous tasks, particularly complicated ones that involve working alone.

In a Swedish study, Åkerstedt found that train engineers repeatedly dozed off for five to sixty seconds while barreling down the tracks, most often in the early-morning hours. They went right past warning lights without noticing they had done so. "In a sleep attack," he explains, "the eyelids feel heavy, you fight it, stare straight ahead and perhaps squint. After a few minutes you lose the battle. Your eyes close, your brain shows low activity and your neck muscles relax. Your head sinks slowly towards your chest. Suddenly you jerk and wake up. You might feel afraid and this perhaps helps you to wake up." The process, he notes, repeats.[33] Two in three Swedish engine drivers, Åkerstedt found, had fallen asleep on the night shift, but only one in six had done so on the day shift.

In Circadian Technologies, Inc.'s 8,000-worker survey, 40 percent of the workers said they fought sleep or briefly nodded off while working at least several times a week. Nearly one-quarter of the workers said this happened as many as several times each shift.[34]

In a study of nearly 800 nurses on all shifts in six community hospitals, Kathryn Lee of the University of California School of Nursing in San Francisco found that about one-third of those who worked night and rotating shifts admitted that they had made mistakes on the job. Only one-sixth of nurses working permanent day or evening shifts did so.

Compared with nurses who never worked nights, those who worked at night or on rotating shifts were at least twice as likely to report that they had had a problem with work performance because of sleepiness, made an error at work because of sleepiness, and struggled to stay awake while taking care of a patient. Their proclivity for errors did not stop at the hospital door. Night and rotating shift nurses also were at least twice as likely to report struggling to stay awake while driving a car and driving off the road because of sleepiness.[35]

The potential for errors by sleep-deprived doctors-in-training aroused widespread public attention after the 1984 death of eighteen-year-old Libby Zion in a New York hospital. In February 1995, a jury in a malpractice suit brought by Zion's family divided blame for her death equally between the young woman herself, who allegedly had used cocaine, and the two sleep-deprived residents who treated her.

The investigation into Zion's death prompted New York in 1989 to pass the first, and still only, state law regulating the grueling work schedules of resident physicians. The law limits their work to eighty hours per week, with no more than twenty-four consecutive hours on duty. State health department inspectors who made surprise visits to twelve New York hospitals in 1998, however, found pervasive violations of this law.[36]

"I got hurt on the job."

Simon Folkard and his colleagues at the University of Wales at Swansea analyzed all 4,645 injury incidents reported in a year on a rotating three-shift system at a large engineering company, where workers performed the same tasks on all shifts. The relative risk of sustaining an injury, they found, was 23 percent higher on the night shift than on the morning shift, which had the lowest incidence. Employees whose work was self-paced were 82 percent more likely to suffer a serious injury on the night shift than the morning shift.[37]

Medical students and resident physicians proved twice as likely to suffer accidental needle-sticks or other exposure to patients' blood at night as in the day, reports Deborah Parks of the University of Texas Medical School in Houston. She and her colleagues examined all such incidents reported in their medical center between 1993 and 1998.[38] Such exposure puts these workers at higher risk of developing HIV or other blood-borne infections.

Our bodies are designed for maximum tolerance of heavy physical and strenuous labor in the daytime, another reason we are more likely to suffer injuries when we attempt such work at night.

The high risk times for shift workers, according to chronobiologist Martin Moore-Ede of Circadian Technologies, Inc., in Cambridge, Massachusetts, are between 1 A.M. and 6 A.M., the first two night shifts after working days or after several days off, the early hours of the day shift, near the end of any shift, times when activity levels are high in the immediate work area, and driving home after the night shift.[39]

Social factors affect error rates, too. At a mining company, errors always shot up on Sunday night. Most of the workers lived in small, closely knit communities and chose to attend church Sunday morning, Timothy Monk discovered, sacrificing sleep to be with their families. Educating workers about the need to nap before starting work on Sunday night boosted safety rates.[40]

"The job gets harder instead of easier as I get older."

Older workers usually earn more money and move to quieter neighborhoods. Their children no longer live at home. Despite these advantages, and despite many years on the job, they may continue to sleep poorly, perhaps even worse. This problem occurs because people never really adjust to sleeping in the daytime. Further, even in day workers, sleep deteriorates with age. While younger workers complain more about trouble falling asleep, older persons complain more about trouble staying asleep, and about difficulty returning to sleep when they awaken. In terms of sleep, says Moore-Ede, "what a twenty-year-old can get away with may not be possible at forty or fifty."[41]

Nearly 76 million Americans will be aged fifty and over in 2000. That number will grow to 115 million by 2020, according to U.S. Census Bureau projections, so the number of older shift workers also will climb dramatically.

"I'm under a lot of stress."

Despite the huge numbers of people working at nontraditional hours, society still views day work as the norm. While telemarketers, thankfully, don't call in the middle of the night, this fact offers no consolation to those besieged by such calls when trying to sleep in the daytime. Changing the time you sleep, eat, and even relax is stressful in itself. The resulting fatigue, digestive upsets, and irritability further heighten stress. Disruptions in body clocks may trigger depression in susceptible persons. Some reports suggest shift workers suffer from both anxiety and depression more often than permanent day workers do.

"Work is hard on my spouse and family."

Family mental health and well-being may suffer, too. This is an important health concern not only for individuals but for employers concerned about absenteeism and lost productivity, and for society as a whole. "Rotating shift work is a contagious disease that infects those around you," one shift worker asserts. It's stressful for you to juggle marital and family demands, and stressful for your spouse and children to try to adjust to your changing schedule.

Your partner may be interested in sex when you want only to sleep. Half the shift workers in one study called life on the night shift "sexless." Only one in ten said that about other shifts.

You might have to work on holidays and weekends. You might miss helping kids with homework and seeing their baseball games or track meets. You can't take your kids to the zoo at night. Indeed, you might see them mostly when they are in bed, asleep.

More than one in four couples in the United States in which both partners work at paid jobs include at least one spouse who works other than a fixed daytime schedule, according to sociologist Harriet Presser of the University of Maryland. When children under age fourteen are in the home, nearly one-third of these couples include one partner with odd hours. More than half of two-income couples include at least one spouse who works weekends. The television sitcom family where both spouses work only on weekdays and only in the daytime is a minority.

Couples in which one partner works at night have higher rates of divorce and separation, Presser's research shows. Couples with children who have been married fewer than five years, she found, have a six times higher likelihood of separation or divorce five years later when men work nights, compared to couples in which men work days. Night-working women married more than five years have a three times higher likelihood of divorce or separation.[42]

Typically, both spouses work different hours with no overlap. This situation increases the time that at least one parent can take care of the children. Indeed, a national study of such couples showed that each parent serves as the primary caretaker while the other works. That's a plus, as it means both parents, fathers in particular, can take a greater role in child care. The downside is that there is little time for both parents, as well as their children, to be awake together. Child care is a big concern for all working parents. Nation-wide, only about 10 percent of businesses offer on-site child care.

Early morning, late evening, weekend, or twenty-four-hour child care for employees is still a rarity, but national child-care providers are beginning to see a business opportunity here. Car manufacturers, hospitals, casinos, and others have found such services a good way to reduce turnover. Some pro-grams offer night-working parents the option of keeping their preschoolers up for part of the night so that parents and children can go home together in the morning and sleep on the same schedule.[43]

"Work is hard on my social life."

This is another mental health concern. Shift workers complain far more than day workers about not having time for friends, organizations, cultural events, and hobbies, all activities that enrich the quality of life. Friends, unless they work the same shift, may not be available when you are. You have less prime time open for socializing in the evenings and weekends.

Shift-work schedules do give more free time in the day for outdoor activi-ties such as biking and gardening, as well as for shopping when stores are less crowded. Persons who enjoy solitary hobbies, such as woodworking or sewing, like shift work better than those who favor group activities, such as golfing or playing cards. "The social and domestic factors," says Timothy Monk, "are at least as important in a person's ability to cope with shift work as the biological ones are."[44]

Female Shift Workers Face Added Health Problems

"My periods are irregular."

In Kathryn Lee's study of nearly 800 female nurses on all shifts, nurses who worked night or rotating shifts reported more menstrual-cycle irregularities than those on other shifts. While nurses as a group generally are healthy, the night and rotating-shift nurses suffered more health problems overall than those on other shifts.[45]

In another study, sixty-eight healthy nurses under age forty reported nor-mal menstrual cycles when working only on the day shift. But more than half told Susan Labyak of the University of North Carolina that rotating shift-work schedules made their menstrual cycles longer, shorter, or more irregular, increased menstrual pain, or altered menstrual flow. In the general popula-tion, only about one woman in five reports variable cycles.[46] Female flight attendants report irregular menstrual cycles more often than do women with unchanging work schedules.

"I had a problem pregnancy."

Female shift workers may have a slightly increased risk of having difficulty getting pregnant, of having a miscarriage or preterm birth, and of having babies with a lower than average birth weight.[47] One report combining several studies of attempts to conceive by more than 10,000 European women found those who rotated shifts were up to twice as likely as those who worked only in the day to report delays of nine months or more.[48]

Canadian researchers found that female shift workers had miscarriages two to four times as often as day workers, with the risk highest in those who worked fixed evening shifts. Exposure to chemicals or other physical factors in the workplace was not a factor.[49] A study of more than 3,300 Norwegian women who continued working past their third month of pregnancy found that shift work doubled the risk of developing preeclampsia in those who already had one or more children. This disorder may retard the baby's growth and lead to premature delivery.[50] Chinese researchers found 900 female shift workers at three textile mills had double the risk of having a small or premature baby as day workers did.[51] There is no evidence that birth defects are higher in babies born to female shift workers.[52]

The reasons for the problems that do occur are unclear. Hormonal upsets, caused directly by schedule changes or resulting from disturbed sleep or stress, are thought to be involved. These studies are important because they involve thousands of women holding a variety of jobs. Certainly, women should not be denied any employment opportunity because of their sex. But existence of these problems urgently demands further study and development of effective preventive strategies.

"I never have time for myself."

This is another mental health concern. Working mothers handle 60 percent of a couple's child-rearing activities, Cornell University researchers found. Keith Bryant and Cathleen Zick added the amount of time parents in two-parent, two-children families spent in child care. They included primary child-care activities such as bathing, dressing, teaching, supervising, counseling, driving, and feeding children, as well as time spent with children while cooking, doing housework, or engaging in hobbies, and so forth. Finally, they added what many parents call "quality" time: playing together, watching TV, or sharing meals. The total came to 7.5 hours a day, almost the equivalent of a full-time job in itself.[53]

Women do most of the housework, even when they also have full-time jobs, spending about fifteen hours a week more than men on this task, sociologist Arlie Hochschild reports in her book *The Second Shift*. Women workers complain more than men of being "overtired, sick, and emotionally drained," Hochschild says. "These women talked about sleep," she writes, "the way a hungry person talks about food."[54]

University of Michigan researcher Sanjiv Gupta, who analyzed reports from 8,200 men and women, found that additional children had no effect on the time men spent on housework, excluding child care. For women, however, each additional child added more than three hours of housework a week, plus still more time for child care.[55]

Does Shift Work Shorten Your Life?

"Shift work takes ten years off your life," workers often assert. Some sound resigned, even fatalistic. Others seem to be embracing a heroic stance. They're saying, "I'm tough, I can handle this job, and I'm going to beat the odds."

Although shift workers experience increased rates of some disorders, there is no proof that they die sooner than persons working only in the daytime. Such studies are virtually impossible to do. Persons who develop serious health problems may drop out of shift work early, leaving those who remain a healthier-than-expected population. Few people work on shift schedules their entire lives. Moreover, shift workers' higher rates of smoking and alcohol use may be more critical than their job schedules in affecting their longevity.

Laboratory studies keeping insects, mice, hamsters, and other animals on schedules that mimic shift work raise some worrisome concerns. At Northwestern University, for example, researchers studied Syrian hamsters prone to die early from heart disease. Half the hamsters lived on a schedule where days and nights remained constant, with twelve hours of light and twelve hours of dark. The others lived on a schedule in which their days and nights flip-flopped on a weekly basis. Plamen Penev and his colleagues recorded how long each animal lived. The hamsters on the shift-work schedule had an 11 percent shorter life span.[56]

Regardless of their work schedules, humans follow much more diverse schedules than laboratory animals. While it is apparent that chronic disruptions in body clocks may have adverse effects, the hope is that persons who build healthy behaviors into their lives, get enough sleep, eat right, exercise, and manage stress effectively can avoid or reduce the toll shift work may take on their health.

Some Chrono "Types" Manage Shift Work Better

Human resources managers would love to have tests that accurately predict which job applicants are likely to make the best shift workers. This is an area of considerable research interest. The current state of the art suggests that certain individual characteristics make it easier for some people to adapt to shift work than others.

Owls manage better than larks. Owls adapt more easily to varied schedules, and prove more alert at night. They also sleep better in the daytime.[57] Extreme owls, persons who would prefer not to go to sleep before 3 or 4 A.M., may thrive on fixed night-work schedules. Being a bartender or a night-shift emergency room physician, for example, would be ideal for these persons. (See page 43 for the Owl/Lark Self-Test.)

Louise Miller, a teacher who once worked split shifts, explores opportunities for jobs at nontraditional hours in her book *Careers for Night Owls & Other Insomniacs.*[58] Miller describes a slew of careers in transportation, hospitality, health care, communications, entertainment, and security and social services, and details education and training requirements and average earnings. She also profiles individual workers, pointing out both the advantages and disadvantages of nontraditional hours. For most jobs, she includes a "what it takes" section, with questions to help readers decide if the work described is right for them.

Daily temperature range may affect ease of adaptation. Body temperature in some persons hovers around a single degree. In others, it ranges between about 96° F and 100° F. Those with a narrow range appear to manage slow rotation schedules better, at least as young adults. After age forty-five or so, they report more trouble sleeping in the daytime when working at night, and more health problems overall. Persons whose body temperature has a wide range do better on rapid rotations, where the aim is not to adapt. (See the section on Speed of Rotation, on page 184.)

Having a long free-running clock is a plus. Some of us, if left on our own, have an innate clock that runs close to twenty-five hours, while others cycle nearer to twenty-four hours. The internal clock generally runs longest in adolescence and gradually moves closer to twenty-four hours as we get older. People with longer free-running clocks tend to be owls, who generally find it easier to adapt to schedule changes than do larks.

Having more "adaptive" rhythms also speeds adjustment. After several days on a shift, some workers outpace others in rapidity of adaptation. Individuals vary considerably. Sleep, meals, exercise, stress, and other factors may impinge on adjustment for any one person from one shift change to the next. Research is in progress to develop strategies to rev up balky clocks.

Youth generally helps. Younger persons adapt more easily to schedule changes, and especially to evening and night shifts, than workers over forty-five. Older persons wake up earlier in the morning, however, and may do better than younger workers at jobs that start extremely early.

Flexible sleepers have an advantage. Persons who can sleep well even if it's noisy or there's light in the room, and who nod off easily, usually sleep better and longer than persons who need a dark, quiet room, a special pillow, or have other requirements.

Short sleepers adapt better than long sleepers. Persons who need little sleep, under six hours, say, stand a better chance of getting it when working shifts than persons who need nine hours or more.

Physically fit persons adapt better than couch potatoes. Persons who are in good shape generally sleep better and have more stamina. Short exercise breaks at work can improve alertness for the rest of the shift.

Extroverts may adapt faster than introverts. While these traits are not, strictly speaking, part of our chronotype, they're linked to it. Outgoing persons often have more flexible sleep habits and are more likely to "go with the flow." Introverts often like night work, however, and feel it offers more freedom to do the job their own way. They often do especially well on fixed night shifts.

Forward Rotations Easier on Body

Eight-hour shifts that rotate forward around the clock—mornings to evenings to nights—are easier on the body than shifts that rotate backward. Forward rotations sustain our natural tendency to stay up later, permitting body clocks to move in the same direction as the work schedule. Such rotations in essence make the day longer. In this they mimic westward travel. On a forward rotation, a worker might go to sleep at 11 P.M. while on the morning shift, 3 A.M. while on the evening shift, and 9 A.M. while on the night shift.

On eight-hour backward rotations, workers have a bedtime that is progressively earlier, and beyond the range to which the body easily adapts. A worker who goes to sleep at 11 P.M. while on the morning shift would likely be attempting sleep at 9 A.M. immediately after rotating to the night shift.

In both directions the night shift is the toughest, and exposure to morning sunlight on the way home invariably undermines adaptation.

All studies to date find that the majority of workers overwhelmingly favor forward schedules. Younger workers, however, often prefer the backward direction because its longest break is eight hours longer than that on a forward rotation. There is no more time off, however. Shorter breaks in the schedule simply are proportionately shorter. In 1999, work sites in the United States using eight-hour shifts included 29 percent rotating forward, 18 percent rotating backward, and 53 percent on fixed shifts, according to a *Shift-Work Alert* survey of 500 round-the-clock companies.

Best Speed of Rotation Still Debated

U.S. workers most often rotate on a weekly basis, spending five to seven days on a shift, while those in many European countries rotate more rapidly, spending only two to four days on a shift.

Spending more time on a shift or working on a fixed shift theoretically permits workers to achieve some adaptation after a few days. In reality, however, morning sun exposure after a night shift counters this benefit. If workers revert to a traditional daytime schedule on days off, as most do, they will reverse any gain.

Spending less time on a night shift theoretically will prevent rhythms from changing and keep workers locked into a daytime schedule. On a morning or evening shift, workers can sleep at the same time and at the right time, that is, at night. They also have some evenings free every week for social activities. When working the night shift, however, they will be much sleepier than they are when working other shifts. Since they do it only for a few days, they may avoid building up a serious sleep debt. The drawback is that they are liable to make more mistakes at night, a particularly worrisome issue for workers in safety-sensitive jobs, such as nuclear power plant operators and intensive-care nurses.

The impact of length of time on a shift remains a concern. The nature of the task to be performed may be the deciding factor. Research suggests that the risk of errors jumps after the sixth or seventh hour on the job. Performance also slides after four or five days in a row on a twelve-hour shift. The crucial issue may not be the number of hours people work in a shift so much as the times of day at which they work.

Workers on fixed night shifts report just as many sleep problems as those on rotating shifts. Still, there are exceptions: one night nurse who lived alone chose to keep the same hours on days off, gardening at night under bright lights in her backyard.

Some shift-work specialists contend that workers should spend less time when working nights than when working at other times, a thirty-hour week, for instance, instead of forty hours. Time between rotations is an issue, too, with more time needed to catch up on sleep after a rotation on the night shift. All of these considerations make for complicated scheduling, a task improved in recent years with the aid of computers.

Bright Light May Speed Clock Resetting

Exposure to daylight that night-shift workers get on their way home from work keeps body clocks oriented to a daytime schedule. Exposure to a few hours of appropriately timed bright artificial light—and to appropriately timed darkness—may help these workers adapt faster to their schedule changes. The light, it is hoped, will trick the brain into thinking night is day and day is night.

Shift workers might get light in the workplace, receiving exposure early in the night shift, for example, to reduce the normal fall in alertness that occurs when temperature is lowest. Or workers might use lights at home in advance to prepare for a schedule change.

Shifting workers' exposure to darkness may be just as crucial for altering their rhythms as getting light at the right time. Charmane Eastman, a leading researcher in this field, showed that night workers can avoid conflicting cues from sunlight by wearing dark goggles on their way home from work. They also need to sleep at consistent times after the night shift, she says, and to light-proof their bedrooms for day sleep by covering windows with black plastic or other protective material.

In a study simulating work-schedule changes, volunteers who previously stayed awake in the daytime and slept at night flip-flopped their activities. For five consecutive nights, they received three hours of exposure to high- or medium-intensity light immediately before their temperature low point, or they stayed in constant low-intensity light. The brightest light was equivalent to daylight about a half hour after dawn; the medium, closer to light like that in many shopping malls; and the low, to ordinary room lighting. The volunteers were required to go outside after the night shift, to mimic the travel-home time in which shift workers ordinarily are exposed to natural light. At these times, they wore large dark sunglasses with top and side shields.

Eastman and her student Stacia Martin found that nearly all the subjects adapted faster after receiving high- and medium-intensity light. The low point of their body temperature cycle quickly moved to the time they were sleeping. They slept better in the daytime and felt less fatigue when working at night than subjects exposed only to low-intensity light. The finding that the medium-intensity light was as effective as the high-intensity light is a practical one. Although brighter than most ordinary room light, it generally proves less disturbing to the eye than high-intensity light. Medium-intensity light causes less glare on computer monitors, and is less expensive to run.[59]

The sunglasses used in these studies are not readily available for use by shift workers. Most ordinary sunglasses do not block light from the sides, Eastman says, and transmit 10 percent or more light. Seven percent or less light transmission is preferable. For the present, she advises workers to wear the darkest glasses possible and to minimize the time they spend outdoors on the way home.

One of the more dramatic uses of bright light in the workplace is at the National Aeronautics and Space Administration (NASA) Johnson Space Center in Houston, Texas. Quarters where astronauts are quarantined for one week prior to orbital flights contain glass ceilings with banks of high-intensity lights that create an indoor daylight zone. Exposure is timed to preadapt crew members to their in-flight shift-work schedules.

NASA also uses bright lights for its ground-control teams. In one study, eight Mission Control workers at NASA's Marshall Space Flight Center in Huntsville, Alabama, received exposure to several hours of bright light in advance of a mission to get them in sync with the astronauts' schedules. They received additional light while the mission was in progress to help maintain the shift in their rhythms, as well as light after the mission was over to help them return to their normal schedules. These workers rated their work speed, concentration, and alertness on duty much higher than did a comparable group of ten workers who did not receive light exposure. Karen Stewart, who designed and supervised the study, said the workers who received light treatment also slept better at home. NASA's workers, of course, were highly motivated to comply with the necessary routine, which required them to wear dark welder's goggles when going out into daylight. Further, such missions occur only a few times a year and last just a few weeks.[60]

Trials of light in more conventional settings show the difficulties of translating research studies into practical strategies for ordinary shift workers. Exxon Chemical, for example, tried bright lights in control rooms at two different plants in the early 1990s. The thirteen workers participating in one study said they found it easier to stay awake on the night shift but did not sleep longer at home. They had more trouble adjusting to days off. On balance, the majority vetoed further use of the lights. San Diego Gas & Electric installed bright lights in two control rooms in 1993 and, after tinkering with various light levels, continued to use them. According to a report in *ShiftWork Alert*, some workers at this company say they feel more alert while working at night and sleep better on their days off.[61]

Can Melatonin Help Shift Workers?

A pill that could reset body clocks would be a boon to shift workers. Whether the hormone melatonin can serve this role is a hot area of investigation.

Melatonin normally surges into the bloodstream around 9 P.M., but it did not begin until three hours after sleep started, six hours later than it should have, in workers ending a week on the night shift who participated in a study at Oregon Health Sciences University. When sleep and hormone rhythms are out of sync, says Robert Sack, who directed the study, both sleep quality and daytime alertness suffer.

The researchers wondered if giving night workers melatonin in pill form shortly before they went to sleep in the morning would reset their body clocks faster. Introducing melatonin into the bloodstream at this time, researchers hoped, might trick the brain into thinking it was night. Nurses and hospital clerical staff participated in a four-week study. All worked seven consecutive ten-hour night shifts and then had a full week off before returning to night work. For the two work weeks, all took identical capsules just before bedtime, at night or in the morning. In one of the weeks, the capsules contained a small dose of melatonin, 0.5 milligrams. In the other, the capsules contained an inactive substance, a placebo. The subjects did not know which was which. In the weeks off work, all subjects slept at night; some took a placebo and some got no treatment at all.

In four of twenty-four subjects, rhythms shifted by about three hours in the right direction with melatonin. Most of the others showed rhythm shifts, too, with no treatment or with the placebo. This finding counters the still prevailing notion that most people never adapt to night work. The dark winter mornings in Portland, Oregon, where the study was conducted, may have made it easier for the workers to adapt, too.

Rhythm shifts can occur on their own, Sack suggests, but there may be wide variation among workers and even in the same person from one time to the next, depending on the individual's own chronotype, and factors such as the nature of the schedule and the amount of bright-light exposure the person receives. The situation is analogous to jet lag, where some people have more trouble than others, and where even the same person might have mild jet lag one trip and severe jet lag on another. Melatonin may help those workers who do not shift fully on their own.

Without sophisticated tests, you can't tell whether your melatonin rhythms shift when you change work hours. If you're a terrible sleeper, you may want to consider trying a low dose of melatonin. Some studies suggest melatonin benefits sleep even without shifting rhythms. If you work nights, the right time to take it is after you get home, an hour or so before you plan to go to sleep. (For more on melatonin, see chapter 4: "How Your Body Clock Works.")

Lawsuits May Force Workplace Changes

In 1991 a jury found the McDonald's Corporation liable for letting a sleepy employee get behind the wheel after a night shift. The eighteen-year-old worker fell asleep and hit another car head on, killing himself and seriously injuring the other driver. The jury decided that McDonald's knew, or should have known, that he would be a danger to himself and others while operating a motor vehicle.[62]

In 1996 the Federal Highway Administration shut down George Transfer, Inc., a Baltimore, Maryland, trucking firm after fining it more than $400,000 in three years for failing to correct numerous safety violations. These included 232 instances of requiring or permitting drivers to falsify logs aimed at keeping tired truckers off the road. The firm soon filed for bankruptcy.

Some shift workers have sued employers under the Americans with Disabilities Act (ADA), charging that poor work schedules harmed their health. In one landmark case, the Missouri Court of Appeals affirmed a lower court's award of more than $400,000 to a railroad worker who claimed he developed heart disease and gastritis as a result of poor work schedules and noisy, badly heated dormitory sleeping rooms provided by his employer, the Norfolk & Western Railway.[63]

In some other cases employers have prevailed, showing that the fired workers could no longer perform the job for which they were hired, which included working at night.

Lawsuits involving errors triggered by poor schedules may prompt changes that benefit both public safety and the health of individual workers.

Timewise Tips for Employers

Round-the-clock companies could take a lead in helping workers cope better with shift work. An optimal shift system is in a company's best interest, as it promotes higher employee morale, lower job turnover, higher productivity, fewer mistakes, and less absenteeism. Employers could take the following steps:

Adopt schedules that rotate forward around the clock, at a frequency tailored to local circumstances and acceptable to workers.

Educate workers about body clocks and strategies for coping with shift work. A host of shift-work consultation companies offers this service.

Target sleep, diet, exercise, smoking, and other areas of special concern to shift workers in employee health programs.

Provide round-the-clock cafeteria service, or at least offer healthy snacks in vending machines, and in a pleasant environment.

Offer cross-training, so that people can do a variety of tasks each shift, a tactic that fosters alertness.

Install exercise equipment for workers to use on breaks, or even on the job, while waiting for phone calls, for example.

Offer frequent breaks in jobs that demand high alertness. Card dealers in gambling casinos get a ten- to fifteen-minute break each hour to ensure they stay sharp, according to a report from the National Institute for Occupational Safety and Health.[64] Air-traffic controllers and others in safety-sensitive jobs need frequent breaks.

Permit on-site napping. Provide cots, space, and management's blessing for nap rooms, to be used on breaks, or before or after work. Nap breaks are required by law for workers on some schedules in Japan and in some European countries. In Japan, for example, nurses working a nine-hour shift get an hour to sleep in the second half of the shift. Quiet rooms are provided, and nurses receive their regular hourly rate. Shift-work experts propose legalizing naps for all workers whose alertness is critical to public safety.

Address needs of workers' families, by providing informational programs and home calendars and by scheduling events, such as company picnics, at times convenient for workers on all shifts.

Offer child-care services for extended hours, including weekends.

Timewise Tips for Employees

If you work outside of daytime hours, use these strategies to foster better performance and health on and off the job:

Do your most boring tasks early, and your most interesting ones toward the end of your shift. Stand up and stretch frequently; walk around if possible. A few minutes of vigorous exercise rapidly boosts alertness. Talk to coworkers, and listen to radio talk-shows if you can to stay alert. Try to schedule breaks for your foggiest times.

Nap on breaks. The character George in the TV show *Seinfeld* once built a napping compartment into the underside of his desk. Real-life workers saw this as a great idea. Try to persuade your employer to offer nap rooms, especially for persons working long hours and at night. As a last resort, nap in your car. Even a ten-minute nap boosts alertness. Napping for up to twenty minutes is unlikely to leave you groggy when you awaken. Use a wristwatch alarm, and plan to take five minutes or so before returning to work to come back to full alertness.

Plan both what and when you eat. Avoid snacking on fatty foods. Nibble on fruits and vegetables instead. If planning to sleep right after your shift, eat lightly. Cereal would be a good choice. If planning to stay awake for several hours longer, make your first post-shift meal high in protein and carbohydrates to boost energy.

Use caffeine judiciously. Two cups of regular coffee or two cans of caffeinated soda at the start of a night shift will boost alertness throughout the shift, according to Mark Muehlbach and James Walsh of St. Luke's Hospital in Chesterfield, Missouri. The researchers gave thirty volunteers either caffeinated or decaf coffee before each of five consecutive nights performing a computer task simulating assembly-line work. The caffeine-drinkers proved faster at quality-control inspections and at repairing or discarding faulty products. Both groups slept equally well and equally long during the day, not surprising because the amount of caffeine consumed was burned before they went to sleep.[65]

If you work at night and rotate forward around the clock, wear the darkest sunglasses you can find that still permit you to see well as you drive home. If rotating backward, spend fifteen minutes or more outdoors after work. If drowsy, nap for fifteen minutes before driving home, or get a ride.

Do not smoke at bedtime. Nicotine is a stimulant and disrupts sleep.

Avoid fluids right before daytime sleep. The bladder fills four times faster in the day than at night. You likely will feel the need to urinate sooner and more often after consuming fluids in the daytime than at night.

Protect your sleep. Darken the room, wear eyeshades and earplugs, unplug the phone, disconnect the doorbell (post a sign saying "day sleeper"), and consider sleeping in the basement or another room removed from family noise. If you cannot sleep at night, try to sleep between 9 A.M. and 3 P.M. Avoid sleeping in the late afternoon and early evening when temperature normally is highest, as higher temperatures make sleep more restless. If working at night, take a brief nap before leaving home. If you spend most of your days off catching up on sleep, you are not getting enough sleep the rest of the time. Noise the equivalent of murmured speech disturbs sleep. "Don't rage against noise; organize quiet," says David Morgan, author of *Sleep Secrets for Shift Workers & People with Off-Beat Schedules*. He suggests rewards for quiet kids.[66]

Consider sleeping pills. Troubled sleepers may benefit from using such pills occasionally. Even merely having them in the medicine cabinet may diminish anxiety about getting a decent amount of sleep. (See also page 349.)

If you are pregnant, make a special effort to get enough sleep and eat regular, well-balanced meals. If nausea is a problem, eat smaller but more frequent meals. Consider the added risks of exposure to chemicals, loud noise, or heavy lifting, possible reasons for exploring a job change. Tell your obstetrician about your work schedule so that he or she can be especially alert to shift work–related problems.

Keep your spouse or partner in the loop. Mark your work days on a kitchen calendar, schedule special "dates," leave notes on a family bulletin board, tape television programs or rent movies to watch as a family, ask a spouse or friend to videotape your child's soccer game or performance in the school play. Try to trade shifts so you can attend special events. Aim to join your family for at least one meal a day.

Beef up home security. This tactic may ease worries about your family's safety at night while you are at work. Install an alarm system, get a dog, add outdoor lights.

Exercise regularly. Walk, jog, bike, or engage in similar activity for thirty minutes three times a week, shortly before or after work, whatever schedule you are on. This will aid general physical fitness and heart health, as well as help synchronize body clocks.

Make sure your doctor knows about your work schedule. If you take medications for any illness, timing makes a difference. When you change schedules, it's not always possible to take medications at the same time with respect to sleep, meals, and activities. If you are supposed to take a medication at bedtime, how do you handle a day off after working on the night shift, for example, when you sleep in the morning and then again that night? If your medication is supposed to be taken at night before sleep, should you take it at night when you stay awake?

Some illnesses are more sensitive to time shifts than others and require a partnership between you and your doctor to organize your schedule in a way that minimizes problems. If you have *diabetes*, you need to consider the times and composition of meals and snacks, and the times you take medication on different work schedules. Diabetics who take three or more insulin shots a day probably are able to control their blood sugar levels better when eating and sleeping at odd hours than those who take only a single shot. If you have *epilepsy*, you need to be especially attentive to getting enough sleep to avert seizures. If you have *narcolepsy*, you need a job with varied activity to enhance your alertness and diminish your likelihood of sleep attacks; you also need to avoid driving. If you have *asthma*, you need to anticipate a higher likelihood of asthma attacks on the night shift and talk with your doctor about possibly altering the type of medication you take or the time you take it. If you suffer from *depression*, you need to weigh shift work carefully, as frequent schedule changes may worsen this disorder.

Study. Visit Circadian Technologies' Web site, www.shiftwork.com.

Summing Up

Highly visible events, such as a near meltdown at a power plant and a train derailment, may affect thousands of lives and undermine the safety and well-being of surrounding communities. More frequent events, such as fender-benders on the way home from work and minor injuries on the job, get little attention from the media. "In financial terms, and in an accounting of human misery," chronobiologists Julie Carrier and Timothy Monk assert, "it is quite possible that the sum total of the frequent small events is as important to society as that of the occasional dramatic ones."[67]

Persons who manage shift work well and are happy in their jobs also may be the ones most suited for this type of work and most likely to remain healthy. Employees and employers both profit when individual needs match those of the job, and when work schedules are designed to maximize both job performance and workers' health and quality of life off the job.

A Time to Heal

Tuning in to your body clocks provides a new and powerful tool to help you stay healthy, recover faster when you get sick, and live well, even if you have a chronic illness. The following chapter, "Sickness and Health from A to (Nearly) Z," details important recent advances to help you in your everyday life. It includes:

- *Self-tests,* to help you identify problems needing a doctor's attention.
- *ChronoDiaries,* to record your symptoms patterns, rate their intensity, identify activities that may have triggered them, describe treatment you tried, and note how well it worked.
- *Timewise Tips,* practical pointers focused on timing of medication, sleep, and other activities that apply to your specific illness.
- *Anytime Tips,* health advice on diet, exercise, smoking, stress management, and other issues relevant to your specific illness.
- *Personal stories,* to highlight the emotional impact of illness.

Keep Your Own Chronorecord

Charting your own body rhythms is a good first step in health maintenance and disease prevention. You need only a few simple tools.

With a pencil and paper, you can chart

- your mood across the day
- your alertness across the day
- your wake/sleep cycle, and the time and type of disturbances of sleep
- what you eat and when you eat it
- symptoms of pain, fatigue, urinary frequency, or other health problems over the day, and, if you are female, across your menstrual cycle. If you have a chronic illness, you also can keep tabs on symptoms over the year.

With the addition of a wristwatch you can chart

- your heart rate
- your breathing rate

With the addition of a thermometer you can chart

- body temperature over the day
- if you are female, body temperature across your menstrual cycle

With the addition of a blood pressure cuff you can chart

- blood pressure over the day

If you have a chronic illness such as asthma or diabetes, inexpensive tools will make self-monitoring easier. Your doctor, pharmacist, or other health provider will tell you about them and instruct you in their use.

You need to understand your illness and how to manage it. Using a computer at home or in your local public library, you now can access a vast amount of medical information via the Internet. Many health sites offer information that once was easily available only to doctors or persons with access to medical libraries. You can find reliable resources by searching PUBMED, the National Library of Medicine's consumer database (www.medlineplus.gov), and visiting excellent health sites maintained by the federal government, institutions such as the Mayo Clinic, Johns Hopkins, and the American Medical Association, as well as many national news organizations.

Many consumer health groups, such as the American Heart Association and the Arthritis Foundation, offer information and support to individuals and their families by mail and online. These often include online and community support groups, where you can learn from others coping with the same illness. You'll find Web site addresses for key organizations for specific illnesses in the next chapter.

Make your doctor your key resource person, your expert adviser, but take charge of your own care. Only you can make daily decisions on when to take medications, how to interpret symptoms, how to adapt to physical limitations, and when to report changes to your doctor. (See illustrations on pages 195–96.)

Educate Your Doctor

Talk to your doctor about

- when your symptoms occur
- when to get blood drawn and undergo other tests

THE WORST OF TIMES

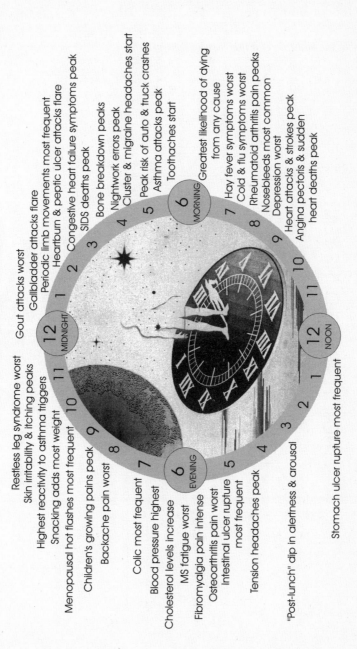

- Gout attacks flare — 12 MIDNIGHT
- Gallbladder attacks flare
- Periodic limb movements most frequent — 1
- Heartburn & peptic ulcer attacks flare
- Congestive heart failure symptoms peak — 2
- SIDS deaths peak
- Bone breakdown peaks — 3
- Nightwork errors peak
- Cluster & migraine headaches start — 4
- Peak risk of auto & truck crashes
- Asthma attacks peak — 5
- Toothaches start
- Greatest likelihood of dying from any cause — 6 MORNING
- Hay fever symptoms worst — 7
- Cold & flu symptoms worst
- Rheumatoid arthritis pain peaks — 8
- Nosebleeds most common
- Depression worst — 9
- Heart attacks & strokes peak
- Angina pectoris & sudden heart deaths peak — 10
- 11
- Stomach ulcer rupture most frequent — 12 NOON
- "Post-lunch" dip in alertness & arousal — 1
- 2
- Tension headaches peak — 3
- Intestinal ulcer rupture most frequent — 4
- Osteoarthritis pain worst — 5
- Fibromyalgia pain intense
- MS fatigue worst
- Cholesterol levels increase
- Blood pressure highest — 6 EVENING
- Colic most frequent — 7
- Backache pain worst — 8
- Children's growing pains peak — 9
- Menopausal hot flashes most frequent — 10
- Snacking adds most weight
- Highest reactivity to asthma triggers — 11
- Skin irritability & itching peaks
- Restless leg syndrome worst

HEALTH AROUND THE YEAR

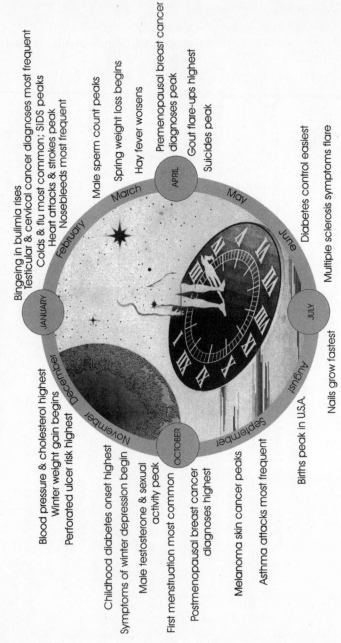

Bingeing in bulimia rises
Testicular & cervical cancer diagnoses most frequent
Colds & flu most common; SIDS peaks
Heart attacks & strokes peak
Nosebleeds most frequent

Male sperm count peaks
Spring weight loss begins
Hay fever worsens
Premenopausal breast cancer diagnoses peak
Gout flare-ups highest
Suicides peak

Diabetes control easiest
Multiple sclerosis symptoms flare

Nails grow fastest

Births peak in U.S.A.

Asthma attacks most frequent

Melanoma skin cancer peaks

Postmenopausal breast cancer diagnoses highest

First menstruation most common

Male testosterone & sexual activity peak

Symptoms of winter depression begin

Childhood diabetes onset highest

Blood pressure & cholesterol highest
Winter weight gain begins
Perforated ulcer risk highest

JANUARY
February
March
APRIL
May
June
JULY
August
September
OCTOBER
November
December

- when to take prescribed medication. If your medication doesn't work as well as expected or causes unwanted side effects, ask whether it might help to change the time you take it.
- whether chronotherapies are available for your illness.

While most physicians unfortunately know little about chronobiology, and still less about chronotherapy, your questions may prompt your doctor to explore the topic further. To facilitate that, you'll find an extensive list of scientific articles to share with your doctor at the back of the book. We've also included suggestions for further information that has References for Physicians and Other Health Care Providers and useful terms for online searches. (See page 406.)

You Need the Right Medicine at the Right Time

Three out of four doctor visits yield prescriptions. An estimated 2.8 billion prescriptions were dispensed in the United States in 1999. Amazingly, as many as 50 percent of people don't take their medicines as prescribed, the United States Food and Drug Administration (FDA) reports.[1] Even when patients follow their doctors' advice scrupulously, medications sometimes do not work as well as expected, or they cause adverse side effects. The person may be taking the right drug in the right dose. It may be only the timing that is wrong.[2]

When you get a prescription, your doctor will tell you whether to take your medication before, with, or after meals, once a day or more often. Your doctor may write the prescription, "b.i.d." or "t.i.d.," for instance, using the Latin abbreviations for "twice a day" and "three times a day." In such cases, you take your medicines in equal intervals across your waking day.

With some medicines, the doctor may specify a time, such as "when you wake up" or "at bedtime." Some medicines, such as sleeping pills, have a time-bound use, but most do not. The general theory behind the design of most pill, capsule, and skin-patch medications still is a homeostatic one: to provide constant levels of the therapy at all times, exerting a uniform effect on the body. This is a fruitless goal. The body's only true constancy is its inconstancy. The body may handle the same dose of the same medication in different ways at different times of day.[3]

When and what you eat, for example, may alter how speedily your body absorbs medications. Since many bodily functions slow down overnight, including the emptying of the stomach, drugs you take orally in the evening move into the bloodstream more slowly than those you take in the morning. Your kidneys, which help eliminate drugs from the body, work more slowly at night, too, the reason you urinate less frequently then. Some drugs thus stay in your body longer at night. The body secretes a vast array of different hormones around the clock, and many alter drug absorption.

Sleep itself modifies both the symptoms of many illnesses and the way the body processes drugs. "The sleeping patient is still a patient," internist Eugene Robin of Harvard Medical School reminded colleagues in the 1950s. "His disease not only goes on while he sleeps but indeed may progress in an entirely different fashion from its progression during the waking state."[4]

Best Time to Take Most Medicines Not Known

In recent years, many once-a-day medications have come on the market. Most aim simply to promote even blood and tissue levels of a drug around the clock. When you take them, you probably get more of the drug than you need at some times, and less than you need at others.

Manufacturers often advise taking once-a-day drugs in the morning. You might assume that these medications are more effective or safer if taken then, but there is no scientific rationale for this time at all. The designation of a specific time is simply a function of FDA administrative regulations. In granting its approval to market a drug, the FDA specifies a dosing time based upon the time patients took the medication in premarketing studies conducted to demonstrate efficacy and safety.

Standardization of a morning dosing time is a matter of custom and convenience. In any large study, more people are likely to be near a bathroom or kitchen where they can get a glass of water to take a pill at 8 A.M. than at other times of day.

If you were to ask your doctor if you could take a once-a-day medication at any hour that suited you, you might be told that time doesn't matter, so long as you take your medication regularly. Recent studies challenge this view. We report these studies in the following chapter and elsewhere in this book. Chronotherapy research shows medications work better and are safer when they are tailored to body time: you get more of the drug when you need it most or tolerate it best, and less when you need it less or tolerate it poorly.

Finding Best Time Proves Daunting Task

"Every system in the body has active chronobiological mechanisms," observed Gerald Sokol, a scientist in the FDA's division of oncology and pulmonary products.[5] "This activity at every level of the species creates individual susceptibilities to pharmacological agents. We know that early morning is the most dangerous time for persons with heart disease, and night for those with asthma. So we need drugs that maintain activity at those times.

"The field is wide-open for research," he said, "particularly for cancer chemotherapy, where we operate on the frontier of maximal potential toxicity."

Designing randomized clinical trials to assess chronobiological issues poses enormous technical challenges, Sokol said. In such trials, volunteer subjects have equal odds of taking the drug or drugs under study, or a placebo for comparison. Receptivity to different drugs may vary not only across the day but by the season. For women, the effects of some drugs vary by time of their menstrual cycle. Men and women in general may respond differently, and the old differently from the young.

Studies of drugs try to address the equivalency of all variables except the one under study. When the variables increase, Sokol said, the number of patients needed to show statistical significance also increases. A present-day premarketing randomized trial to show the efficacy and safety of a single drug now requires at least one hundred patients, and researchers often find it hard to recruit them. "Chronobiological trials," Sokol said, "may require three hundred patients.

"We would have to develop a system of statistics sensitive to this whole spectrum of variabilities," Sokol said. "The FDA has enormous difficulty doing basic chocolate and vanilla kinds of studies. To address all of the data that would have to be analyzed to address chronobiological issues would represent orders of magnitude of increased complexity."

Some Chronotherapies Are Already Available

Some medications already on the market deliver varying amounts of a drug at different times, thanks to their built-in design. To earn FDA approval, their manufacturers had to take into account rhythms in drug requirements for specific diseases, or the nature of the toxicity of the drugs themselves. They then were able to devise chronobiological medications and to develop a successful strategy for testing their efficacy and safety at multiple times over the day.

Typical present-day drug studies represent an old-fashioned approach to clinical design, according to Gordon Amidon of the University of Michigan.[6] "There is no *a priori* reason to think equal dosing is best," he said. "The opposite more likely is true." It might be better to take one-third of a day's medication in the morning, he said, and two-thirds in the evening. One way to determine optimum dosing would be to give a drug by mouth or intravenously at different dose rates and times, while measuring pharmacological responses to see which rate or time works best. Drugs could be delivered over various time periods: a day, a week, a month, or even years.

Matching a drug to specific characteristics of the person taking the drug might improve treatment further, said Amidon, who is Charles Walgreen Jr. professor of pharmacy and pharmaceutics at the University of Michigan. Your doctor might assess your responses to known marker compounds, add details about your genetic makeup, allergies, and health status—including results of round-the-clock ambulatory monitoring, or your daily symptom diaries—and then project how well you're likely to respond to a particular drug if you take it at different times. Your comprehensive health profile could be downloaded onto a wallet-sized scanable card, miniaturized to wear on jewelry, or even implanted in a tooth for easy access in emergencies.

The delivery of drugs at varying rates over time requires sophisticated technology. Some of it already exists. Programmable drug delivery pumps able to hold a week's or a month's supply of medication already are being used by persons with cancer, diabetes, and other hard to manage illnesses. Some of these pumps are implantable and easily refilled via external openings, and some are worn outside the body.

Some medications, including contraceptives and antipsychotic agents, now come in forms that can be implanted under the skin, delivering medications for months or even years; such systems could be adapted to release the drugs in a chronobiologic manner.

Skin patches offer another potential way to deliver more or less medication at different times; many are already in use. A dime-sized silicon microchip developed at the Massachusetts Institute of Technology, now undergoing testing, contains reservoirs for multiple chemicals.[7] You might swallow this so-called smart tablet in the morning, when convenient, though it might not release the drugs until you need them later in the day. This microchip also could be implanted under your skin.

Drugs in the future will include many more rhythm-shifting *chronobiotics*, such as melatonin. You may use them to avoid jet lag, hasten adjustment to different hours of work, or simply recover from sleep loss.

Chronobiology and chronotherapy may still be unfamiliar terms, but doctors' and patients' comfort with these concepts is growing. In the next chapter, you'll find reports on many common illnesses, with attention to their circadian or other rhythmic patterns, and current knowledge of existing chronotherapies.

The momentum is building. Chronotherapy is moving into prime time.

Sickness and Health
from A to (Nearly) Z

In the following sections, time of day terms, such as morning and evening, apply to the customary day/night pattern of day-active people. If you work on rotating shifts, on the night shift, or another nontraditional schedule, adapt advice to your personal "day" or "night."

AIDS

Acquired Immunodeficiency Syndrome (AIDS) disrupts daily rhythms in waking energy levels, sleep, body temperature, hormone secretion, and immune system functioning. These changes hold implications for managing daily life, as well as for diagnostic tests and treatment.

AIDS is caused by infection with the human immunodeficiency virus (HIV), a virus not known to have existed until the 1970s. It is transmitted primarily by having unprotected sex with a person who has the virus and sharing needles or syringes with an infected person. HIV-infected women may pass it on to their unborn babies. Effective screening tests now make it highly unlikely that blood transfusions will transmit HIV, as occurred some years ago.

In 1999 about 34 million persons worldwide were living with an HIV infection or with AIDS, according to the United Nations and World Health Organization. AIDS is the last stage of infection with HIV. This virus invades mainly CD4 white blood cells that the body needs to fight infections. HIV turns these cells into factories for churning out more HIV, which then invades other CD4 cells, leaving the factory cells behind to die. Responding to this attack, the body makes more CD4 cells, but it cannot produce them as fast as HIV destroys them. The death of huge numbers of CD4 cells leaves the body with an incompetent immune system, and vulnerable to a variety of "opportunistic" infections, such as pneumocystis pneumonia and a rare type of cancer known as Kaposi's sarcoma. In persons infected with HIV, a CD4 count of 200 or below per cubic milliliter of blood leads to a formal diagnosis of AIDS. (A normal count is 600 to 1,000.) By 1999, AIDS had killed more than 16 million persons. It is the second leading cause of death worldwide for people aged twenty-five to forty-four.

Potent drugs that suppress HIV activity, known as protease inhibitors, first became available in the United States in 1995, rapidly reversing the rising death rate from AIDS. They do not totally eradicate the virus, however, and have to be taken indefinitely. Some people develop a drug-resistant form of the virus.

Current treatment involves a combination of protease inhibitors and other drugs aimed at preventing replication of different stages of the virus, plus drugs designed to prevent opportunistic infections. Many patients take vitamins and other nutritional stimulants to maintain overall good health and promote appetite. They may need still other drugs to treat adverse side effects of other medications.

Fatigue Dampens Quality of Life

More than 50 percent of persons with advanced AIDS report they feel overwhelmed by fatigue, too exhausted to continue working, or even driving a car. They sleep longer and nap more than persons in the early stages of the illness do.[1]

Beyond poor sleep, causes of fatigue in AIDS include anemia, pain, infection and fever, deficiencies of certain hormones or nutrients, depression and anxiety, and even resting too much, without the balance provided by daily activity. Some of these problems respond to specific treatments.[2] (See Mood Disorders, page 296, and Sleep Disorders, page 339.) Fatigue also may be a side effect of medications used to treat AIDS.

Fatigue is even more common in HIV-infected women than in HIV-infected men. One hundred HIV-infected women participated in a two-day study at the School of Nursing at the University of California, San Francisco. None of the women was taking protease inhibitors. All wore a wrist actigraph, a small movement-activated recording device, to monitor their waking activity and the length and nature of their sleep. They also completed a daily diary, rating their fatigue and quality of sleep. The researchers also took blood samples to assess CD4 cell counts.

Kathryn Lee and her colleagues found women with lower CD4 cell counts had more fatigue, and slept more in the daytime. European-American women reported more fatigue than African- or Hispanic-American women did, perhaps reflecting different cultural attitudes toward this symptom. Working women reported more fatigue in the evening than unemployed women.

Mothers with children living at home felt less improvement in their fatigue after a night's sleep than women without children.

Biological time and its disturbances in HIV infections and AIDS must be viewed in the context of the infected person's life. "Results from this study indicate that clinicians caring for women with HIV who report fatigue should not attribute the symptom entirely to physiologic factors such as CD4 cell counts or poor sleep," the researchers asserted. Treatment planning must address sociocultural and home environments as well.[3]

Is Fatigue a Problem for You?

♦ Does fatigue get in the way of your daily activities?
If you have a job, does fatigue slow you down?
If you stopped work, was fatigue a factor?
Is fatigue a concern when driving?
Are you bothered by fatigue more than one hour a day?
Do you fall asleep when you don't intend to?
Are you a restless sleeper?

If you answered "yes" to any of these questions, see Timewise Tips, page 205, and explore possible treatment strategies with your doctor.

Sleep Disturbances Occur Early in HIV-Infection

The need for sleep increases markedly soon after infection with HIV, even in persons with no other obvious symptoms, some studies suggest. Sleep-laboratory studies show newly infected persons get much more deep sleep than they previously did, perhaps part of the body's all-out effort to overcome the infection.[4] Disturbances of sleep by night sweats, along with fever and joint pain, are other early symptoms that may identify people recently infected with HIV, even before their blood antibody tests are positive, which may not occur for as long as six months.[5] Other tests can be used to determine the presence of the HIV virus in the body and the need to begin treatment immediately, before the immune system is affected. The sooner the illness can be detected and treatment started, the longer the person is likely to live.

As the illness progresses, sleep usually deteriorates. People take longer to fall asleep, get less deep sleep, awaken more frequently, and report poorer sleep quality. The architecture of sleep changes, too, with more deep sleep later in the night, possibly reflecting an alteration in the circadian rhythm of body temperature.

One study found the daily peak of body temperature in ten persons infected with the AIDS virus came in the morning or early afternoon, rather than in late afternoon or early evening, as in healthy persons.[6] In some, the temperature rhythm followed a cycle different from that of twenty-four hours. This change may be a marker for other changes in body-clock function.

Persons infected with HIV make more of an immune system chemical called tumor necrosis factor-alpha. This substance is involved in inflammatory responses, and is associated with wasting in persons infected with HIV, as well as persons with cancer. When this chemical is high, people get less of the deeper, more restful stages of sleep.[7]

Persons with AIDS who sleep poorly also have more anxiety and depression, and consume more caffeine than those without sleep complaints. Medications and psychotherapy may improve mood, and cutting back on caffeine may add to that effect. It is worth the effort to make such changes because sleeping better has a global effect on well-being.

Finally, an important reminder: Some people with HIV infections who sleep poorly also have medically curable sleep disorders, such as a breathing disorder, sleep apnea, or periodic limb movements (see page 330). These disorders may even be more frequent in HIV-infected persons than in the general population.[8]

HIV-Infection Changes Immune and Hormone Rhythms

The infection-fighting CD4 white blood cells move in and out of the tissues and organs of the body in a rhythmic manner. Twice as many circulate in the blood at the high point of the cycle at night, as at the low point in the morning.

One of the first effects of an HIV infection is a flattening of the day-night range, sometimes with a change in the peak time, or even a complete obliteration of the CD4 circadian rhythm.[9] In most people, the circadian variation in CD4 numbers is so low that the time of day of blood sampling is not significant. In those who have a large variation in CD4 counts, however, the circadian time of blood sampling may reveal rhythmic patterns, yielding information that may be of possible practical relevance in guiding treatment decisions in the future.

Other types of infection-fighting white blood cells beside CD4 cells fall in number and lose their circadian rhythmicity in persons infected with HIV. The day/night range of circadian rhythms in several indicators of the blood's oxygen-carrying capacity also flattens. These include the total number of red cells, the amount of hemoglobin they contain, and the percentage of total blood volume that red blood cells make up.[10] Researchers suspect that the degree to which such rhythms are obliterated predicts the body's ability to control the infection and fend off progression of the disease.

The amounts of certain hormones the body secretes also change in persons infected with HIV. HIV-infected men, for example, secrete 25 percent more of the stress hormone cortisol than healthy men. This is a natural response to infection. Nonetheless, cortisol's circadian pattern remains unaltered. The same men secrete 50 percent less dehydroepiandrosterone, or DHEA.[11] What DHEA does in humans is as yet unclear, but animal studies suggest it may help fight viral and bacterial infections and cancer.[12] The timing, though not the amount, of growth hormone secretion changes. Since growth hormone plays an important role in tissue repair, a deviation from the normal secretion pattern offers another indicator of AIDS' bodywide assault.[13]

Doctors who treat HIV-infected women say that patients often complain of symptoms worsening in association with menstruation, but there have been no scientific studies so far to document such reports. This complaint is consistent with reports of symptom-worsening at this time of month in many illnesses.

More Research Needed on Medication Timing

So far only one antiviral medication, zidovudine (AZT), has been tested to see if its impact reflects the time it is taken. In one study, a small group of volunteers with HIV took either 100 or 200 milligrams of AZT at noon and at midnight. They then provided blood and urine samples at four-hour intervals around the clock. The researchers found 20 to 25 percent more AZT circulating in the body after the midnight dosing. Of more importance, medication levels varied substantially over the twenty-four-hour study period. Although the subjects took equal amounts of AZT at noon and midnight, there was a two- to fourfold difference in the amount of the drug detected in the blood across the twenty-four hours. These results suggest body rhythms may affect the absorption and therapeutic effects of this and perhaps other AIDS medications, too.[14]

Timewise Tips

Chart rhythms in energy levels using the fatigue diary on page 314. In healthy people, stamina is highest in the late morning. Use the knowledge of your daily pattern to plan activities and rest periods. Try to do your most important tasks first.

Plot your daily medication schedule, integrating it with work, meals, and other activities to be sure you take all doses of your prescribed medications. Find out whether to take medications before, with, or after meals to minimize the likelihood of stomach upsets.

Don't expect to see marked changes in blood drawn to assess CD4 levels at different times of day. The variation over the day is relatively small in most people, and laboratory procedures alone may account for differences from time to time.

Nap or schedule a rest period at a consistent time each day. For most people, whether they have HIV or not, brief midday naps provide the biggest boost in alertness.

Aim for the best possible sleep, by keeping regular hours, avoiding caffeine and alcohol in the evening, and following other good sleep habits. (See Timewise Tips for Good Sleep, page 77.) Discuss sleep problems with your doctor.

Anytime Tips

Continue safe-sex practices. While antiviral drugs have slowed the rate of deaths from HIV-AIDS, new cases of infection are rising, especially among sexually active young people, who often hold overoptimistic views of the drugs' efficacy.

Half of the 44,000 persons newly infected with HIV in the United States in 1998 were under age twenty-five.

Don't self-medicate with St.-John's-wort for depression if you are taking protease inhibitors. This herbal remedy dramatically lowers blood levels of the drug indinavir, National Institutes of Health researchers found. They warn it may affect other protease inhibitors the same way.[15]

Study. Visit the Web sites of the HIV-AIDS Treatment Information Service, sponsored by the U.S. Department of Health and Human Services (www.hivatis.org), John Hopkins University AIDS Service Web site (www.hopkins-aids.edu), or the University of California at San Francisco HIV InSite (http://hivinsite.ucsf.edu/).

ARTHRITIS

Pain, stiffness, and swelling are the hallmark symptoms of arthritis, which is not one but a family of more than one hundred diseases affecting 43 million Americans of all ages, women about twice as often as men.[1] The most common forms, osteoarthritis (OA) and rheumatoid arthritis (RA), both show distinctive circadian patterns of pain. Indeed, pain typically is their most bothersome symptom.

While many people feel stiff for an hour or so after first getting up in the morning, particularly as they get older, persons with OA typically hurt most and have the most trouble moving in the afternoon and evening. Those with RA almost always feel much worse in the morning.[2] This is not simply a function of being relatively immobile all night, but rather of the body's circadian changes. Even persons with RA who stay in bed all day report worse symptoms in the morning.

More than half of those with RA in one study ranked pain as their main source of stress. Some say, "It's terrible and I feel it's never going to get any better," while others assert, "I can't let the pain stand in the way of what I have to do." The former are more passive, more likely to catastrophize, to pray and hope and to view resting as appropriate, while the others employ more adaptive coping strategies, according to pain specialist Jennifer Haythornthwaite of the Johns Hopkins University School of Medicine.[3] Active copers with arthritis pay attention to their own daily pain pattern and participate more fully in their own treatment. They also report a higher overall quality of life.

Osteoarthritis (OA)

Nearly everyone shows signs of OA in later life; that's why it's often called the "wear and tear" disease. When severe, OA can make it hard to open a jar, turn a key, write a note, or manage other everyday tasks. OA attacks cartilage, a smooth and spongy tissue that covers bone ends, absorbs shocks, and enables joints to move freely. When cartilage is damaged, the bone ends may scrape against each other, making movement awkward and painful, particularly in the hips, knees, back, toes, and fingers.

About 21 million Americans have OA. Most report their pain peaks between midafternoon and midevening, usually at about the same time from day to day.[4]

Take Your Medicine before Pain Usually Starts

While there are hundreds of pain-relieving medications on the market, they contain only a handful of different ingredients. These include:

Acetaminophen

You can buy this pain-reliever without a prescription. It rarely has side effects when used as directed; many doctors recommend it as their first choice to ease pain in persons with little or no inflammation. Acetaminophen does not relieve inflammation. *Caution:* If you consume three or more alcoholic drinks a day, don't use this drug or any of the others listed here without your doctor's advice. The alcohol/drug interaction increases the risk of liver damage and stomach bleeding.

Non-Steroidal Anti-Inflammatory Drugs (NSAIDs)

These are the most widely used medications for both OA and RA. They effectively reduce swelling and stiffness, along with pain, but they do have certain significant side effects that pose concern when they are used over the long-term and in high doses.

Aspirin is the best-known NSAID. Even a single dose of aspirin may cause tiny sores in the lining of the stomach, although these sores ordinarily heal quickly without causing pain. The hefty dose of aspirin used for arthritis—

Pain Diary

Name _____

Make seven copies of this chart and fill them in for the coming week. Change times if you work at night. Take this diary with you when you see your doctor.

Day/Date _____

Time of Arising _____ A.M./P.M.

Bedtime _____ A.M./P.M.

Women: Are you menstruating today? Y/N

Time	Pain Severity Low High 1 2 3 4 5	Stiffness Low High 1 2 3 4 5	Swelling Low High 1 2 3 4 5	Activity Restriction Low High 1 2 3 4 5	Treament Used
8 A.M.					
10 A.M.					
NOON					
2 P.M.					
4 P.M.					
6 P.M.					
8 P.M.					
10 P.M.					
MIDNIGHT					

often a dozen or more tablets a day—may cause chronic stomach irritation, however, and lead to painful peptic ulcers.

Taking aspirin in the evening instead of in the morning lowers the amount of damage it causes. In one study, volunteers took aspirin at 10 P.M. on one occasion, and at 10 A.M. on another. Using a device called an endoscope to examine the lining of the stomach, researchers counted the number of small sores that developed in the stomach lining after each dose. Taking aspirin in the evening prompted half as many sores as taking it in the morning.[5] Taking coated aspirin, designed to dissolve after leaving the stomach, reduces the risk of irritation but delays pain relief. Hence, for persons with chronic pain doctors often recommend NSAIDs other than aspirin.

NSAIDs commonly used for arthritis include ibuprofen, ketoprofen, and naproxen. They come in both low over-the-counter doses, and higher doses that require a prescription, in tablets taken one to four times a day. Persons with severe arthritis usually need prescription strengths. Chronotherapy studies show there is a right time and a wrong time to take NSAID medications. Taking them at the right time may help prevent such unpleasant side effects as stomach ulcers and bleeding, indigestion, nausea, headache, anxiety, dizziness, and even liver and kidney damage. Such side effects are not uncommon. Federal studies show about seven in a thousand persons with OA who take NSAIDs for one year develop serious gastrointestinal complications.

Chronotherapy studies typically compare long-acting NSAIDs with a look-alike but inactive pill, or placebo, giving patients one or the other at different times of day. These studies show persons with OA get the most pain relief when they take the active medication four to eight hours prior to the time of day their pain is most intense, rather than waiting until pain flares. Side effects occur two to four times less often when people take these medications at night instead of in the morning.[6]

In the largest of these studies, French scientists recruited more than 500 persons with OA of the hip, the knee, or other joints to participate. The researchers sought to determine the best time to take a long-acting, once-a-day formulation of the NSAID indomethacin. Participants took their medicine at 8 A.M., noon, or 8 P.M. for a week. They assessed their pain intensity every two hours for two days before treatment began and at the end of the treatment week. When taking indomethacin at 8 A.M., they had four times as many complaints of dizzy spells, headaches, anxiety, nausea, stomach pain, and indigestion as when they took the same drug at 8 P.M., the least troublesome time. One in twelve volunteers dropped out of the study, saying they found the side effects intolerable. Two-thirds of those who dropped out did so when they were taking indomethacin in the morning.[7]

Cox-2 Inhibitors

Drugs known as cox-2 inhibitors first came on the market for the treatment of arthritis in the United States in 1999. Like other NSAID medications, these drugs reduce the body's production of an enzyme called cyclo-oxygenase, or cox-1, that figures in the development of pain and inflammation, and thus provide comparable pain relief. Unlike other NSAIDs, these drugs also suppress an enzyme called cox-2, a stomach irritant. They thus may be less likely to cause stomach bleeding, nausea, and other digestive system problems. Low rates of reported side effects in early users of these widely prescribed medications, which include celecoxib (Celebrex) and rofecoxib (Vioxx), suggest they may be safer than traditional NSAIDs,[8] but longer follow-up clearly is needed. The manufacturers of these drugs recommend that they be taken once or twice a day. There were no published studies at press time on how different dosing schedules affect the daily pattern of symptoms.

Timewise Tips for OA

Ask your doctor to time treatment to your particular symptom pattern. Taking your medication four to eight hours before your pain usually is worst may provide the best pain relief.

Ask if you should take the NSAID prescribed for you with a glass of water, or with food or milk, to coat the interior of your stomach and help minimize stomach irritation.

For afternoon pain, take medication at noon. For a few people morning treatment will be better, provided side effects are tolerable.

For evening pain, take medication in midafternoon.

For nighttime pain, take medication with your evening meal. This strategy will help you get the rest you need at night. Pain itself is a notorious sleep disrupter, and sleeping poorly may make your pain more troublesome the next day.

Exercise in late morning, before pain bothers you most. Walking, swimming, biking, and cross-country skiing are among the many low-impact activities that can strengthen muscles, while helping keep joints flexible. Remind yourself: "Motion is lotion." Apply generously.

Rheumatoid Arthritis (RA)

In RA, white blood cells that normally battle unwanted invaders in the body mistakenly attack cells lining the joints, primarily those in the fingers, toes, hands, wrists, elbows, feet, and ankles. The siege inflames tissues and generates pain. The resulting swelling also may cause disability and deformity. Fatigue and fever are other common symptoms. RA may strike at any age but most often first appears between ages thirty and sixty, just when people are most involved in having and rearing children and are most focused on their careers. Some 2.5 million Americans have RA.

The morning peak in swelling, stiffness, and pain in RA is tied to the daily rhythm of cortisol secretion. This hormone is virtually absent from your body overnight, but surges into the bloodstream around the time you normally awaken. Cortisol, the body's key "get up and go" hormone, also fights inflammation. Even though persons with RA awaken with pain, cortisol goes to work fast to subdue it.

Self-ratings of symptoms by persons with RA show the effects of the cortisol's circadian rhythm. One group of British volunteers with RA measured the circumference of their arthritic finger joints to gauge swelling, and checked their hand-grip strength every two to three hours for several consecutive days. They also assessed their pain and stiffness. In the morning, when pain and stiffness were worst, grip strength proved minimal and joint swelling maximal. At night, their hands were 30 percent stronger than in the morning. Moreover, they had three times as much joint pain and swelling between 8 A.M. and 11 A.M. as they did at bedtime.[9] In another study, persons with RA took tests for hand coordination several times a day. They showed best hand dexterity and least pain and stiffness between 5 P.M. and 6 P.M.[10]

Women with RA commonly report that their symptoms worsen just before menstruation, and that they bother them least the week or so after ovulation.[11] Menstrual cycle variations stem from periodic alterations in estrogen and progesterone that alter both tissue inflammation and immune system reactivity. Women who take birth-control pills or use estrogen supplements often report fewer menstrual flare-ups in RA symptoms.

Take Medicine at Night to Prevent Morning Pain

NSAIDs

NSAIDs are widely used for RA as well as for OA. Persons with RA, a more severe disease, usually require higher doses of NSAIDs, and many take them for decades. They are also twice as likely to develop NSAID-induced intestinal bleeding and perforation as persons with OA, according to Gurkirpal Singh and George Triadafilopoulos of Stanford University. The researchers tracked side effects in more than 12,000 OA and RA patients who had used NSAIDs for up to thirty years.[12] Even low doses of these drugs may cause serious side effects in both OA and RA patients. Unfortunately, 80 percent of those who suffered serious gastrointestinal complications had no warning sign. Appropriately timed treatment may lower your risk of such problems. Assess your risk with an online test developed by Singh and his colleagues (www.seniors.org/score/).

Even though RA symptoms are worst in the morning, research going back to the 1970s shows that taking the NSAID indomethacin once a day in the evening controls these symptoms better than taking it once a day in the morning. In the 1970s the eminent British rheumatologist E. C. Huskisson found people complained of fewer side effects when they took this medicine at night rather than in the morning. He reached the right conclusion but for the wrong reason. He surmised that patients simply slept through the side effects, a notion that many physicians still hold today.[13] In fact, biological rhythms in drug absorption and metabolism explain the difference.

More recent studies using newer NSAIDs verify Huskisson's findings. A single NSAID dose, taken in the evening or at bedtime, best controls the morning swelling, stiffness, and pain of RA while causing fewest side effects.[14]

Corticosteroids

If NSAIDs don't control your pain and stiffness, your doctor may prescribe a corticosteroid, a potent synthetic hormone tablet medicine, such as prednisone, prednisolone, methylprednisolone, or triamcinolone. These medications mimic and augment the inflammation-fighting activity of the body's naturally produced cortisol. They can make you feel dramatically better fairly rapidly. The introduction of such medications into the body may turn down or turn off the body's natural cortisol output, however, particularly when they are taken at the wrong times, that is, in the evening or at night. These medications also may have other serious side effects, including bone thinning, bruising, cataracts, weight gain, mood changes, diabetes, and high blood pressure.

In the past thirty years, researchers have examined a host of complex dosing schedules for corticosteroid medications in persons with RA. Patients have taken these medications once a day, twice a day, in the morning, afternoon, evening, or at bedtime, in equal dosages, and in different amounts at various times.

The best way to minimize or avoid their side effects, especially when large doses are involved, is to take them in the morning, in sync with the body's natural production of cortisol. The later in the day these medications are taken, the higher the risk of side effects.

Morning dosing poses problems for persons working odd hours, such as rotating shift workers. Their body rhythms often are out of sync with the hours they work and sleep. If you work outside of daytime hours, you need to work closely with your doctor to find the best time to take medications. If your illness is severe, your doctor may advise you to switch to a more traditional schedule. (See chapter 13: "Clockwatching at Work.")

There are a few exceptions to the morning rule, another good reason to team up with your doctor to determine your best treatment time. In one study, twelve persons with RA took a low dose of prednisolone for four consecutive weeks at 8 A.M., 1 P.M., or 11 P.M. While side effects were infrequent, the benefits of the treatment differed according to the time of day. Hand strength was higher in about two-thirds of the patients when they took the medication at 1 P.M. than when they took it at the other times.[15]

Cox-2 Inhibitors

The recommended dose of these drugs may be higher for persons with RA than for those with OA. With RA, these drugs usually are taken twice a day.

Other Medications

For severe RA, doctors sometimes prescribe medications such as gold, anti-malarials, or penicillamine, designed to slow the course of the disease. They also may use potent medications that suppress the immune system, the same drugs used to treat cancer. Optimal timing has not yet been determined.

Timewise Tips for RA

Ask your doctor to tailor treatment to the time of day that best relieves your pain.

To relieve morning pain and minimize side effects, take long-acting NSAIDs at bedtime.

Take synthetic cortisone-like medications once a day or every other day in the morning.

If a single morning dose of a cortisone-like medication does not provide adequate relief, ask your doctor to consider increasing the dose, or adding a small, early-afternoon dose. With your doctor's supervision, you also might try taking the single dose between noon and 3 P.M. for a week or so, to see if that makes a difference.

Exercise in late afternoon or early evening, when joints are least stiff and swollen. Exercise such as walking and swimming can improve flexibility and brighten mood.

Set an alarm at night to awaken you every two hours to avoid stiffness from sleeping too long in a single position. This tactic lets you sleep with more confidence. People who do this say they awaken only long enough to turn off the alarm and turn over. They then fall back to sleep easily. To avoid waking a bed partner, get an alarm that vibrates under your pillow.[16]

Check hand-grip strength and finger-joint swelling at home at different times of the day, using measuring devices available in pharmacies or from medical supply companies. This habit will help chart the course of your illness and show how well treatment is working. Wide-handled toothbrushes and vegetable peelers, spongy grips for pens and pencils, and similar devices can make it easier to do everyday chores.

If you are a woman whose symptoms flare around the time of menstruation, talk to your doctor about possibly using medications containing female hormones.

Anytime Tips

To modulate pain, take a warm bath or shower, avoid overexertion, pace your activities, and practice relaxation techniques. If pain suddenly worsens, call your doctor.

Write down feelings. Persons with RA who wrote about the most stressful event in their lives for twenty minutes three times a week showed less pain, tenderness, and swelling in affected joints after four months than did equally ill persons with RA who wrote only about their plans for the day, Joshua Smyth of North Dakota State University and his colleagues found. All the patients got comparable and appropriate medical care.[17]

Study. The Arthritis Foundation offers a six-week series of classes that provide basic information about arthritis relaxation techniques for pain and stress management, an overview of medications, an exercise program, and strategies for problem solving. For information, visit the foundation's Web site (www.arthritis.org). Also see the Web site of the National Institute of Arthritis and Musculoskeletal and Skin Diseases (www.nih.gov/niams/healthinfo/).

ASTHMA

Asthma, a chronic lung disorder, is a textbook example of the power of the biological clock. Asthma attacks occur one hundred times more often between 4 A.M. and 6 A.M. than at other hours of the day.[1] Surveys show four in ten persons with asthma awaken with trouble breathing every night, and nearly eight in ten do so at least once a week.[2] Severe asthma attacks, those in which people die, occur most often between midnight and 6 A.M.[3]

With effective control, persons with asthma can live normal, active lives. Jackie Joyner-Kersee and many other Olympic athletes train and compete successfully despite having this illness. Indeed, at least one in six U.S. athletes participating in the 1996 Olympic Games in Atlanta had a history of asthma. Nearly 30 percent of them won team or individual medals.[4]

For unknown reasons, asthma recently has become more common in both the United States and around the world. This fact gives new urgency to finding better treatment. One in every sixteen Americans has asthma, more than 17 million persons.[5] Five million are under age eighteen. Asthma prompts 470,000 hospital admissions in the United States annually, making it the leading reason children are admitted to hospitals in this country and the nation's third leading cause of hospitalizations overall. Asthma kills five thousand Americans every year.[6]

Many of the severe, life-threatening asthma attacks that send people to hospitals could be prevented by managing symptoms better. Tuning in to asthma's rhythmic patterns can help you and your doctor keep your asthma under the best possible control.

Asthma: A Nighttime Sickness

♦ "I was under a lot of stress at work. I thought that was why I kept waking up with trouble breathing. But one night, I couldn't catch my breath. I managed to call 911 on my bedside phone. I vaguely remember the ambulance ride and the emergency room, with all those doctors and nurses hovering above me. I had to stay in the hospital three days. Now I know what is wrong: I have asthma."

—Karen, age 27

"Our son's second-grade teacher told us Thomas hated recess. She thought that was strange. She noticed Thomas couldn't run or climb as well as the other kids, and often couldn't catch his breath. He was draggy around the house, too. We knew it wasn't right for a little boy to be tired all the time. It was the coughing at night that sent us back to the doctor. When Thomas can't sleep, none of us sleep. The doctor told us Thomas has asthma. Once Thomas started taking his medicine, he really perked up."

—Mother of Thomas, age 7

Asthma Has Many Triggers

"Asthma" comes from the Greek word for "panting," its most common symptom. Chest tightness and coughing are also frequent. Most, but not all, people with asthma wheeze.

Asthma makes the small airways of the lungs hypersensitive. When exposed to certain substances or situations, airways swell, muscles around them tighten, and tiny glands lining the airways secrete copious amounts of mucus. As a result, less air gets through. The airways even may collapse, trapping air in the lungs. Breathing *in* is not usually a problem, but breathing *out* often is difficult.

The long list of triggers of asthma includes

- *allergens (substances that affect only persons with specific sensitivities):* These include pollens from grass, ragweed, and trees; mold spores; house dust mites; cockroach debris; skin flakes or dander of dogs, cats, and other warm-blooded pets; bird droppings and feathers; and some foods and food additives.
- *irritants (substances that bother most people to varying degrees):* These include smoke from cigarettes, and fumes from burning wood or paper; aerosols of perfumes, hair spray, cleaning products, paint, and workplace chemicals; and automobile exhaust.

- *situations (events that affect breathing):* These include bouts of colds, flu, and other upper-airway infections; cold weather; exercise, particularly in the cold; and stress.

People exposed to asthma triggers usually first experience mild symptoms lasting less than fifteen minutes. This is called the early asthma reaction. Many hours later, a more severe reaction involving shortness of breath, chest tightness, and wheezing occurs. This so-called late asthma reaction represents an aggravation of the existing airway inflammation that characterizes this disease.

Many persons who could benefit from treatment don't know that they have asthma. If symptoms come and go, you may think you or your child are unusually susceptible to chest colds or allergies. Or you may blame stress, not realizing that tightness in the chest and the accompanying anxiety are the result of asthma, not the cause of it.

Infrequent symptoms make it hard for doctors to recognize asthma, too. A 1997 report from the National Institutes of Health soberly concludes, "undertreatment and inappropriate therapy are major contributors to asthma morbidity (illness) and mortality in the United States."[7]

Why Asthma Peaks at Night

Nighttime flare-ups reflect daily cycles in airway biology, hormone release, and nervous system function.[8]

Airways are most relaxed around 3 P.M. and most constricted around 5 A.M. in everyone, not only in persons with asthma. If you are healthy, your airway function varies only slightly from day to night, a change of perhaps 5 to 8 percent from the daytime high to nighttime low. You won't be aware of this difference. But if you have asthma, your best to worst airway function may vary from day to night by as much as 50 to 60 percent. The greater the daily variation, the more severe asthma typically is, and the more pronounced your symptoms are likely to be.

The impact of sleep on asthma is still poorly understood. Lying down may make asthma worse by compressing airways, allowing fluids to pool in the lungs or letting irritants enter the lungs more easily. Sleep itself makes breathing slow at some times and irregular at others, not a problem for persons in good health but potentially disturbing to those with asthma.

The two key hormones involved in asthma, adrenaline (also called epinephrine) and cortisol, are both produced by the adrenal glands, located just above the kidneys. Both hormones are secreted almost exclusively in the daytime, and in the highest amounts at the start of the daily activity cycle. They are virtually absent from your bloodstream at night. Adrenaline keeps muscles of the airways relaxed so breathing is easiest in the daytime. At night, the muscles around the airways constrict, making breathing difficult. Cortisol reduces swelling of the airways in the daytime. At night, swelling escalates, further compromising airway function.

Day-night differences in the functioning of the body's nervous system add to the effects of adrenaline and cortisol by fostering relaxation of airway muscles in the daytime and tightening airway muscles at night.

Physicians Still in the Dark on Nighttime Pattern

"I have observed the fit always to happen after sleep in the night when the nerves are filled with windy spirits," John Floyer, a British physician, wrote in 1698.[9] "Sleep favours asthma," Henry Salter, another British physician, observed in 1859.[10] But only one out of four physicians correctly identified asthma's nighttime pattern in a Gallup survey conducted for the American Medical Association in 1996.[11]

Lacking knowledge of circadian rhythms, most doctors think nighttime attacks follow nighttime exposure to environmental triggers, such as dust mites or mold spores on pillows or blankets, or pet danders in bedrooms. Some attribute nighttime flare-ups to asthma medications that don't last through the night. Some think sleep alone makes asthma worse. Some feel nighttime reactions are a delayed response to daytime triggers. Some believe that reports showing attacks increase at night are skewed by the inclusion in some studies of subjects with a history of nighttime symptoms. And some concede that some patients deteriorate at night but believe relatively few patients do so.

Asthma experts are trying to change these beliefs.

In 1997, a National Heart, Lung, and Blood Institute (NHLBI) panel defined asthma as a chronic inflammatory disorder of the airways, and said reducing inflammation is a prime goal of treatment. "In susceptible individuals," the panel said, "this inflammation causes recurrent episodes of wheezing, breathlessness, chest tightness, and cough, *particularly at night and in the early morning.*"[12] (The italics are ours.) This report signals a whole new spin on how specialists in the field view asthma. They now see it primarily as a nighttime disease, not a daytime disease. They recognize that nighttime symptoms in asthma are not a sometime event; they are the main event.

In 1998 another NHLBI group of experts looked specifically at the impact of circadian rhythms and sleep on asthma. "Chronotherapeutic strategies," meeting chairperson Richard Martin said, "are important to the efficacious treatment of nocturnal asthma."[13] Treatment of nighttime symptoms may improve daytime asthma, too. Asthma that occurs in the daytime reflects a response to a specific trigger. How often asthma attacks occur at night and how much airway functioning varies from day to night are now regarded as the key criteria that determine asthma's severity.[14]

Attacks Vary over Menstrual Cycle

About one in three women with asthma, particularly if she has moderate to severe asthma, finds that symptoms increase right before or while she menstruates. The risk of life-threatening asthma crises rises at these times, too. Three out of four adults who require hospital treatment for severe asthma attacks are women. Most hospitalizations in menstrual-age women occur in the days just before or after the start of their menstrual period. Shifts over the month in levels of the hormones estrogen and progesterone may serve as asthma triggers.[15] Progesterone, for example, known to relax airway muscles, falls just before menstruation.

Most physicians do not know about these menstrual-cycle changes. The latest National Heart, Lung, and Blood Institute's *Guidelines for the Diagnosis and Management of Asthma*, published in 1997, fails to mention menstrual-cycle variations in asthma.[16] So does an otherwise excellent book for patients, the *American Medical Association Essential Guide to Asthma*, published in 1998.[17]

If you are a woman with asthma, follow the advice under Timewise Tips (page 222), and keep a menstrual symptom diary. (See page 329.) Take the diary with you when you see your doctor.

Attacks Vary by Season

Environmental triggers account for seasonal patterns. In spring and summer, grass and tree pollens are major triggers. Autumn is ragweed season, and in winter cold weather and cold and influenza viruses exert more influence.

Better Results, Fewer Side Effects with Timed Dosing

Medications for asthma fall into two main categories: *reliever medications* provide quick relief from asthma attacks by relaxing airway muscles and opening airways, while *maintainer medications* are taken daily to reduce persistent inflammation and swelling.

Of the hundreds of available asthma medications of both types, some are inhaled while others are taken orally in pill, capsule, or liquid form, or injected. Pilot studies of skin patches worn only at night are in progress. Some commonly prescribed asthma medications work better and are safer when taken at certain times of day. We describe here circadian issues for the most widely used categories of asthma maintainer medications.

Theophylline Medications

Theophylline is particularly effective for nighttime asthma. It works by reducing the severity of airway inflammation, relaxing the muscles of the airways, and stimulating the breathing center in the brain. Some theophylline

Breathing Diary

Name _____

See a doctor if you

- wake up with trouble breathing
- often feel short of breath and lack stamina
- breathe noisily
- feel tightness or aching in your chest
- cough for more than a week
- cough after exercise, crying, or laughing
- have trouble taking a deep breath
- have persistent trouble with mucus

Photocopy this page, and keep track of trouble breathing for at least three days in a row. Take this diary with you when you see your doctor.

Day/Date _____

Time of Arising _____ A.M./P.M.

Bedtime _____ A.M./P.M.

Women: Are you menstruating today? Y/N

Day/Date A.M./P.M.	Wheeze A.M./P.M.	Cough A.M./P.M.	Activity (Sports, Sleep, etc.) A.M./P.M.	Awakened by Asthma?	Possible Trigger	Medication Use, If Any
Sample Mon. 7/3/00	7:30 a.m.	No	Running for bus	no	Exercise	None

products are taken every twelve hours and some only once a day. Such schedules appear to cover the whole day, but that may not be so, as the body absorbs, uses, and excretes drugs faster or slower at different times.

Some brands of theophylline are absorbed in different amounts or at different rates depending on when they are taken. In one study, researchers found children absorbed their 8 A.M. dose of a twice-a-day medication rapidly, and the drug worked for 12 hours. When they took the same dose of the same drug at 8 P.M., it was absorbed too slowly to ward off nighttime attacks. In another study, people absorbed two to three times more of another widely used theophylline medication when they took it only in the evening than when they took it only in the morning. That particular medication is safe if taken in the morning but may be harmful if taken in the evening.[18]

Unfortunately, few brands have been evaluated with regard to time of day of dosing. To use most of these medications, you currently have to rely on a trial and error approach to find a product or dose that works for you.

This situation is changing. Some pharmaceutical companies now offer medications that work in synchrony with asthma's day-night pattern. The first theophylline chronotherapy for asthma was introduced in the United States in 1989 under the brand name Uniphyl. This medication is taken as a single pill in the evening. Uniphyl's drug-release technology ensures that drug levels peak overnight when theophylline is most needed to improve lung functioning. One study comparing this medication to twice-a-day forms of theophylline showed that it cut in half the number of nights disturbed by asthma.[19]

Airway Dilator Medications

These are the most commonly used asthma medications. They relax the muscles of the airways and make breathing easier. Sustained-action tablet medications, such as Proventil Repetabs and Volmax, relieve nighttime breathing distress, although they sometimes cause agitation. These 12-hour tablets work well as chronotherapies. Doctors may prescribe twice the dose to be taken at night as in the morning. A once-a-day tablet chronotherapy, bambuterol, is sold in Europe. Airway dilator medications also come in inhaled formulations. The original ones, including the commonly used medication albuterol, last four to six hours, not long enough to avert nighttime asthma. Newer inhaled drugs, such as salmeterol and formoterol, taken at bedtime, last twelve hours.[20]

Corticosteroids

These synthetic hormones mimic and augment the inflammation-fighting activity of the body's naturally produced cortisol. They can make you feel dramatically better rapidly. But they may curb the body's natural cortisol output, particularly if taken in the evening or at night. They also can exert serious side effects, including bone thinning, bruising, cataracts, weight gain, mood changes, diabetes, and high blood pressure if taken for prolonged periods of time, especially in high doses.

Researchers are trying to find the best time to take corticosteroids to treat asthma. In one study, adults with hard-to-control asthma took either the synthetic hormone prednisone, or a look-alike but inactive substance, once a day, at 8 A.M., 3 P.M., or 8 P.M. Richard Martin of the National Jewish Medical and Research Center in Denver and his colleagues gave their volunteers 50 milligrams of the medication, a dose thought large enough to reduce swelling and inflammation at any time. They measured the volunteers' airway function around the clock and withdrew samples of lung fluid at 4 A.M. The 3 P.M. dose was the only one that both made breathing better and significantly reduced airway swelling during the critical overnight period. Treatment with this presumably powerful medication at other times of the day was totally ineffective.[21]

Some drugs developed with timing in mind already are in use. A synthetic corticosteroid tablet medication, Dutimelan 8-15, was first marketed in Europe two decades ago, by the Italian pharmaceutical company Hoechst-Italy. The drug's name describes the times it is to be taken, 8 A.M. and 3 P.M., or 0800 and 1500 on a twenty-four-hour clock. Giving the drug at the start of the daily activity period and midway through it reduces nighttime asthma attacks while minimizing the risk of unwanted side effects common to this type of medication. This product is not sold yet in the United States.[22]

In this country, doctors typically prescribe tablet corticosteroid medications for asthma in once-a-day morning dosing. This timing lowers the risk of side effects. Yet it ignores the evidence that these drugs work best when taken in the early afternoon. Some doctors who realize that asthma is likely to worsen at night recommend bedtime dosing, a strategy that may sound logical but is a mistake. Studies clearly show that nighttime dosing of this type of medication is ineffective and increases the risk of side effects.

Inhaled Corticosteroid Medications

Doctors prescribe these drugs to control airway inflammation. Many doctors assume that all of the inhaled medication reaches the lungs and that the risk of side effects is low. Numerous studies show, however, that a small amount of every inhaled corticosteroid dose usually makes its way into the body. The user may swallow a residual amount that remains in the mouth after treatment, or minute amounts may enter the bloodstream in the lungs. Use of inhaled corticosteroids in the evening, especially in high doses, may result in some of the same types of side effects as occur when these medications are taken in tablet form.

Richard Martin and his colleagues evaluated the efficacy of inhaled triamcinolone at different times of day. Taken once a day at the best circadian time, 3 P.M., it was just as effective as the same dose, divided into four smaller doses and inhaled at four times across the day.[23] Unfortunately, 3 P.M. is not an ideal time to take medicine, as many patients are at work or in school at this time. Because convenience often affects how well patients follow treatment plans, the researchers are trying to find drug formulations and doses that will enable patients to take their medicine at a better time, such as around dinnertime. These studies still are in progress.

Timewise Tips

Keep track of your symptoms. If you have asthma, suspect you may, or wonder if your child does, record when the symptoms occur, and possible triggers. Use the breathing diary on page 219 and take it with you when you see your doctor. This information will help the doctor devise the best treatment.

See your doctor in the morning. Try to schedule visits early in the day. Airway function at this time is the best indicator of your overnight condition.

Take breathing tests in the morning. To decide if you have asthma, or to monitor ongoing treatment, your doctor needs to know how much air you can breathe, and how rapidly you can move air in and out of your lungs. Persons with asthma have a reduced capacity to expel air rapidly from their lungs. In a typical exam, the doctor will ask you to inhale deeply and then exhale rapidly and forcefully, using a spirometer. This device measures the volume of air you expel per second. You'll then inhale an aerosol medication called a bronchodilator, which relaxes the muscles of the airways, and then take the test again. If you have asthma, you'll be able to expel air better from the lungs the second time. People with other lung diseases, such as bronchitis and emphysema, show little or no improvement. Time of day alters results of this test. If you see your doctor in the afternoon, improvement in lung function after taking a bronchodilator might not be apparent. Afternoon test results may lead your doctor to underestimate the severity of your illness.

Tell your doctor if you sleep poorly, even if you are not aware of trouble breathing. Asthma itself disturbs sleep, and some medications used to treat asthma also disturb sleep. Your doctor may suggest a change in the dose or type of medication to avert this problem.

Try to avoid morning rush-hour traffic. If auto exhausts bother you, try to arrange to go to work earlier or later, create a flextime schedule, or work from home one or more days a week.

Exercise in the afternoon, when airways are most open and least sensitive to environmental agents and breathing is easiest. Skip outdoor exercise when air quality is poor.

Use plastic covers on your pillows and mattress to seal off dust and similar asthma triggers while you sleep.

Cut back on housecleaning. Let someone else do dust-raising chores. If that's not possible, wait to vacuum and run the dryer until afternoon.

Keep pets out of your sleeping area.

If you experience heartburn, a burning sensation in the stomach and esophagus, particularly in the evening or at night, elevate the head of your bed on six- to eight-inch wooden blocks. Let your doctor know. It may be a side effect of medications for asthma or it may be one of the triggering factors for night-time asthma. (See page 274.)

Anytime Tips

Make asthma prevention guidelines part of your daily life. Some steps you can take: avoid foods or animals to which you are sensitive, install an air conditioner and dehumidifier in your home, and don't smoke or linger around people who do.

Use a peak flow meter at home to assess the rate at which you can expel air forcefully from your lungs. Do this self-test morning and evening for several consecutive days every month, or as your doctor advises. This tactic will show how stable your asthma is and how well your medications are working. Devices for home use are small enough to fit in a pocket or purse, available at most drug stores, and cost from $10 to $25. If you are a woman with premenstrual asthma, your diary may show you that your breathing capacity begins to decline the day or two before a symptom flare-up. Many women use reliever medications more frequently at this time. Your doctor will need to see the regularity of this pattern, and may adjust your daily medication to control symptoms better at that time of month.

Don't start tinkering with your medication schedule on your own. Discuss timing with your doctor, and make changes only with medical supervision.

Fill out your breathing diary before you change your medication schedule. Fill it out again after you follow the new schedule for a week or so. This tactic will let you and your doctor see if timing makes a difference.

Study. Visit the Web sites of the Asthma and Allergy Foundation of America (www.aafa.org) and the American Medical Association (www.ama-assn.org/asthma).

BACK PAIN

The typical case of back pain is worst in the evening. That's because gravity makes the small bones, or vertebrae, in the spinal column collapse slightly over the course of a day. This causes pressure on nerves coming off the spinal cord, which travel through canals behind each of the vertebrae.[1]

Lying down allows vertebrae to separate slightly, relieving pressure on nerves, and easing pain. This fact also explains why you are tallest by a fraction of an inch in the morning, and shortest at bedtime.

Half the U.S. population reports having had back pain in the past year. Four in five American adults will have this problem at some point in their lives. Elite athletes suffer this agony along with ordinary mortals. After more than sixteen years without missing a baseball game, Baltimore Orioles' Iron

Man Cal Ripken was sidelined twice by lower back pain in the 1999 season. Back pain is second only to headaches as Americans' most frequently reported cause of pain. It is a major cause of disability as well.

Back Pain: A Glitch in Human Design

If humans walked on four feet like other mammals, we'd probably escape back pain. Upright posture means your lower back bears the majority of your weight, the reason back pain most often strikes this area. You may feel pain not only in your lower back but also in areas served by nerves traveling through that area, including your buttocks and legs. Back pain is a symptom, not a disease.

The immediate trigger isn't always apparent. Being overweight, habitually slouching, or bending over paperwork all day may be contributors. Stress can make muscles tighten. An unaccustomed activity such as shoveling snow may strain muscles. Injury from a fall or car crash may spark muscle spasms, which can be excruciating. They are a powerful message to stop moving, lest you cause further harm.

Osteoarthritis Causes Most Back Pain

Osteoarthritis affects most people aged fifty and over. (See page 207.) Common consequences of this disorder include both thinning of disks, rounded pillows that separate the vertebrae and serve as shock absorbers, and disintegration of cartilage, a protective tissue that normally keeps vertebrae from grinding against each other. When these events occur, movement becomes painful.

Disks sometimes bulge, causing pressure on the spinal cord. They might rupture, losing some of their inner cushioning. These "herniated" disks commonly are called "slipped" disks, although they don't really move out of place. Without their protection, vertebrae compress nerve fibers.

In a Canadian study, volunteers with degenerative disk disease assessed their own pain every few hours for a week. Their pain was 50 percent more intense at 8 P.M. than in the morning, when it was least severe.[2]

Morning Back Pain Linked with Rare Condition

Back pain that hurts most in the morning is so unusual that timing is an important diagnostic clue. Its cause often is a specific type of arthritis called ankylosing spondylitis (AS). Persons with AS in one study reported twice as much back pain and eight times as much stiffness between 6 A.M. and 9 A.M. as they did between noon and 3 P.M., the calmest time. Their symptoms flared again between 7 P.M. and 9 P.M., though somewhat less strongly than in the morning.[3]

Nine out of ten persons who develop AS are men, typically between the ages of twenty and forty. It is an inherited disorder in which the immune system turns on itself, causing swelling and damage in ligaments and tendons, mainly those around bones and joints in the spine. It restricts movement and may cause the vertebrae to fuse, producing a rigid spine. If it affects ribs and hampers breathing, it may even be life-threatening. It also may cause inflammation in the hips, shoulders, and knees.

AS often starts with a dull ache deep in the buttocks, sometimes only on one side, or in the lower back. This pain is often intermittent at first, and then becomes more frequent and constant. The pain may be less troubling than the stiffness. Because the symptoms are common to many back conditions, the diagnosis may take a while; that's why it's useful to pay attention to the time symptoms occur. AS varies with the seasons, too. Symptoms appear for the first time in winter twelve times more often than they do in summer; recurrences are more frequent in winter, too.[4]

Take Your Medicine before Pain Usually Starts

Nonsteroidal anti-inflammatory drugs, or NSAIDs, are the mainstays of treatment for back pain. NSAIDs include aspirin, ibuprofen, ketoprofen, and naproxen. While studies of these drugs show they provide the most pain relief for most types of OA when taken four to eight hours prior to the time pain is most intense, studies specifically in persons with common types of back pain suggest that taking these drugs in the morning may offer better pain control and more flexibility. Persons with AS may get the most relief when taking NSAIDs around noon. Since NSAIDs have a higher risk of stomach irritation when taken early in the day, try taking them later and see how you do. Ask your doctor or pharmacist if your particular medication should be taken with food.

Timewise Tips

Lie down in midafternoon to give vertebrae a chance to spread apart. This tactic may ease evening pain. Use this time to perform gentle stretching exercises.

If taking NSAIDs, use trial and error to find the best time of day to relieve your symptoms. Avoid taking NSAIDs in the morning if possible.

Use the Pain Diary on page 208 to record your pain pattern.

Anytime Tips

Apply ice to new injuries for about twenty minutes several times a day. This measure may reduce swelling. Put ice in an ice bag or wrap ice in a towel. After a few days, switch to heat treatment.

Use warmth on tight muscles. Try a heating pad, or take a warm bath or shower.

Use a back brace as infrequently as possible. It may offer support when doing heavy lifting or when pain is severe, but habitual usage may make back muscles weaker.

Exercise regularly. Exercise will strengthen your back and supporting muscles in your abdomen, helping to prevent pain. Try these exercises: On hands and knees, round and raise your back, then lower and arch it. On your back, bring knees to the chest. Illustrated books with back exercises abound; this information also is widely available on the Internet.

For persistent pain, see your doctor. About nine out of ten episodes of back pain resolve in about six weeks regardless of treatment. Physical therapy may help restore function, particularly as pain moves past the usual healing period of three to six months.

Study. Visit the Web site of the Arthritis Foundation (www.arthritis.org).

CANCER

Cycles ranging from hours to years influence the abnormal growth of cells that characterize cancer, which is not one disease, but rather, a group of diseases. Chronotherapies, treatments geared to body rhythms, can improve both treatment outcomes and quality of life. Research findings suggest that *when* people with cancer receive drug treatment, and possibly surgery and radiation as well, is at least as critical a determinant of how well they do as the dose or type of treatment they receive.

Chronotherapies may permit higher, potentially more helpful, doses of anticancer medications than now are standard. They also may reduce hair loss and other unwanted side effects. Furthermore, the time during the menstrual cycle when women undergo surgery for breast cancer may govern the procedure's success. Certain cancers are more likely to be detected at some times of the year than at others.

Although such findings percolate slowly into medical practice, any measure that boosts the effectiveness of existing treatments is an important advance in itself. No one disputes the pressing need for further progress: cancer ranks second only to heart disease as the leading cause of death in the United States. According to the American Cancer Society, more than

1,200,000 Americans are newly diagnosed with cancer annually, and 550,000 persons in this country die of cancer each year.[1]

Cancer Cells Multiply Too Fast

Some cells reproduce themselves as often as every twelve, eight, or six hours, with shorter cycles particularly prominent in aggressive cancer and often as the disease advances. This rapid turnover usually, though not always, seen in cancer cells contrasts with the prominent twenty-four-hour life cycle of most other cells of the body.

A cancer may start in any type of cell, forming a mass called the *primary tumor.* Cancer cells then invade surrounding tissues, They may spread, or *metastasize,* traveling to distant body sites where they form *secondary tumors.* As their numbers grow, they scarf up oxygen and nutrients that normal cells need and release chemicals that damage or kill those cells.

It typically takes months to years for cancer to make itself known. An easy way to remember some key warning signs of cancer is to think of the word "caution."

- **C**hange in bowel or bladder habits
- **A** sore that does not heal
- **U**nusual bleeding or discharge
- **T**hickening or lump in the breast or elsewhere
- **I**ndigestion or difficulty swallowing
- **O**bvious change in a wart or mole
- **N**agging cough or hoarseness

To treat cancer, doctors may surgically remove tumors if they can be located and are accessible, shrink or destroy tumors with radiation, or use various types of medications. Some anticancer drugs kill cancer cells directly, while others contain hormones to deter tumor growth or block hormones that foster such growth. Most research in chronotherapy has focused on improving drug treatment.

Anticancer Drugs Kill Both Cancer Cells and Normal Cells

While drugs that seek out and destroy only cancer cells would be ideal, such drugs have yet to be developed. Studies of more than thirty anticancer medications, primarily in laboratory animals, show some of these drugs vary by more than 50 percent in the severity of their side effects at different times of day. When given these medications at some times of day, all or most of a group of healthy animals remained well. At other times, some animals got sick, and some died. Most drugs cause the greatest amount of damage to both cancer cells and normal cells if taken at the time when the cells the drugs target are actively multiplying. They cause the least damage if taken when these cells are resting.[2]

In order to determine the best times to give anticancer drugs to people, the researchers next gave them to animals with cancer. They gave some animals these drugs at the circadian time when least damage to healthy cells was expected, and they gave others equal doses spread out over the day, the way doctors currently prescribe most medications. The results were quite startling: tumor size fell by 60 to 70 percent and cancer cure rates rose by about 100 percent on average with chronotherapy, in comparison to conventional treatment. Giving drugs at the right time also caused fewer side effects.[3]

Although most present-day anticancer drugs destroy proportionately more rapidly reproducing cancer cells than slower-to-reproduce healthy cells, they also wreak havoc on healthy cells that multiply rapidly. These include cells in the hair follicles, bone marrow, and digestive tract. This explains why persons receiving chemotherapy often lose their hair, have lower red and white blood cell counts, and suffer nausea and diarrhea. Giving anticancer medications at the best circadian time enables doctors both to minimize these and other side effects and to use higher doses to treat cancer as aggressively as possible.

The principle here may seem straightforward, but there are many potential snags: not all normal cells reproduce at the same time. Circadian rhythms, though similar from one person to the next, still vary in important ways among individuals depending on their daily sleep/wake schedules and perhaps even the stages of their cancers.

Furthermore, some types of healthy cells are more vulnerable to certain drugs than to others, and the body responds to various anticancer medications in different ways at different times of day. Thus, there is no single treatment time that uniformly yields the best results. Cisplatin and oxaliplatin, used to treat tumors of the bladder, ovary, and lung, for example, are best tolerated when administered in the late afternoon and early evening. By contrast, 5-fluorouracil, the mainstay of treatment for cancers of the intestine, colon, and rectum, is best tolerated in the middle of sleep.

Anticancer drugs work on the border of safety, with only a thin line separating the dose that helps from the dose that harms. Doctors often employ multiple drugs with different methods of action in an attempt to kill the most tumor cells. Devising treatment schedules is a complex business.

Additional practical considerations govern the timing of treatment. Ours is a daytime world. Although hospitals are open around the clock, most activities are organized around a daytime schedule. Most cancer medications are given by infusion, that is, in a liquid form delivered through a needle inserted in a vein. They then circulate through the body via the bloodstream or lymphatic system, the transport system for white blood cells that fight infection and other diseases.

Having staff available to give infusions in the evening and at night would involve a drastic change in scheduling. The development and refinement of portable mechanical pumps that automatically dispense medication at the right time, however, removes this particular barrier. Use of these devices allows patients to receive treatment in their own homes, markedly cutting treatment costs. The first such pump became available only in 1984.

How Timed Medication Dosing Works

A growing body of research demonstrates the clear benefits of timed treatment for several cancers. This section describes only a small sample. It focuses on chronotherapy for colorectal cancer as a model of how doctors employ chronotherapy and assess its utility.

Colorectal Cancer

The third most common cancer and cause of cancer death in the United States, colorectal cancer is diagnosed in about 130,000 Americans annually. Rectal bleeding, blood in the stool, and a change in bowel habits are typical signs and symptoms. While surgery often cures these cancers when they are small and confined to one location, those that have spread resist treatment. The amount of medicine patients can take is limited by the severity of drug-induced side effects. Fewer than one in ten persons with colorectal cancer that has spread is alive five years later.[4]

Starting in the early 1990s, Francis Lévi and his colleagues at the Hôpital Paul Brousse in Paris, France, began treating people with advanced colorectal cancer with a combination of two or three potent anticancer medications. They synchronized drug delivery with the body's circadian rhythms.[5] Their laboratory studies showed two of the drugs caused the least damage to normal cells midway through sleep, while the other produced the least damage midway through waking hours: 4 A.M. and 4 P.M. in most people. They programmed a wearable computerized pump to deliver a higher dose of the appropriate drugs to the patients' bloodstream at these times, and a lower dose at other times.

The patients received their treatment in their homes or in the community while going about their usual activities. The computerized pump, which is about the size of a tape recorder, has multiple compartments for various drugs, with ample room to hold the four- to five-day supply the patients got every two to three weeks. The pump even contains a modem. If necessary, doctors will modify the dose or rate of drug delivery over the phone.

By 1999, 1,500 patients had completed chronotherapy with the drug 5-fluorouracil, the prime treatment for this type of cancer, along with leucovorin, with or without oxaliplatin. Oxaliplatin, not yet available in the

United States, has side effects that many patients cannot tolerate for long. With chronotherapy, however, they were able to continue to take it and even to take a larger dose more often. Their tumors shrank more, enabling doctors to surgically remove some that previously had been deemed inoperable. The patients also experienced fewer digestive upsets and other side effects than people with comparable illness who received conventional therapy infused in a constant amount at a steady rate.[6]

"These are the best results available worldwide for the treatment of metastatic colorectal cancer," Lévi told us when we visited his clinic in Paris in 1998. "At first nobody believed the findings. Some doctors still think the improvements come from the drugs, not the schedule."[7] Since the patients who participated in the first studies and received chronotherapy usually had the most advanced cancer, it will take more time to see if chronotherapy also adds years to their lives.

One Patient's Story

◆ Jean Cayzac, a fit-looking seventy-year-old we met in Lévi's clinic, was the first person to use high-dose chronotherapy. Diagnosed with colorectal cancer in 1990, he first received chronotherapy in 1992, after his cancer spread to his liver, again in 1994 after the cancer showed up in his lung, and again after subsequent recurrences, sixty-five courses of drug treatment in all. He also had surgery four times to remove tumors.

At the time of our visit in 1998, Cayzac was taking anticancer drugs once a week, three weeks a month, still on a chronotherapy schedule. About fifty other persons with colorectal cancer also receive chronic treatment, a new approach that aims to keep remaining tumors as small as possible for as long as possible.

A waiter for forty years, Cayzac enjoyed his retirement, riding his bicycle about twenty-five miles a day, even while he received his treatment. "I know I still have cancer," he said, "but I feel well."

When colorectal cancer has spread, the five-year survival rate is only 8 percent. Jean Cayzac lived with his cancer for a decade and died of it in January 2000.

Cancer specialists at thirty-five medical centers in Europe and Canada began a large clinical trial in 1998 in 554 patients to compare three-drug chronotherapy for advanced metastatic colorectal cancer with the present standard treatment. They will assess the response rate and side effects of both types of treatment. They also will assess each patient's quality of life, often a determinant of whether a person is willing to continue therapy, and they will track long-term survival.[8] Similar studies of breast cancer and pancreatic cancer are in progress.

Cancer of the Ovaries

This cancer causes more deaths than any other cancer of the female reproductive system. It takes the lives of about 14,000 women in the United States annually, the American Cancer Society reports.[9]

The first study of chronotherapy for any cancer, conducted in the early 1980s, compared different treatment schedules for two commonly used anti-cancer drugs in thirty-one women whose cancer of the ovaries was so advanced that surgery was not an option. One month the women took the drugs adriamycin in the morning and cisplatin in the evening, and the next month they took the same doses of the same drugs in reverse order. They alternated mornings and evenings for the two drugs for eight months or more.

William Hrushesky of New York's Albany Medical College and his colleagues at the University of Minnesota found that when the women took adriamycin in the morning and cisplatin in the evening, they did much better. They developed fewer infections and problems with bleeding, so they needed fewer transfusions. Fewer of them had side effects severe enough to make doctors lower their medication dose or delay their next treatment.[10]

This study, conducted in a hospital, was both costly and labor intensive. With the present-day availability of computerized pumps, it could be repeated in a community setting, although it has not been done so far. French researchers found that women with advanced ovarian cancer had deeply altered daily patterns of secretion of the hormone cortisol, a strong marker of body rhythms. This finding, they said, implies that doctors should not give treatment at a uniform time, but instead should key it to an individual patient's circadian rhythms.[11]

Childhood Leukemia

In a Canadian study, 118 children who had been treated for a cancer of white blood cells, acute lymphoblastic leukemia, and were doing well, with their cancer in remission, took a daily maintenance dose of their medication at home. The children received their treatment between 1976 and 1984. Since there was no evidence then suggesting that timing mattered, the doctors told the children's parents to give the drug when convenient but consistently at the same time.

Georges Rivard and his colleagues at the University of Montreal followed the children until 1991. They found that children who took their medicine in the evening were nearly three times less likely to relapse than those who took it in the morning. The evening group had a nearly 20 percent higher survival rate, too.[12]

In 1997, Danish researchers reported a similar study of nearly 300 children with the same illness treated with the same medications. They, too, found that children taking their maintenance medication in the evening had a higher likelihood of staying well. They also found that whether or not the children took their medication with food made no difference, a question the earlier study was not able to answer. They advised colleagues to recommend an evening schedule for maintenance therapy for the drugs used in this study.[13]

Although the best timing may be different for other medications, present-day treatment provides an 80 percent cure rate for this type of cancer, one of the field's best success stories. About 2,000 children in the United States develop this cancer annually.

Rhythms Affect Breast Cancer Detection

Although heart disease kills more women, breast cancer is the disease women fear most. It is the most common cancer in women, aside from skin cancer. The first symptoms of breast cancer typically include a lump that feels different from surrounding tissue, swelling in the breast or underarm area, skin irritation or dimpling, nipple pain or retraction (turning inward), redness or scaliness of the nipple or breast skin, or a discharge other than breast milk. Eight in ten breast cancers are first discovered by the women themselves. To boost the odds of finding breast cancer in its earliest, most treatable stage, doctors urge women to examine their breasts monthly.

Breast cancers grow more rapidly at some times of year than at other times, perhaps because of annual cycles in female hormone activity or seasonal changes in melatonin secretion. Premenopausal women discover their own breast cancers twice as often in late spring and early summer as in winter. Postmenopausal women detect their own breast cancers most frequently in the fall.[14] These patterns suggest that young women should examine their breasts with extra diligence in the spring and also schedule their mammograms then, and that older women should follow suit in the fall.

Time of the menstrual cycle also influences the accuracy of a mammogram, a test that uses low-dose X rays to detect breast abnormalities. In premenopausal women, breast tissue is less dense before ovulation, that is, in the first two weeks of the cycle, making it easier to see abnormalities in a mammogram then. Although breast tissue generally is less dense in postmenopausal women, density may increase in those who use replacement hormones on days they take progestin. They thus should schedule mammograms at other times. (See chapter 11: "Time for Sex.")

It may be possible to detect breast tumors at an early stage by monitoring breast temperature over the menstrual cycle. Since cancer cells are more active than normal cells, they also generate more heat, making nearby tissue warmer than normal, according to Scottish researchers. Hugh Simpson of the Glasgow Royal Infirmary and his colleagues developed a "chronobra" that automatically monitors and records breast skin temperature. They compared temperature changes in women with breast cancer and healthy women, and in the affected breast and healthy breast in the same woman. They found breast surface temperature to be higher by about 0.5° F in the affected breasts before ovulation, and not to rise as much as normal after ovulation. Further work is needed before the chronobra enters general use.[15]

Does the Time of Breast Cancer Surgery Affect Survival?

This question is one of the most contentious in chronobiology.

In premenopausal women, the hormone estrogen rises in the first half of the twenty-eight-day menstrual cycle, the two weeks before ovulation. Estrogen falls just before ovulation, when the hormone progesterone starts to rise. After ovulation, in week three, estrogen rises again and both hormones reach their monthly high. Then both fall before menstruation. These vastly different hormonal states affect many biological functions, including the activity of the body's immune system, rates of tumor growth, and the likelihood that large numbers of tumor cells will escape in surgery and circulate through the rest of the body.

The first study to explore whether these hormonal ups and downs altered the results of breast cancer surgery was published in 1989.[16] This study and fifteen others conducted since then, involving more than 5,000 women with breast cancer, show that those whose breast surgery is performed in the week or ten days after ovulation live longer on average than women who undergo surgery earlier or later in the month.[17] A nearly equal number of studies, involving about the same number of women, show the time of the menstrual cycle has no impact on the outcome of surgery.

In this climate of confusion, most surgeons today still schedule biopsies, lumpectomies, and mastectomies for breast cancer at all times of the woman's menstrual cycle.

Two cancer specialists who reviewed all published studies on menstrual timing of surgery in 1998 found great differences in the quality of the research methods. Some studies relied only on women's recall of the date of their last menstrual period before surgery. Some asked the date before the operation, and others as long as several months afterward. Some measured estrogen and progesterone levels in blood or urine to estimate menstrual stage.

Some simply divided the cycle into two parts, before and after the presumed day of ovulation, based on an average twenty-eight-day cycle, although many women have shorter or longer cycles. Some did not verify that ovulation actually occurred. Some did not record the start of the next menstruation, a better indicator of when ovulation took place than an estimate based on counting two weeks forward from menstruation. Some studies included women who took birth control pills and thus did not ovulate. Some included women with irregular cycles.

Some of the women first had a surgical biopsy, and then surgery to remove their cancer several days later. Others had both procedures at the same time. The various studies also included different types of surgery from a lumpectomy to a partial or more extensive mastectomy. Some of the women received radiation, drug treatment, or additional surgery.

"The data are unfortunately, in sum, inadequate to be able to tell a young woman with breast cancer, with adequate certainty, when in her menstrual cycle to have her cancer biopsied and/or resected [removed]," concluded the doctors who conducted this review, Andreas Hagen of the University Medical Center Benjamin Franklin in Berlin, Germany, and William Hrushesky, now at the Stratton Veterans Administration Medical Center in Albany, New York.[18]

A National Cancer Institute–sponsored study that began in 1996 may help resolve these concerns. The study is called "Correlation of Menstrual Cycle Phase at Time of Primary Surgery with 5-Year Disease-Free Survival in Women with Stage I or Stage II Breast Cancer."

Researchers at nearly 100 medical centers in the United States, Canada, and Europe hope to recruit 884 women with breast cancer by 2002. They are recruiting women with regular cycles ranging from twenty-one to thirty-five days, who do not use birth control pills. As women will enter the study at all phases of the menstrual cycle, surgery will be scheduled at all phases, too, according to Clive Grant of the Mayo Clinic, one of the principal investigators for this project. "We didn't think the existing data were strong enough for a true controlled study where women would be randomly assigned to surgery at different times, and some might have to wait for perhaps two weeks," Grant said. "We think a randomized registration study should answer the key questions."

Women who elect to have surgery at a specific phase of their cycle will not be eligible for this study. The researchers will ask the women to report the date of their last period. They also will perform blood tests to assess circulating hormones at the time of the biopsy and within a day of surgery if it is performed at a later date. The researchers will query the women six months after surgery to see if they also received chemotherapy and will follow the women for the next ten years.

They will analyze results according to whether women were in the follicular or luteal phase of their cycle, that is, in a pre-ovulatory or post-ovulatory phase, at the time of surgery. The blood tests serve as the "gold standard" for making this determination, Grant said. Although some women may have a biopsy at one phase of their cycle and a lumpectomy or mastectomy at another, the researchers will analyze data from these women separately, he said. The researchers expect to issue progress reports, watching particularly for early evidence of a significant difference in the recurrence of breast cancer according to the time of surgery.

Many chronobiologists contend that assessing the best time for breast cancer surgery requires a determination of the exact menstrual cycle day to do the surgery. Grouping the results of surgery into two week periods before and after ovulation is unlikely to be sensitve enough to determine when surgery is best, as the optimal time window may be only a few days. "The National Cancer Institute sponsorship of this multi-center study is very important," said Erhard Haus of the University of Minnesota and president of the American Association for Medical Chronobiology and Chronotherapeutics, "but it is likely that further detailed studies will be needed to truly answer the question."

Answers can't come too soon for the 185,000 American women diagnosed with breast cancer each year, hundreds of thousands more worldwide, and their families.

Does the Time of Radiation Therapy Make a Difference?

Radiation therapy can shrink or even eliminate some tumors. Animal studies suggest that radiation may kill more or less cancer cells at different times of day. Astonishingly little research has explored this issue in humans. One study conducted in India in 1976 found that radiation therapy was more successful for mouth and facial tumors if given at the daily peak of the tumor's temperature.[19] The matter merits further investigation.

Timewise Tips

Women: examine your breasts monthly the week after menstruation, or at the same time of month if you no longer menstruate, and get regular Pap smears and mammograms.

Men: examine your testicles monthly for lumps or swelling. If you are over age fifty, you should get a prostate-specific antigen blood test and digital rectal examination for prostate cancer yearly.

Everyone: practice good health habits to minimize your cancer risk. Don't smoke and drink only in moderation. Eat a healthy diet, low in animal fat, with plenty of grains, fruits, and vegetables. Wear sunscreens. Practice regular self-exams of skin and mouth.

Talk to your doctor about preventive strategies and specific tests appropriate for your age, family history, and general health.

To learn more about studies recruiting patients with various cancers, visit the Web site of the National Cancer Institute (www.clinicaltrials.gov). Type "chronotherapy" in the search window to learn about those in which chronotherapy is an option.

For reliable information on cancer prevention and treatment, visit the Web sites of the American Cancer Society (www.cancer.org), the National Cancer Institute (www.cancer.gov/), and the Pubmed database of the National Library of Medicine (www.medlineplus.gov).

Study. To learn more about chronotherapy for cancer, visit William Hrushesky's Web site (www.rpi.edu/~hrushw). Visit the Web site of the Association for Cancer Online Resources (www.acor.org), for access to electronic mailing lists for persons with cancer and their families.

COLDS AND FLU

Crumpled tissues provide a good gauge of cold and flu symptoms, even beyond the familiar "runny nose." Volunteers infected with these two viral infections use the greatest number of tissues between 8 and 11 A.M., and the fewest between 5 and 8 P.M. The morning tissue count often is double that of the afternoon. Subjects also produce the most mucus in the morning. These findings come from research studies in which a brigade of masked and gloved technicians count and weigh used tissues to assess symptom severity.[1]

A cold is a minor infection of the nose and throat. The flu tends to be more severe and to cause a longer list of symptoms. Sneezing, sinus congestion, sore throat, headaches, and muscle aches in both a cold and the flu prove worse in the morning than in the afternoon.

When flu strikes, however, the tissue count could even stand in for a thermometer, as body temperature also is disproportionately higher in the morning than later in the day. Healthy children and adults typically awaken with their body temperature close to 97° F. With a cold or the flu, morning temperature may be higher than 99° F. If you think that body temperature of 98.6° F is normal, you might not be concerned. But 98.6° F first thing in the morning indicates fever. Fevers may run as high as 100° F to 103° F in adults, and often go even higher in children.

The morning peak in cold and flu symptoms reflects daily rhythms in key bodily functions. Symptoms build up overnight chiefly because the hormone cortisol, a key inflammation fighter, is missing then. Cortisol's secretion surges around the time you normally awaken. After it goes to work, cold and flu symptoms ease up. Nasal passages also normally shrink at night and relax and open in the daytime.

In British studies, cold sufferers who rated themselves from "drowsy" to "alert" across the day felt about as alert as usual. Persons with flu felt drowsier than usual, a decline of about 20 percent from their normal levels of alertness. The dip in their alertness, moreover, proved most striking early in the morning.

Even coughing has a circadian rhythm. In one study, cold sufferers wore small microphones and tape recorders for sixty hours. They coughed several hundred times more often in the middle of the day than at night or in the morning. Coughing, a natural response to airway irritation, helps rid air passages of excessive secretion and mucus from infected tissues. By midday, when airways are most open, the presence of these excess secretions is most noticeable.

Colds and flu also have seasonal rhythms. Colds are cold-weather illnesses. Cold season in the United States runs from about September to May, while flu typically attacks between December and March. Flu is not a trivial illness. In an average year, it kills 20,000 Americans. Older persons are at highest risk.

Cause of Colds No Mystery

Colds and flu are spread by viruses that come in contact with the lining of the nose. While sneezing can transmit these viruses, direct contact is the usual mode of transmission. A person with a cold sneezes into his hand, say, and then touches a doorknob that you touch before touching your own nose. When people around you have colds, you're likely to catch one, too.

Colds aren't caused by going outside without a coat. Stress, often blamed, may in fact disrupt sleep, leading to exhaustion, irritability, and depression. It also may suppress the body's immune system, possibly making you more susceptible to viruses. This fact may explain why colds surge in college students at exam time.

There's a good reason for calling colds "common." They are the leading reason Americans visit doctors. Adults average two to four colds a year, while children average six to eight. If your child gets a cold, there's a 40 percent chance that you'll be sniffling soon.

Medications Can Ease Cold Symptoms

Americans spend two billion dollars annually to relieve the discomfort of colds. Hundreds of different products exist, prompting uncertainty about which ones to take when, and for which symptoms. Most do not require a prescription. Read labels carefully to determine which products contain ingredients for your specific symptoms. If you have nasal congestion, for example, a pain reliever won't help. If you aren't coughing, cough suppressants offer you no benefit.

It's often said that colds last about a week if you treat them and seven days if you don't. Flu symptoms may hang on longer, perhaps up to three weeks. While colds and flu go away by themselves, there's no need to suffer unnecessarily.

Different types of cold and flu medications include:

Pain Relievers

Many doctors say acetaminophen is the drug of choice for muscle aches and headaches associated with colds and flu. Acetaminophen is less likely to upset the stomach than aspirin and other nonsteroidal anti-inflammatory drugs (NSAIDs), but you can further reduce your risk of stomach irritation by not taking any of these drugs in the morning. (See Arthritis, page 207.) Don't give aspirin to children or teenagers. Its use is linked with Reye syndrome, a rare but potentially fatal illness. Use acetaminophen instead.

Combination Remedies

These may contain as many as six different ingredients alleged to relieve nasal stuffiness, calm scratchy throats, get rid of headaches, and ease other cold symptoms. Many products sold over the counter are promoted for bedtime or morning use. These are not true chronotherapies, however, as they are not tailored to the circadian rhythms of symptoms. The day/night distinction reflects the nature of the side effects of the ingredients they contain. The nighttime products contain relatively higher doses of antihistamines and lower doses of decongestants, while for the daytime products, the opposite is true. Both substances help dry up swollen tissues. Antihistamines in these over-the-counter products induce drowsiness, a side effect that is desirable when you want to sleep. These include brompheniramine, chlorpheniramine, and diphenhydramine. Decongestants, on the other hand, may cause agitation, nervousness, and insomnia. Their side effects may be acceptable in the daytime, particularly if you are feeling drowsy. Decongestants include pseudophedrine and phenylephrine; talk to your doctor before using these substances if you have heart disease or high blood pressure.

Decongestant Sprays

These medications work fast to open nasal passages. Don't use them for more than three consecutive days. Their continued use creates an alternating cycle of relief and rebound, and may leave you stuffier than before you started. These medications contain stimulants. Some people find they disturb their sleep if used near bedtime. Older persons, in particular, may experience urinary urgency.

Cough Suppressants

Medications containing dextromethorphan may relieve a dry cough. If you have excessive phlegm, you may do better with the expectorant guaifenesin. Sometimes, it's useful to cough at night. Coughing is a natural reflex to clear the lungs. For severe dry cough, codeine-containing medications, available only by prescription, may be more helpful. When used in the evening, they are particularly useful in controlling bouts of coughing that keep you from sleeping.

Ipratropium Bromide

Aerosol nasal sprays containing this prescription drug are particularly useful in drying up runny nasal discharge, a symptom that is particularly bothersome in the morning. Since these sprays work quickly, they can be used upon awakening as well as at other times of day, if needed.

Corticosteroids

Anti-inflammatory aerosol sprays or drops containing corticosteroids lessen swelling and make breathing easier, especially at night. Tablet corticosteroids, however, generally are not indicated for colds or flu.

Antibiotics

Don't ask your doctor to prescribe antibiotics. These drugs kill bacteria. They don't help cold and flu symptoms, which are caused by viruses. Using antibiotics if you don't need them may prompt your body to develop resistance to various strains of bacteria, rendering these medications useless in the future when you really do need them.

Alternative Remedies

Vitamin C, herbal remedies, zinc lozenges, echinacea, chicken soup. . . . Your best friend or your mother may urge you to try one or more of a long list of cold and flu remedies. "Evidence for zinc and echinacea, the current top two alternative cold cures," according to *Consumer Reports on Health,* "is still rather long on anecdotes and short on science."[2] Take unsubstantiated claims with the proverbial grain of salt.

On the Horizon

While hundreds of different viruses cause colds, about half are caused by members of the Rhinovirus family (*Rhino* is Greek for nose). Scientists have reported recent progress in developing a drug targeted broadly against many rhinoviruses. Since this drug, if successful, would combat the causes of colds rather than simply cold symptoms, it would represent a major advance in treatment.

Medications Can Ease Flu Symptoms

If you've got symptoms such as muscle aches and fever, it's always wise to call your doctor. Two drugs, amantidine and rimantidine, commonly are prescribed to help inactivate the invading flu virus. These drugs don't combat all flu strains, however, and may have side effects such as agitation and insomnia that some people can't tolerate. Two new drugs, oseltamivir phosphate (Tamiflu) and zanamivir (Relenza), may shorten the duration of the flu if started in the first two days after symptoms appear. Flu shots remain the first line of defense against this illness.

Try to Get Your Flu Shot in the Morning

Scientists try to predict which flu viruses are likely to be most active in any given year. Manufacturers then develop vaccines against the three expected to be most common. Because scientists must select the specific viruses about nine months in advance, and because viruses may change over time, vaccine effectiveness varies from year to year.

Flu shots are given in the United States in the fall so the body will build up sufficient levels of virus-fighting antibodies by the time the winter flu season is in full swing. Shots need to be repeated from year to year because both immunity declines in the year following vaccination and viruses change.

The U.S. Centers for Disease Control and Prevention (CDCP) recommends flu shots for everyone over age sixty-five, health care personnel, and persons with illnesses that make them particularly susceptible to infections.[3] Flu shots protect as many as 90 percent of healthy young adults who get them. In older persons they may be less effective in preventing flu, but they make the illness less severe and reduce the risk of serious complications, such as pneumonia, and even heart attacks.

About one in three persons who get flu shots have some soreness at the vaccination site afterward. Although it usually lasts only a day or two, you may be able to reduce your odds of soreness by getting your shot in the morning. The second best time is late afternoon. Two studies show arm soreness is up to four times more common in persons who get their shots between about noon and 3 P.M. than in those who get them earlier or later.[4]

Fewer than 10 percent of persons who get flu shots experience mild side effects, such as headache or low-grade fever. These symptoms typically last for about a day. The time the shot is given does not appear to make a difference here. Whether time of day influences the efficacy of flu shots is not yet clear. Studies to date show conflicting results.

Timewise Tips

When taking your temperature, keep daily rhythms in mind. A reading of 98.6° F or higher on awakening in the morning indicates fever.

When taking medicines, choose ingredients for their effects on specific symptoms and side effects at different times of day. Taking twelve-hour nonprescription antihistamines at bedtime may both help you sleep and improve your breathing in the morning. New nonsedating antihistamines, now available only by prescription, improve nasal symptoms without causing daytime drowsiness or affecting nighttime sleep.

Avoid contact with those who are ill in the first three days of a cold or the flu. If you are sick, stay home. Contagion peaks early in these illnesses.

Anytime Tips

Wash hands frequently, and try to avoid touching your nose, eyes, and mouth. This practice will help avoid spreading infection.

Feed a cold and starve a fever. Or is it starve a cold and feed a fever? If you can't remember, you're not alone. The fact that you can't remember suggests neither approach has worked perfectly for you in the past. If you're sick, especially if you experience nausea or vomiting, you won't feel much like eating. The best approach is to listen to your body. Drink plenty of fluids, especially warm ones, which help keep nasal passages open.

Use exercise, relaxation, and other stress-reduction techniques year-round. Some studies show stress weakens the body's immune system, possibly making people more susceptible to colds and flu. Good health is a good defense against colds and the flu.

COLIC

About half of all babies suffer bouts of fussiness and crying that last more than three hours, almost always starting between 5 P.M. and 8 P.M., and ending by midnight.[1] This behavior usually appears in the first three months of life, and then fades. Folk names for it reflect this predictable pattern. The Chinese call it "100 Days Crying," the Vietnamese, "3 Months plus 10 Days Crying," and the Japanese, "Evening Crying." About 90 percent of colic episodes begin when the baby is awake, and about 90 percent conclude when the baby falls asleep.

Colicky babies often draw their legs to their abdomens, curl their toes, and clench their fists. The effort of crying may make them alternately flushed and pale. Often the crying begins or ends with a bowel movement or passing of gas, leading parents to conclude that what or how the baby was fed is to blame. Breast-fed and bottle-fed babies appear equally likely to develop colic, although foods the mother eats or type of formula still may cause stomach upsets.

Colic may reflect a discrepancy between the new baby's still immature daily melatonin rhythm and that of its surroundings. Once the baby regularly secretes melatonin at night, starting at about three months, colic subsides.[2]

Timewise Tips

Set up a shift schedule for nighttime baby care. Then each parent can be assured of at least a few hours of unbroken sleep. Parents also may need to nap at other times.

Try to keep middle-of-the-night feedings short and dull. For crying episodes, try to comfort your baby without taking him or her out of the crib, or providing alerting entertainment.

If the baby cries at all times of the day, see your doctor. The baby may have an ear infection or some other problem that needs medical attention.

Anytime Tips

Always put your baby to sleep on its back. This strategy helps prevent sudden infant death syndrome. (See page 355.)

If you are breast-feeding, pay attention to what you eat and when. Your baby shares your diet. Foods such as broccoli, cabbage, coffee, peppers, and onions bother many babies. Some trial-and-error experimenting may help you avoid likely suspects.

If you are bottle-feeding, talk to the baby's doctor about changing the formula. Many babies have trouble with both cow's milk and soy formulas. They often outgrow these sensitivities within a few months, but until then you may need to try different products to find one that is well tolerated.

Try repetitive noise and vibration, time-honored approaches to calm a colicky baby. Try a rocking chair, or mechanical swing, or, if it is not too late at night, a car ride. Some babies quiet down when placed in an infant seat near a running dishwasher or dryer.

Massage the baby's tummy gently with oil or lotion.

Put the baby, tummy down, on a warm hot-water bottle in your lap. Bounce your knees gently, while patting the baby on the back.

Give the baby two tablespoons of weak herbal tea, if your doctor approves. One study showed chamomile tea, given up to three times a day for a week, eased colic in six of ten babies with this problem, while sugar-water, a placebo, helped only three in ten.[3]

Study. Visit the Web site of the American Academy of Pediatrics (www.aap.org).

CONSTIPATION

Although regularity is a prime indicator of circadian harmony, some people worry too much about regularity of their bowel movements (BMs). They may think they are constipated, or irregular, if they do not have a BM every day.

But regularity for some people means having BMs twice a day, and for others, twice a week. Both are normal. Your doctor probably would define constipation as having fewer BMs than is usual for you, especially if passing them takes a long time, is difficult, or causes pain or bleeding.

Constipation is the most common gastrointestinal complaint in the United States. It prompts some 2.5 million visits to doctors annually in this country, although most people treat it themselves. Americans spend $725 million on laxatives each year.[1] Constipation may occur at any age, but is most common in persons aged sixty-five and older.

Bowel Activity Is Cyclic

BMs usually show a time-of-day pattern. Two out of three people customarily have BMs in the morning before breakfast, or within two or three hours after the morning meal. Because digestive and other bodily functions slow down at night, BMs are rare between 1 A.M. and 5 A.M.[2]

Many women report changes in bowel habits across the menstrual cycle. One woman in three reports more frequent constipation and hard stools after ovulation, that is, in the second half of the menstrual cycle. The sex hormone progesterone, which reaches its peak about a week after ovulation, exerts a constipating effect. After menstruation begins, progesterone plunges, inducing loose stools or diarrhea in some women.[3]

Menstrual-cycle variation in BMs is even more profound in women who suffer from Crohn's Disease and ulcerative colitis. Both of these chronic inflammatory bowel disorders cause abdominal pain and diarrhea, problems that usually worsen just before or at the start of a woman's period. Irritable bowel syndrome, a disorder that produces diarrhea in some persons and constipation in others, follows a similar pattern.[4]

Constipation is a common complaint in pregnancy, when the heavy uterus compresses the intestines, as well as right after childbirth, when dramatic hormonal changes occur.

What Causes Constipation?

Disruptions in meal timing, meal content, and daily activities all contribute to constipation. As people get older, particularly if they live alone, they may lose interest in food. If they stop eating regularly, they probably don't consume enough fiber. Fiber is the part of fruits, vegetables, and grains that the body cannot digest. It adds bulk to stools.

People who don't eat regularly also may not drink enough fluids, needed to prevent hard, dry stools and make BMs easier. Many older persons find cooking and grocery shopping a chore. Concerned about spoilage of fresh fruits and vegetables, they often buy fewer of them, opting for convenience foods that often are low in fiber. If they have problems with their teeth or with swallowing, they may choose soft, processed foods that lack fiber. Dairy products, eggs, and sweets high in refined sugars also may be constipating.

Other changes in daily routines, such as leading a sedentary lifestyle or having an illness that requires bed rest, slow body metabolism and foster constipation. Travel can do it, too, by disrupting normal meal schedules and introducing unfamiliar foods. Constipation also may be a symptom of some illnesses beyond those of the digestive tract, such as stroke and spinal cord injuries.

Misusing laxatives and enemas also may contribute to this problem. The body starts to rely on their use to trigger BMs, and stops working on its own. Older persons also take more medicines, some of which cause constipation as a side effect. These include some antidepressants, antacids containing aluminum or calcium, antihistamines, diuretics, high blood pressure drugs, and antiparkinsonian drugs.

Get More Fiber, More Fluids, Eat Regular Meals

The best way to prevent and treat constipation is to increase fiber and fluid intake, and make regular exercise and mealtimes part of daily life. Most people following these guidelines do not need laxatives. These medicines are most useful in circumstances such as travel, illness, menstrual cycle flare-ups, and sluggish bowels that sometimes develop with aging.

Different types of laxatives are on the market:

Bulking agents soften stools so they are easy to pass and stimulate intestinal contractions. They include bran, psyllium, methylcellulose, and calcium polycarbophil.

Stimulant laxatives cause the walls of the intestine to contract strongly to expel stools. They include senna, cascara, phenolphthalein, bisacodyl, and castor oil. If taken orally at bedtime, a stimulant laxative generally induces a BM within six to twelve hours, in synchrony with the body's normal rhythm of elimination.[5] Suppository stimulant laxatives work more quickly, so they can be taken in the morning.

Stool softeners attract water to stools, facilitating elimination. They include docusate and mineral oil. *Caution:* If mineral oil is used consistently, it may interfere with uptake of vitamins from foods.

Timewise Tips

Do not ignore the urge to have a BM. If constipation is a problem for you, plan for an undisturbed visit to the toilet at the time of day your BMs usually occur.

Organize daily life to include regular mealtimes and exercise.

If you are a woman with severe menstrual constipation, you may find bulk-forming laxatives helpful in the last two weeks of your menstrual cycle. Women with severe symptoms may benefit from medications that prevent ovulation, reducing hormone shifts, and thus blunting menstrual flare-ups.[6]

Anytime Tips

Add more fiber to your diet, including beans, bran, whole grains, fresh fruits, and vegetables. Dried fruit such as apricots, prunes, and figs are high in fiber. Americans eat only about 5 to 20 grams of fiber daily on average. The American Dietetic Association recommends 20 to 35 grams daily.

Drink one to two quarts of liquids daily. If you have heart, blood vessel, or kidney problems, consult your doctor about your appropriate fluid intake. Water and unsweetened fruit juices are ideal drinks.[7] They add fluid to the colon and bulk to stools, making BMs softer and easier to pass. Some people find milk constipating. Go easy on coffee and soft drinks containing caffeine as they have a dehydrating effect.

If you develop a significant or persistent change in bowel habits, see your doctor.

Study. Visit the Web site of the American College of Gastroenterology (www.acg.gi.org).

DIABETES

Diabetes mellitus, or sugar diabetes, disrupts the way the body handles sugar, its chief source of energy. Biological rhythms regulate every step of this process.

Sugar comes from the foods you consume. When you eat, the body converts the carbohydrates, fats, and proteins in foods into a simple sugar called glucose that enters your bloodstream. An organ behind the stomach called the pancreas secretes insulin, enabling cells to take up glucose to fuel their work. Extra glucose goes to the liver, where it is stored for future use. As the cells use up glucose, the liver releases a new supply. These events take place automatically, ensuring that cells get the amount they need.

In diabetes, the body's system of checks and balances fails, causing too much glucose to circulate. This oversupply may cause numerous health problems, including heart attacks, strokes, blindness, and lowered ability to function sexually. About 16 million Americans have diabetes. Those who manage their diabetes well can avoid complications and live normal lives.

What Goes Wrong in Diabetes?

Persons with diabetes may produce too little insulin or no insulin, or their bodies may not make proper use of the insulin produced. There are three main types:

Insulin-dependent, or Type I: This is the more severe form of diabetes, and usually first appears in childhood or early adulthood. Here, the pancreas makes too little insulin. Persons with this form of diabetes, about 10 percent of Americans with the disorder, require several daily injections of insulin. Scientists suspect that exposure to a virus triggers this type of diabetes in persons with an inherited susceptibility to it.

Noninsulin-dependent, or Type II: This form of diabetes usually develops in persons over age thirty, particularly those who are severely overweight. The excess weight boosts the body's need for glucose, but the supply may not keep up with the demand. This prompts the pancreas to go into high gear and manufacture more insulin. That works for a while, but eventually the overworked pancreas shuts down. This type of diabetes often can be controlled by diet, weight loss, and, in some instances, medications taken orally to stimulate insulin release from the pancreas and more efficient use of glucose by the cells.

Pregnancy-related: Some women develop diabetes in pregnancy. While the disorder goes away afterward, these women have a higher risk of developing Type II diabetes later in life. Women who already have diabetes and are considering pregnancy need to work with their doctors to decrease their own risk of complications and ensure good health for their babies.

Daily Rhythms Alter Blood Sugar Control

The pancreas secretes insulin in response to food intake. The amount secreted, however, varies in a circadian manner, with the highest levels around 6 A.M., and the lowest around 6 P.M. The pancreas also releases insulin 50 percent faster in the morning.[1] This means that even if you eat the same foods at different times of day, the amount of insulin you secrete varies.

If you are healthy and eat a three-ounce chocolate bar in the morning, your blood sugar concentration returns to normal in about ninety minutes. In the afternoon, this process takes two hours or longer. In persons over age forty-five, time-of-day differences become more extreme.[2]

Cells also vary in the efficiency with which they handle insulin at different times of day. In one study, researchers gave the same amount of insulin to volunteers at either 8 A.M. or 5 P.M. The morning insulin shot reduced glucose 40 percent more than the afternoon one did.[3]

These findings suggest why diabetes is hard to treat. People differ from day to day in what, when, and how much they eat, how active they are, and how much stress they experience, all factors that alter the body's need for glucose. It is tricky to take insulin in a manner that mimics what the body ordinarily does automatically, and with great precision. Too little insulin allows blood glucose levels to get too high—hyperglycemia—producing symptoms such as excessive urination and thirst. Too much insulin makes blood glucose fall too low—hypoglycemia—which triggers sweating, dizziness, weakness, and faintness.

Menstrual Cycle Affects Diabetes

Many healthy women crave carbohydrates just before or after their menstrual period starts, a hint that blood sugar regulation varies over the month. One survey of 406 insulin-dependent women with diabetes found that nearly 70 percent experienced substantial changes in their blood sugar level near the time of menstruation. Those with cravings for sweets reported greater difficulty controlling their blood sugar levels at this time.[4]

Diabetes May Be Harder to Manage in Winter

Blood sugar regulation also varies over the year, with more precision in summer than in winter. Yet blood glucose levels are higher in winter than in summer, making winter theoretically a more difficult time for persons with diabetes. These facts also may help explain why even people without diabetes tend to gain weight in the winter, and find it easier to lose weight in the summer.

Several studies show insulin-dependent, or Type I diabetes, is diagnosed in children 50 percent more often in the fall and winter than in the summer.[5] The higher winter glucose levels may serve to unmask the children's susceptibility. The higher likelihood of viral infections in the winter also may increase the risk of diabetes in those susceptible to it, including pregnant women, their unborn babies, and young children.[6]

Timed Dosing of Insulin Improves Control of Type I Diabetes

Some persons with insulin-dependent Type I diabetes experience an abrupt rise in the level of glucose in their blood, or in their need for insulin, or both, between 6 A.M. and 8 A.M. This so-called dawn phenomenon occurs as a reaction to the nighttime surge in growth hormone, and in conjunction with the morning surge in the hormones cortisol and adrenaline. Before the nature of this predictable response was understood, patients might have taken a large amount of insulin to compensate for the morning rise in glucose. Now, their doctors may suggest they increase their insulin dose the night before to prevent or minimize this change.[7]

Recognition of circadian variations in the level or need for glucose also permits persons with diabetes to approximate a more normal rhythm with timed dosing of insulin. Most people need less insulin to maintain their target blood sugar level at night, for example, than in the morning.

Maintaining tight control, that is, as normal a blood sugar level as possible, may reduce your risk of developing heart disease, nerve damage, and other complications from your illness. Proper monitoring requires checking blood glucose levels several times a day, typically with finger sticks, and possibly taking four or more injections.

A wrist-worn device, undergoing testing in 1999, eliminates finger sticks. The GlucoWatch uses a painless, constant, low-level electrical current to transport glucose across the skin where it can be measured. The device sounds an alarm if glucose drops below a designated level. A study of the device in ninety-two persons with diabetes suggests that the ease and accuracy of automatic monitoring may further aid control.[8]

Different forms of insulin make tight control easier today than in the past. They differ in how soon the insulin starts working, how long after being taken it works the hardest, and how long it stays in the body. A person might take a shorter-acting insulin right before eating, for example, and a longer-acting insulin at bedtime. Attention to diet and exercise also are key parts of every treatment regimen.

A battery-operated insulin pump worn on the body provides insulin automatically and continuously through a needle in the abdomen. Although the pump may give wearers better control and more flexibility in choosing when to eat and exercise than intermittent injections, it still does not provide insulin in a chronobiologic manner. It is designed to provide a steady dose of insulin, not more or less as the body requires at different times. Development of a pump that meets this need would be a major advance in diabetes treatment.

Diet, Exercise, Drugs Improve Type II Diabetes

Since obesity is the prime cause of Type II diabetes, weight loss often reduces or eliminates this disorder. Dieting works best when combined with exercise, which helps the body make more efficient use of glucose. Diet and exercise may reduce or avert the need for medication.

Medication sometimes is necessary, however. Some of the most widely used types are described below. These drugs may be prescribed for use alone or in combination. None has been systematically researched for dosing-time differences in effectiveness.

- Glipizide, glyburide, and several others known as sulfonylureas work primarily to stimulate the pancreas to release more insulin. Manufacturers recommend that people with diabetes take these medicines once a day with breakfast.
- Metformin increases the use of insulin by cells and tissues. It usually is taken just before meals.
- Acarbose delays absorption of glucose into the blood after eating to keep sugar levels from rising too high. It also is taken just before meals.

Timewise Tips

Regularize your life. If you have diabetes, your aim is to keep blood sugar levels in a normal range. Eat, exercise, and sleep at about the same times each day. Eat about the same amount of food each day, and avoid skipping meals, or having large meals, as too much or too little food puts blood sugar levels on a roller-coaster path. Have a snack about a half-hour before exercising.

Keep a diary to record your blood sugar levels. Your doctor or diabetes educator will tell you when and how often to take measurements.

If you work odd hours, or rotate shifts, work with your doctor to devise a medication and meal schedule that shifts when your work hours do. If you take insulin, try to avoid having to get up from sleep to give yourself a shot. Center your diet on foods such as eggs, vegetables, and fruits that you enjoy at all times, instead of foods that you regard as "breakfast only" or "dinner only." To mentally expand meal options, change meal names to "first meal," "second meal," and so on. You may need to divide your daily food intake into frequent small snacks. After starting a new work schedule, try to be more diligent than most shift workers about sticking to new hours on days off. If you cannot control your diabetes successfully with these measures, you'd be wise to transfer to a fixed shift, or to seek a job with more regular hours.

If you take insulin, be attentive to temporal patterns in insulin reactions and in abnormal blood sugar values. These may be expressions of your own body rhythms. They require appropriate dose adjustments.

If you are female, monitor your glucose levels carefully the week before your period, as well as while it is in progress. If sugar levels consistently change over your menstrual cycle, inform your doctor. Be sensitive to food cravings around menstruation, and try to avoid consuming extra sweets and carbohydrate-rich foods.

Check your blood pressure regularly at home around the clock. Diabetes often raises blood pressure at night, not detectable in daytime visits to the doctor's office. Use the Blood Pressure Diary on page 289, and take it with you when you see your doctor. Also follow Timewise Tips for high blood pressure and heart disease prevention.

If you experience nerve pain that disturbs your sleep, ask your doctor about taking gabapentin (Neurontin). Recent research suggests use of this medication reduces pain and improves sleep.[9] Other new medications can relieve other diabetes-caused pain.

Anytime Tips

Learn your cholesterol levels. Persons with diabetes often develop high cholesterol, increasing their risk of heart disease and stroke. A low-saturated-fat, low-cholesterol diet will help you keep your cholesterol down.

Wear easily accessible emergency medical information, such as a bracelet or necklace. Be sure family and coworkers know how to help you in an emergency, and always carry a source of sugar to use if your blood sugar level falls too low after you take insulin.

Learn stress management techniques, which will help avoid surges of hormones that boost glucose levels.

Study. Visit the Web sites of the American Diabetes Association (www.diabetes.org) and the National Diabetes Information Clearinghouse (www.niddk.nih.gov/health/diabetes/ndic.htm).

EPILEPSY

In the majority of persons with the brain disorder epilepsy, seizures recur at predictable times of day. About half of those with epilepsy experience seizures mainly in waking hours. About one-quarter have them mainly in sleep. In the others, timing is less consistent; their seizures strike both day and night.

In most women, seizure activity intensifies at times of hormone shifts in the menstrual cycle, as well as in pregnancy and at menopause. Seizures in men also reflect hormonal influence. With present-day medications, most persons with epilepsy can live full and productive lives. Growing attention to daily and monthly biological rhythms offers the hope of even better seizure control.

What Goes Wrong in Epilepsy?

In epilepsy, sudden and intense bursts of electrical energy disrupt the normal low-level electrical signals brain cells use to communicate with one another. This neurological lightning bolt may cause unconsciousness or confusion and jerky muscle movements. It may also distort the senses, making a person smell strange odors or hear peculiar sounds, for example.

Seizures may be *partial*, affecting one area of the brain, or *generalized*, affecting nerve cells brainwide. Partial seizures are both the most common and most difficult to treat. Seizures usually last from a few seconds to a few minutes, but when severe, they may last a half-hour or longer. After a seizure, a person may have a headache and feel fatigued and confused.

Sleep deprivation, fatigue, stress, and skipping meals or doses of prescribed medications often trigger seizures. Body clock-disrupting experiences that typically accompany jet travel or changes in shift work schedules also make seizures more likely.

Some people who experience seizures in the daytime feel a sense of unease or discomfort called an aura when the seizure starts. Some see flickering lights or sunbursts. This experience may have prompted artist Vincent van Gogh, diagnosed with epilepsy in his lifetime, to paint works such as *The Starry Night*. The painting shows a pulsating moon and huge stars shimmering in a roiling sky above the rooftops of a small village. About 5 percent of persons with epilepsy have a heightened sensitivity to pulsing light. Viewing video games, flashing strobe lights, or sunlight sparkling on water may trigger their seizures. These experiences do *not* trigger seizures in everyone with epilepsy.[1]

Brain injury before or at the time of birth, head injury of the type experienced by boxers or by motorcyclists involved in a crash, nutritional deficiencies, some genetic and infectious diseases, brain tumors, and some poisons are among the known causes of epilepsy. The reason remains a mystery in about half of all cases, according to the National Institute of Neurological Disorders and Stroke (NINDS).

An estimated 2.5 million Americans of all ages now live with epilepsy, and 181,000 persons, both children and adults, are newly diagnosed with it every year. An estimated one million Americans have seizures that do not respond to treatment with existing medications.[2] Prolonged seizures may damage the brain and even be fatal. Three-time Olympic gold medal-winning track star Florence Griffith Joyner died at age thirty-eight in 1998 after suffering a seizure in her sleep.

Sex Hormones Alter Epilepsy in Women

Life cycle events that are under the control of reproductive hormones are critical times for women with epilepsy. Yet "the role of hormones as a contributing cause or treatment for epilepsy has received very little systematic investigation," according to the Epilepsy Foundation. "Despite the fact that half the people who have epilepsy are women," the foundation said in 1997 when it announced a campaign to address women's issues, "practically all the research in this condition has involved men."[3] That situation is changing today.

Puberty
The seizures that young children sometimes experience when they have a high fever do not constitute epilepsy. Such seizures may recur with later bouts of severe colds or the flu, but they usually diminish or disappear after puberty.

Recurring seizures that characterize epilepsy, which are not linked to a fever, sometimes first appear in girls around the time they begin to menstruate.

Menstrual Cycle

Eight in ten women with epilepsy have seizures more often at specific times in the menstrual cycle.[4] The primary female sex hormones, estrogen and progesterone, both act on cells in the temporal lobe of the brain, an area where partial seizures often originate. Estrogen excites brain nerve cell activity, while progesterone slows it. Seizures therefore often increase when estrogen is at its monthly high, around ovulation, and when progesterone is at its monthly low, just before the start of menstruation and while bleeding is in progress.

In one study, 184 women with epilepsy charted their seizures across the menstrual cycle. These women had a severe form of epilepsy, *intractable complex partial seizures*. Researchers at the Beth Israel Deaconess Medical Center in Boston, Massachusetts, also used blood tests to determine when the women ovulated. Andrew Herzog and his colleagues found that these women collectively had nearly 3,000 seizures in a single cycle. Most of those who ovulated had more seizures than usual at ovulation, and most of the total group had more seizures at menstruation. One-third of the women had at least double their average daily number of seizures at these vulnerable times.[5]

Some antiepileptic drugs make birth control pills less effective by hastening the breakdown of contraceptive hormones. For this reason, doctors may advise women with epilepsy to use birth control pills containing a higher dose of estrogen. Use of oral contraceptives also may affect the doctor's selection of anticonvulsant medication.

Pregnancy

More than nine in ten women with epilepsy have normal, healthy babies. Sadly, however, women with epilepsy are more likely than healthy women to have stillborn babies, or to give birth prematurely. Their babies more often have delays in development. The risk of taking anticonvulsant drugs while pregnant must be balanced against the risks to both mother and baby of not taking them.

The body absorbs, uses, and excretes these drugs differently in pregnancy. Blood levels sometimes go too high, inducing side effects, or too low, triggering more seizures. In an Australian study, over 40 percent of women with epilepsy had more seizures while pregnant, although about 10 percent had fewer seizures. Women who had had epilepsy longer before becoming pregnant proved most likely to deteriorate. Many were taking a lower than usual dose of their anticonvulsant medications to reduce the risk of harm to their babies.[6]

All women of child-bearing age now are advised to take 0.4 milligrams of folic acid daily before becoming pregnant to reduce their risk of a birth defect that involves incomplete closure of the spinal cord, *spina bifida*. Folic acid is particularly important for women with epilepsy as their babies are at greater risk of this disorder than those of healthy women.

Menopause

At the start of menopause, when estrogen levels fluctuate, women with epilepsy often report experiencing more seizures. After menopause, when estrogen production stops, the frequency of seizures may fall. Women using estrogen replacement therapy, however, may experience an increase in seizures, researchers found in a study at New York Presbyterian Hospital and Cornell University's Weill Medical College. Cynthia Harden and her colleagues urge women with epilepsy and their doctors to carefully weigh the benefits and risk of this type of therapy.[7]

In a study at the University of Maryland School of Medicine, Fariha Abbasi and her colleagues found that menopausal women using hormone replacement therapy who took progestin, a synthetic form of progesterone, in addition to estrogen were significantly less likely to report that their seizures worsened than women who took estrogen alone.[8]

Sex Hormones May Alter Epilepsy in Men, Too

Men with epilepsy frequently have lower than normal levels of male sex hormones, including the chief male sex hormone, testosterone. In men, as in women, certain anticonvulsant drugs may clear reproductive hormones from the bloodstream faster than the body can replace them. The deficiency of testosterone may contribute to difficulty with sexual arousal and fertility and also may increase the frequency of seizures, some research suggests.

Hormone replacement therapy using testosterone along with a medication that inhibits its breakdown by anticonvulsant drugs may improve control of seizures in some men with epilepsy, Boston researcher Andrew Herzog reports.[9]

Sleep Laboratory Studies Aid Diagnosis and Treatment

Why seizures occur mainly or exclusively in sleep in some people with epilepsy is not yet clear. Seizures commonly occur in the nondreaming state of sleep, the state in which brain activity least resembles that of wakefulness. In the sleep laboratory, doctors simultaneously record brain activity and monitor the sleeper via a video camera. This technique helps identify the particular type and number of seizures. It is especially valuable in showing small repetitive movements that are not otherwise easily detected. If you are to have a sleep study, your doctor may ask you to forgo sleep beforehand, and to not take your medications that day so that the severity of your seizures will be more obvious.[10]

Time of Dosing May Alter Efficacy of Antiepilepsy Drugs

More than twenty antiseizure medications (also called anticonvulsant or antiepilepsy drugs) currently are available in the United States. They are the primary treatment for epilepsy. Your doctor's prescription will depend on the type and severity of seizures you have. It may take some trial and error effort to find the drug or drugs that work best for you, while causing the least drowsiness, dizziness, or other side effects. So-called new generation antiepilepsy drugs are said to provide better control of seizures with fewer side effects. Some are specifically designed not to interfere with the activity of other drugs, including birth control pills. They include gabapentin (Neurontin), lamotrigine (Lamictal), topiramate (Topamax), tiagabine (Gabatril), levetiracetam (Keppra), and oxcarbazepine (Trileptal).

None of the newer medications and only two of the older ones, valproate and phenytoin, now sold as generics as well as by brand name, have been studied with regard to how they work when taken at different times of the day or in different phases of the menstrual cycle. Whether the findings in valproate and phenytoin can be generalized to other antiepilepsy drugs is not known; the results do raise issues, however, that urgently need further study.

Studies of valproate show that people absorb it more slowly and less efficiently when they take it in the evening than in the morning.[11] This finding is of concern because protection against seizures usually is needed most in NREM sleep, the state that dominates the first half of a night's sleep.

Research on phenytoin shows this medication breaks down faster and leaves the body sooner in the week before menstruation and when menstruation is under way than at other times of the month. Women using this medication thus have less protection against seizures at the time of month their risk of seizures rises.[12]

Better appreciation for menstrual cycle patterns in seizures has prompted changes in the treatment of women with epilepsy. If you are a premenopausal woman with epilepsy, your doctor may suggest that you have blood tests to determine the level of your anticonvulsant medication every week for one to two cycles. He or she also may suggest that you use either natural or synthetic progesterone premenstrually, or possibly throughout the month. Additionally, your doctor may prescribe a higher dose of your medication for times of the month that you have more seizures than usual.

If medications fail to control seizure activity, an implantable device, the vagus nerve stimulator, delivers a mild electrical pulse that may bring relief. Its action inhibits abnormal electrical activity in the brain. When seizures are severe and do not respond to other treatment, surgery to remove abnormal brain tissue may be necessary.

Timewise Tips

Men and women: use the Sleep/Wake Diary (page 353) to record the times your seizures occur. Extend the diary to cover a full month. Indicate seizures with a "Z" and anticonvulsant medication with "AC." Devise your own code for missed medication, excessive fatigue, illness, stress, and other relevant events. Take your diaries with you when you see your doctor.

Women: use the Menstrual Cycle Diary (page 329) to track your cycles for several months. Determine your date of ovulation reliably by using a home urine test kit that measures monthly shifts in hormone levels. Such kits are widely available in pharmacies. As on the Sleep/Wake Diary, indicate seizures with a "Z" and anticonvulsant medication with "AC." Devise your own code for missed medication, excessive fatigue, illness, stress, and other relevant events. Take your diaries with you when you see your doctor.

Men: use any monthly calendar with room for notes to track your seizure pattern. Take the calendar with you when you see your doctor.

Everyone: if your seizures occur primarily in sleep or just after awakening, talk to your doctor about the possibility of increasing your bedtime medication dose. Caution: do not change the dose or timing of your medication on your own.

Study. Visit the Web sites of the Epilepsy Foundation (www.efa.org) and the National Institute of Neurological Disorders and Stroke (www.nih.ninds.gov).

FIBROMYALGIA

Fibromyalgia (FM) follows a daily pain pattern similar to that of osteo-arthritis. Persons with FM suffer from muscle pain at specific locations in the body, known as *tender points.* They often feel stiff and achy when they awaken, then improve, and then worsen again as the day wears on. Many sleep poorly and feel fatigued in the daytime. Fatigue sometimes is more of a problem than pain.

"Until the mid-1980s, FM was virtually unheard of," the Arthritis Foundation reports.[1] Biological rhythm studies and other research turned up objective physical evidence that helps distinguish FM from other disorders that prompt similar complaints of pain, such as the chronic fatigue syndrome. An estimated five million Americans have FM. Most are women, who typically are diagnosed in their forties. FM may not be a new disorder, but simply one that previously got little attention. The high frequency of this disorder in women, combined with the difficulty of assessing pain, once led many physicians to dismiss FM as a hysterical complaint.

New awareness of stigmatizing sexual stereotypes is breaking down such attitudes. Physicians also know more about FM today. In the 1990s the American College of Rheumatology developed an FM pain symptom inventory and guidelines for physicians to use in diagnosing the disorder. The tender points most often reported by persons with FM include the neck, spine, shoulders, and hips. Some persons describe their pain as aching, radiating, gnawing, shooting, or burning.

Body Clocks May Be out of Sync in FM

Daily rhythms in mental performance in persons with FM may differ from those in healthy persons. In one study, matched groups of persons with and without FM took a complex computer test mimicking an office job in which a person has to do several things at once. The participants had to perform memory and math tasks at the same time, track a moving cursor, and tell two tones apart. The healthy group loved the challenge, Kimberly Cote and Harvey Moldofsky of the University of Toronto Centre for Sleep and Chronobiology found. "But the FM patients hated it," Moldofsky said. "They found the fast pace frustrating." Persons with FM responded more slowly than the others, although they proved equally accurate.[2]

Those with FM also suffer from nonrestorative sleep, not simply a vague complaint but one tied to a distinctive brain-wave pattern called *alpha/delta sleep*, in which alpha waves characteristic of wakefulness disrupt delta waves of deep sleep.[3] Sleep in those with FM differs from that in persons with a psychiatric illness called *somatoform pain disorder*, which involves a preoccupation with pain despite a lack of evidence to explain it.

In a clever demonstration that sleep loss itself may cause FM-type symptoms, Martha Lentz and Carol Landis of the University of Washington used a buzzer to disrupt deep sleep in healthy midlife women for three nights in a row. With each day, the women reported increasing muscle aches, tiredness, fatigue, and reduced vigor. After the third night, simply stroking their skin with a cotton-tipped swab made the skin red, leading the researchers to suggest that missed sleep may boost susceptibility to an inflammatory response.[4]

Women with FM had to agree to stop taking pain relievers and sleeping pills to take part in another sleep study these researchers conducted. Surprisingly, neither the women's pain nor their sleep got worse, according to objective measures. But they complained more about sleeping poorly. Disturbed perception of sleep may be another facet of this illness.[5]

In other studies, researchers have found abnormalities in a variety of daily hormone rhythms in persons with FM. They may secrete cortisol too early or in too little quantities. They also may secrete too little growth hormone, which adults need to maintain and repair muscles. This hormone normally is secreted in a series of bursts in deep sleep at the beginning of the night. If persons with FM get less of this type of sleep than healthy persons, they may also secrete less growth hormone. Some research suggests that giving growth hormone to persons with FM who do not make enough of it may reduce their pain. This therapy costs about $1,500 a month, however, out of reach for most people.[6]

Recognition that sleep is disturbed in persons with FM prompts the question of whether improving sleep would ease the pain. Happily, some research suggests that this is indeed the case.

Some persons with FM report that their symptoms worsen in winter and improve in the spring, much as in persons with a type of depression called seasonal affective disorder, or SAD. (See page 297.) Researchers attempted to realign rhythms in this group by using the same type of bright-light therapy that often helps those with SAD. Unfortunately, the studies done so far don't show any benefits from light treatment for pain, sleep, or mood in those with FM.[7]

Timewise Tips

Practice good sleep hygiene by getting enough sleep and getting up around the same time each day, including days off. If your sleep is disturbed, keep a sleep/wake diary. (See page 353.)

Keep a pain diary. (See page 208.)

Exercise in late morning and early afternoon, when pain bothers you least. Walking, swimming, biking, and cross-country skiing are among the many low-impact activities that can improve muscle fitness.

Use nonsteroidal anti-inflammatory drugs (NSAIDs) to relieve acute pain and swelling. While there have been no studies of the timing of NSAIDs specifically in FM, studies of these medications in osteoarthritis and rheumatoid arthritis suggest they cause fewer side effects if taken in the afternoon or evening. (See Arthritis, page 206.)

Anytime Tips

Talk to your doctor about taking antidepressant medications, which may both improve the quality of sleep and reduce pain.

To modulate pain, take a warm bath or shower, avoid overexertion, pace your activities, and practice relaxation techniques.

Study. Visit the Web sites of the Arthritis Foundation (www.arthritis.org) and the National Institute of Arthritis and Musculoskeletal and Skin Diseases (www.nih.gov/niams/healthinfo/fibrofs.htm).

GALLBLADDER ATTACKS

Gallbladder attacks may occur two to three times more often between 11 P.M. and 3 A.M. than at midday, the least frequent time.

This finding comes from a single study of fifty persons undergoing surgery for removal of gallstones.[1] The timing of gallbladder attacks, not yet rigorously investigated, may provide an important clue to help distinguish such attacks from other causes of pain in the upper right portion of the abdomen.

The gallbladder serves as a storage bin for chemicals produced by the liver to digest fats, vitamins, and other components of foods. Gallbladder attacks typically are episodic, and may last from a few minutes to several hours. The pain reflects inflammation in the lining of the gallbladder, or the presence of gallstones that block small passageways between the gallbladder and the liver or pancreas. The "stones" represent clumps of cholesterol, calcium, or other chemicals that commonly build up when people habitually consume large amounts of cholesterol. Someone who polishes off a pint or more of ice cream every night, for example, is a good candidate for gallstones.

An estimated one in ten Americans has gallstones. Most have few or no symptoms. One in three persons who experiences a gallbladder attack never has another. Surgery is not always necessary. Medications may be sufficient to dissolve gallstones.

Timewise Tips

Pay attention to the timing and anatomical location of any recurrent pain. It may help your doctor target the cause sooner.

Pay attention to when and what you eat. Avoid high-fat foods. Eat a well-balanced diet low in fat.

Study. Visit the Web site of the American College of Gastroenterology (www.acg.gi.org).

GOUT

Excruciating pain and swelling in the big toe, almost always starting at night or during sleep,[1] are the usual first indications of gout, a form of arthritis most common in men aged forty and older. Attacks also are more common in the spring than at other times of year.[2]

Gout occurs when excess uric acid, a bodily waste product, remains in the blood and accumulates in and around joints. Gout once was called the disease of kings, because it's linked with high consumption of protein-rich foods, such as bacon, liver, salmon, and turkey, and alcoholic beverages, items once enjoyed in large portions mainly by the wealthy.

A Physician Describes His Own Symptoms

◆ "The victim goes to bed and sleeps in good health. About two o'clock in the morning he is awakened by a severe pain in the great toe; more rarely in the heel, ankle or instep. . . . The pain which was at first moderate, becomes more intense. . . . So exquisite and lively meanwhile is the feeling of the part affected, that it cannot bear the weight of bedclothes nor the jar of a person walking into the room."[3]

—Thomas Sydenham, 1850

While the inflammation usually goes away without treatment in a week or so, attacks may recur if the underlying cause is not remedied. Some people with gout produce too much uric acid, a problem treated with drugs that control its buildup. Others do not excrete uric acid properly. In this instance, drugs that hasten its removal in the urine are used.

Timewise Tips

Use nonsteroidal anti-inflammatory drugs (NSAIDs) to relieve acute pain and swelling. While there have been no studies of the timing of NSAIDs specifically in gout, studies of these medications in osteoarthritis and rheumatoid arthritis suggest they are most effective and least likely to cause stomach irritation and other side effects if taken in the afternoon or evening. (See Arthritis, page 206.)

Pay attention to when and what you eat. Avoid consuming large portions of protein-rich foods that trigger attacks, such as bacon, liver, salmon, and turkey. Drink only in moderation.

Study. Visit the Web site of the Arthritis Foundation (www.arthritis.org).

GROWING PAINS

Pain occurs more often in children than many adults suspect. In any given month, a typical, normal, otherwise healthy child averages about four bouts of pain related to normal injuries and diseases, plus one episode of achy pain, according to Patricia McGrath of the University of Western Ontario Child Health Research Institute.[1]

The achy pains primarily involve stomachaches and headaches. But an estimated 15 percent of schoolchildren report deep pains in their legs and calves in the evening or at night.[2] The pains, which are comparable to leg cramps in adults, may be severe enough to keep a child from falling asleep, or to cause waking at night.[3] Growing pains also may occur in the afternoon after heavy exercise or when a child is overly fatigued.[4]

These so-called growing pains take their name from those who suffer from them, growing children. The name does not describe their cause. The process of growing, so far as is known, does not cause pain. The elementary school years when these pains most often occur are not even the time of most rapid growth and development. Infancy and adolescence far outpace these years in that regard.

There is no evidence that growing pains, despite the tears they may prompt, have any medical consequences. They eventually fade away.

Timewise Tips

Reassure your child that growing pains don't last long.

Teach your child that he or she can make the pain go away sooner and hurt less. Reading, listening to music, and playing with toys are effective strategies for active distraction, helping reduce fear and anxiety. Younger children often benefit from simple stretches and guided imagery, following suggestions such as "Let's take an imaginary walk through the zoo."

If your child complains of severe or persistent pain, consult your doctor. Children, sadly, sometimes do develop painful illnesses such as cancer or arthritis. Children who experience persistent pain without any evidence of injury or underlying disease may benefit from pain-relieving medications along with psychological support.

Study. Visit the Web site of the American Academy of Pediatrics (www. aap.org).

HAY FEVER

Hay fever typically worsens at night and peaks in severity in the morning. Persons with hay fever, also called *allergic rhinitis*, commonly wake up sneezing, with an itchy and stuffed or runny nose, and swollen puffy eyes. Despite the disorder's name, fever is not part of the picture. As the chart on page 261 graphically shows, hay fever symptoms last for several hours. Fortunately, treatment targeting this daily rhythm often can provide substantial relief.[1]

What Causes Hay Fever?

A lot more than hay, it turns out. A great variety of airborne pollens, molds, and other substances in the environment may trigger it. Hay fever flares in some people only in certain seasons: tree pollens set it off in the spring, grass pollens in the summer, and ragweed and other weed pollens in both the summer and fall. Such persons are said to have *seasonal rhinitis*. Others experience symptoms year-round. Triggers for *perennial rhinitis* include mold spores,

The Nose Has Its Own Clock

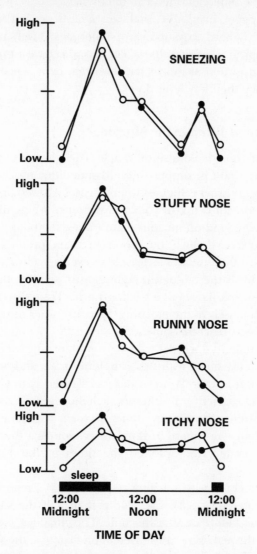

This chart shows daily patterns of symptoms reported by nearly 800 day-active persons with hay fever before they started taking medication. Study participants rated sneezing twice as intense in the morning as in the evening.[2]

house dust mites, and animal dander. Exposure to cigarette smoke, automobile exhausts, industrial chemicals, and other irritants may further aggravate hay fever.

About one in ten persons with hay fever suffers only seasonal allergies. The rest have symptoms year-round, and one-third of them also experience seasonal flare-ups. About one in five adults in the United States and four in ten children have hay fever. While people don't "outgrow" allergies, symptoms may fade with time. Allergies often run in families.[3]

The specific trigger, or *allergen*, that causes hay fever in those who have it year-round often is hard to pinpoint. As allergens travel via air, you can't escape them simply by staying indoors. Persons who have asthma, sinusitis, or other breathing disorders as well as hay fever may experience a worsening of that problem when their hay fever flares.

Why Are Symptoms Worst in the Morning?

Airways are most constricted around 5 A.M. The hormones adrenaline and cortisol, both important in suppressing inflammation, are at their daily lows at night. Swelling of tissues is highest when cortisol is lowest, in your rest span, and least when cortisol is up, in your active hours. When allergen particles enter your nose and land on mucous membranes, the body recognizes them as invaders. It mounts a defense, but it overreacts and produces too much histamine, a chemical that initiates a cascade of events leading to an inflammatory response. This is the biological equivalent of sending the whole town's fire engines to put out flames in a backyard grill. Tissues swell and itch, and they do so most intensely in the morning. Mucous tissues near the nose in the throat, eyes, and ears react the same way.

Two medical students documented persistent morning sneezing by secretly keeping tabs on a classmate with this symptom for six and one-half months. Their first-year class at Case Western Reserve University in Cleveland, Ohio, attended lectures together for four hours each morning, six days a week. They took turns recording the precise time of their classmate's sneezes and counted more than one sneeze in rapid succession as a single event. When the school year ended, they plotted the times of the 118 sneezes they had noted.

"The subject sneezed with startling regularity," they reported, "in a short time interval centered at 8:20 A.M." More than half the sneezes occurred within ten minutes before or after this time. The circadian sneezing persisted from November through May and shifted immediately to the same clock hour following the daylight saving time change. Startled but amused when told of the study, their classmate agreed to share her medical, allergy, and sneeze histories. The student researchers, Arthur Grant and Eric Roter, ruled out exposure to perfumes, light, and other factors as causes of the sneezes. They concluded that an underlying circadian process was the most likely explanation.[4]

The worsening of symptoms in the early morning helps explain why hay fever is a significant cause of school and work absences. A survey of over 4,000 adults with hay fever conducted in 1999 for the Children's Hospital of Pittsburgh found that the disorder hampered many aspects of daily life. The majority of respondents said they had to avoid spending time outdoors, cleaning their homes and other daily chores, and physical exercise or sports. Even those who took medication ranked loss of taste and smell, difficulty concentrating, and fatigue as moderately severe.[5] The fatigue, sometimes attributed to side effects of medication, also reflects poor sleep resulting from nasal congestion.[6] About 75 percent of hay fever sufferers complain of difficulty sleeping.[7]

T-i-m-e Spells Relief

Studies performed to date show clear benefits of timed treatment in persons whose symptoms show a pronounced daily pattern. In selecting a particular type of drug or drugs for you, your doctor will take into account the nature and severity of your specific symptoms. If you use over-the-counter hay fever remedies, read labels carefully, as different products contain ingredients that serve different purposes and have side effects that may help or disrupt sleep and alertness depending on when you take them. Here's what is now known about types of medications commonly used to treat hay fever:

Antihistamines

This type of medication helps control sneezing and a stuffy or runny nose. Antihistamines that you can purchase without a prescription have fatigue as a major side effect. Thus, they are best taken at bedtime, as they may help you sleep. You should not take them in the daytime if you expect to drive or engage in other activities demanding alertness. Over-the-counter antihistamines generally work for periods ranging from four to twelve hours.

New nonsedating antihistamines that require a prescription can be used in the daytime without making you sleepy. They are designed to be taken once or twice a day. Taking a once-a-day antihistamine in the evening produces better control of morning symptoms than does taking the same medication once a day in the morning. The twenty-four-hour antihistamines exert their peak action twelve hours after they are taken, so an evening dose goes to work when it is needed most.[8]

Decongestants

These medications reduce nasal stuffiness but don't affect sneezing, runny nose, or nasal itching. Doctors often recommend them for persons with hay fever year-round for whom stuffiness is the predominant symptom. Prescription decongestant tablet and nasal spray medications usually ease nasal congestion for about twelve hours. Although there have been no studies to assess the best time to take them, these drugs are known to have a stimulating effect and thus may be more appropriate for daytime use. If taken at bedtime they may disrupt sleep and aggravate urinary and prostate problems. (See Urinary

Disorders, page 362.) They also may raise blood pressure. If you have high blood pressure, talk to your doctor before using them.

Decongestants also are available in over-the-counter topical aerosol sprays or drops. Caution: do not use these formulations for more than a few days. Doing so may produce tolerance, not only making the drugs less effective but also causing congestion to worsen.

Anticholinergics

These prescription medications, generally delivered via an aerosol spray, suppress production of mucous and other watery secretions in nasal and sinus tissues. They help dry up a runny nose but don't affect sneezing and nasal itching. Again, no studies have been conducted to determine optimal timing. Studies of the treatment of asthma with related medications, however, suggest bedtime dosing may work better than morning dosing to relieve morning symptoms.

Cromolyn Sodium

This over-the-counter medication, delivered in spray form, is designed to prevent rather than treat hay fever symptoms. It inhibits the release of histamine and other inflammation-causing substances. The best time to use it has not been studied.

Corticosteroids

These medications, available only by prescription, reduce inflammation and congestion of nasal and sinus tissues. They're usually given in a form that is inhaled one to four times a day and has infrequent side effects.

Doctors sometimes prescribe tablet corticosteroids for persons with severe hay fever. Proper timing is critical here to prevent side effects such as suppression of normal cortisol secretion, mood changes, and weight gain. These drugs work best and are safest when taken in the morning right after awakening, in synchrony with the body's normal peak production of cortisol.

If people don't obtain relief with once-a-day or alternate-day morning dosing, doctors sometimes suggest a one-week course of once-a-day dosing in the midafternoon, about eight to nine hours after awakening. Midafternoon dosing of this type of medication works well in the treatment of other inflammatory diseases such as *asthma* (see page 220) and *arthritis* (see page 212).

Eye Drops

Eye drops containing an antihistamine can ease eye redness, itching, and watering. Avoid wearing contact lenses when these symptoms flare.

Timewise Tips

Schedule doctor visits at the time of day your symptoms (or those of your child) are worst. That will help the doctor make a more accurate assessment of symptom severity. Schedule allergy skin tests in the later afternoon, when they are likely to be most accurate. (See Skin Disorders, page 334.)

Adapt the Breathing Diary (page 219) to your symptoms. Record when symptoms occur, and take the diary with you when you see your doctor. If you have hay fever year-round, try keeping a symptom diary a few days in each season. Knowing your own pattern may help you plan trips and other activities at that time of year.

Tell your doctor if you experience daytime fatigue or sleep poorly. Nasal stuffiness can make sleep restless. Some medications used to treat hay fever may disturb sleep. Your doctor may change the dose or type of medication to help you sleep better.

If you have seasonal allergies, stay indoors in an air-conditioned environment and drive in an air-conditioned car when pollen counts are high.

Review Timewise Tips and Anytime Tips for asthma (pages 222 and 223) and adapt tactics for daily coping to your symptom pattern.

Study. Visit the Web site of the Asthma and Allergy Foundation of America (www.aafa.org).

HEADACHES

Some headaches derive their name from the time they occur.

Alarm-clock headaches awaken people from sleep. They include *migraines* and *cluster headaches,* which strike in episodic bursts. Many women experience *menstrual migraines* just before or while having their periods.

Morning headaches occur in persons with sleep apnea, a disorder in which breathing repeatedly stops in sleep, causing the amount of oxygen that reaches the brain to plunge dangerously low. *Morning-after headaches* may strike if you've had too much to drink the night before. They reflect in part alcohol's sleep-disruptive effects.

Sleeping late may trigger *caffeine-withdrawal headaches* in habitual coffee-drinkers. *Performance-day headaches* afflict jittery actors and musicians. Indeed, such headaches are so common that they go by many names. *Preacher's headache* occurs in some members of the clergy on days they deliver sermons. Students sometimes report *exam-day headaches* just after waking up. Parents often are amazed by how quickly such headaches disappear after they agree to let their child stay home. Harried workers, trying to pack all their chores into their days off, may develop *weekend headaches.* As these examples suggest, *tension headaches* may erupt reliably at certain times of the day or days of the week, or in specific situations that cause the sufferer to feel unusual stress. Some people reliably get headaches the day *after* a stressful event.

Sleeping too little or too much, skipping meals, and traveling rapidly across multiple time zones may prompt headaches, too, perhaps by jarring body rhythms out of their usual synchrony.

Biological-rhythms research offers new understanding of the causes of some common types of headaches, and new approaches to headache treatment.

Almost everyone gets headaches now and then. Most go away on their own with simple, common-sense treatment: you stop what you're doing; rest in a quiet, dark place, apply ice or heat, maybe take aspirin or acetaminophen. Americans spend half a billion dollars on drugstore headache remedies annually. Some 45 million Americans suffer from recurring or chronic headaches that interfere with school, work, and family life, according to the National Institute of Neurological and Communicative Disorders and Stroke.[1]

How Does It Hurt?

♦ Like most pain, that of headaches is hard to assess. Pounding, stabbing, throbbing, splitting, nagging. . . . Headache sufferers often offer graphic descriptions.

"When I have a headache, I feel as if someone has put a pane of cloudy glass between me and the world. The pain feels like a small animal with big teeth gnawing on the side of my head."

—Katy, age 38

"It feels like I am in a marching band and my head is the drum."

—Adam, age 11

A nineteenth-century etching by George Cruikshank pictures a hapless headache sufferer under siege by small devils. The demons assault his ears with a trumpet and off-key tunes, while attacking his skull with a hammer, drill, corkscrew, and red-hot poker. Stone Age healers actually did drill holes in skulls, perhaps attempts to relieve headaches.

Migraines

Most migraines involve dull, throbbing pain on one side of the head. The word migraine, in fact, comes from the Greek *hemicrania*, which means "half the head." One in five sufferers may have a warning that a migraine is developing, often a heightened sensitivity to light or sound. Some see flashing lights or zigzag lines or feel queasy. This warning, called an aura, may precede the headache by several hours.

Migraine Warnings

◆ "Occasionally, I see a cobalt-blue flash the night before I get a headache. Even without the flash, I know when I am going to wake up with a migraine. I call it being in Migraine Alley."

—Katy

In one study, fifteen chronic migraine sufferers kept daily diaries for five months, reporting 211 headaches. Three out of four migraine attacks began between 6 A.M. and noon.[2] Migraines usually last a few hours, but may drag on for several days, even weeks. Sleep laboratory studies show the "alarm clock" attacks that awaken people in the morning often start in or soon after REM sleep, a time when heart rate and blood pressure are highly variable.[3] For migraines that occur in the daytime, a nap sometimes proves a good antidote. About 23 million Americans, including young children, suffer from migraines. The tendency to get them runs in families. In susceptible persons, blood vessels appear to overreact to various triggers. These include

- stress, particularly that involving disruptions in your daily schedule and time pressures
- changes in weather, humidity, or altitude
- missing a meal
- consuming certain foods or food additives. Foods include yogurt, nuts, lima beans, chocolate, aged cheeses, and red wine. Food additives include nitrates and nitrites used in processed meats, yellow food coloring, and monosodium glutamate.
- in women, shifts in reproductive hormone levels

Migraines and other headaches involve spasms of the small blood vessels of the brain and head. When these spasms reduce the flow of blood to the brain, arteries within the brain open wider to make sure the brain gets the oxygen it needs. Nerve cells spring into action, alerting the brain that something's wrong and, at the same time, mobilizing defenses. The flurry of activity produces the sensation of throbbing pain.

The nerve signals travel on a major pain route traversing the face, scalp, and muscles surrounding blood vessels in the head via chemical messengers, such as serotonin. Studies show that serotonin levels drop when blood vessels swell. Most headache-relieving drugs boost the amount of serotonin in the body. What's especially interesting here is that serotonin also plays a key role in carrying messages to and from the biological clock. These findings reinforce the suspicion that the biological clock is a strong determinant of the timing of headaches.

Menstrual Migraines

The key impact of hormonal shifts on migraines may explain why women get migraines three to four times more often than men.[4] Two-thirds of migraines in women are menstrual migraines, occurring in the four days before a menstrual period, or while a period is in progress, as gynecologist Katharina Dalton documented back in the 1970s. Some women get migraines only at menstruation, when estrogen levels plummet to their monthly low. Dalton distinguished three different daily patterns of menstrual migraines. Attacks associated with water retention occur in the early morning. Those related to stress occur in the evening, she said, and those linked to low blood sugar occur after three or more hours without eating.[5]

Birth-control pills make migraines worse in some women, but better in others. In pregnancy, a time when estrogen levels stay high, many women report that their migraines disappear. Some, however, experience migraines for the first time. Some women also develop migraines immediately after childbirth, when estrogen falls sharply. Migraines usually become less frequent as women grow older, but they sometimes make their first appearance only after menopause.

Cluster Headaches

Cluster headaches, named for their repeated appearances in groups or clusters, start as a minor pain around one eye that eventually spreads to that side of the face. The pain quickly intensifies and becomes excruciating. People often experience reddening and tearing of the eye, a droopy eyelid, and a stuffed nostril on the painful side of the face.

Film Noir

♦ "Suddenly a huge phantom bird sank three talons of its angry claws deeply into my head and face and tried to lift me. No warnings, no preliminary signs. Just wham! A massive, killing pain came over my right eye. . . . In the dark, I moaned, I panted. Ballooned my cheeks, blew out short bursts of air, licked my hot lips, wiped tears that poured out of my right eye, and clawed at my head trying to uproot the fiendish talons from their iron grip. One racking hour later the talons let go."[6]

—Frank Capra, film director and producer

Cluster headaches are six times more frequent in men than in women. They do not run in families. They affect an estimated one million Americans, who reportedly show certain striking physical similarities: the typical cluster patient is a tall, muscular middle-aged man with a square, jutting, or dimpled chin, a craggy face, hazel eyes, and coarse skin.

Two-thirds of cluster-headache attacks always or usually start in sleep, particularly REM sleep. The headaches usually last about thirty minutes, but may recur later in the day, and at the same hours the next day, often for weeks or months. Some people have them several times a day. A very rare type of cluster headache involves repeated brief attacks, usually less than two minutes long, but up to several hundred times a day for several days. Such episodes are most frequent in the morning, starting soon after awakening.[7]

Structural abnormalities of the hypothalamus, the area of the brain that houses the biological clock, may account for the distinctive time patterns of cluster headaches. Using sophisticated brain-imaging techniques to examine persons with cluster headaches while headaches were under way, Peter Goadsby and his colleagues at the Institute of Neurology in London found both increased gray matter and increased blood flow in this area.[8]

After a blitz, cluster headaches may disappear for months or years. Bouts of cluster headaches are more frequent in the spring and fall than in summer and winter, which suggests a link with seasonal hormone changes or changes in hours of daylight.[9] A medication sometimes used for migraines, ergotamine tartrate, often can subdue a cluster headache if taken early in the attack. Some cluster patients benefit from inhaling pure oxygen through a mask for a few minutes.

Tension Headaches

These are the most common type of headaches. About two out of five people, slightly more women than men, say they get tension headaches once or twice a month. Their name comes from accompanying muscle tension in shoulders, neck, face, and scalp. In tension headaches, pain typically starts above the eyes or neck, and then expands into a "hat-band" pattern around the head. Some people liken it to feeling that their head is trapped in a vise.

These usually are daytime headaches, and last about thirty minutes. The pain typically is nagging but mild. Sustained muscle tension is a common trigger.

A Reminder: Stand Up and Stretch!

◆ I'm at the computer all day and get so involved with my work I don't even go to the bathroom. By 5 P.M., my neck is stiff and my head hurts.

Roughly two out of every hundred people suffer from chronic tension headaches. These occur several times a week, last longer, and often include symptoms of nausea and increased sensitivity to light or sound. These symptoms are so similar to those of migraines that some researchers suspect they are migraines in sheep's clothing.

Depression and anxiety often play a key role in triggering tension headaches. Timing often suggests the likely cause.

Anxiety and Headaches

◆ On Friday night, I'd like to go out with my friends, but my mother insists I come for dinner. That's headache time.

I don't have to look at the clock to know when it's time for our daily staff meeting. My headache tells me that.

Studies in which headache sufferers keep daily diaries show that headache-inducing situations often show high consistency for any one person, but vary considerably from one person to another.

People with high levels of education suffer more episodic tension headaches, but not chronic ones, than those who are less educated, according to researchers at the Johns Hopkins University School of Public Health who surveyed more than 13,000 Baltimore-area residents by phone. Headache sufferers miss nearly nine work days a year on average because of their headaches, they found.[10]

Sex and Headaches

The ties between sex and headaches are complex: some people avoid sex because of headaches; others seek sex to relieve headaches; and still others develop headaches following orgasm. When it's "Not tonight dear, I have a headache," stress or anxiety may be the culprit. But when it's "Not tonight dear, I might get a headache," blame exertion and sudden expansion of blood vessels pressing against the scalp. Some people get similar headaches after any vigorous exercise. Such headaches suggest a possible abnormality of blood vessels. If you get them, see your doctor promptly.

The Exploding Head Syndrome

Some people report sudden sensations of flashing lights and/or loud banging noises in the head that rouse them from sleep, a condition dubbed the *exploding head syndrome*. First described in medical writings in the 1920s, this unusual tension headache may occur as often as several times a night, every night, for months on end. A fifty-five-year-old woman reporting this frightening experience also heard a rustling sound, as if made by a fire. Swedish researchers who studied her and others with similar complaints in their sleep laboratory reported that sufferers often were awake, not asleep, at the time the sensations occurred. The researchers found nothing wrong with their patients, other than high levels of stress. Most of the patients reported hectic life situations when their attacks were intense, improvement when things settled down, and recurrences in later stressful times.[11]

Timing May Be Tip-off to Diagnosis

While most headaches have no serious medical consequences, not all are benign. About one in ten are caused by sinusitis, brain tumors, brain injuries, or other diseases. Usually, but not always, these also include other signs, such as ear pain, if Eustachian tubes are blocked, or slurred speech, if a person has had a stroke.

Researchers at the Stanford University Medical School surveyed attendees at a headache clinic. They found forty-nine adults, 9 percent of the clinic's patients, who had suffered for nineteen years on average from headaches that occurred mostly in sleep or just after it. All had tried many different treatments, and some had experienced an adverse reaction to medications they had received.

When evaluated in the sleep laboratory, more than half of these people turned out to have sleep disorders, including obstructive sleep apnea, periodic limb movements (see page 339), fibromyalgia (see page 255), and a type of insomnia related to poor sleep habits (see page 340).

With appropriate treatment, the headaches disappeared in everyone with obstructive sleep apnea and nearly half of those with periodic limb movements. Many persons with fibromyalgia and insomnia reported their headaches occurred less often. Unfortunately, these persons suffered needlessly for many years. "If timing of headaches is neglected," sleep specialist Christian Guilleminault warns, "a correct diagnosis may be missed."[12]

Old and New Medications Ease Headaches

Pain relievers and pain preventers comprise the two main categories.

Pain Relievers

These are taken to abort or cut the pain after headaches start. Aspirin, acetaminophen, and nonsteroidal anti-inflammatory drugs (NSAIDs) are home medicine cabinet staples, and may be sufficient for the majority of headaches. New formulations of these drugs contain caffeine and may offer speedier relief for daytime headaches. Warning: taking headache remedies daily, and then trying to cut back, may cause rebound headaches for a few days. To minimize stomach irritation, avoid taking NSAIDs in high doses in the morning for more than a week.

The newest prescription medications, drugs in the triptan family, include sumatriptan, naratriptan, zolmitriptan, and risotriptan. These drugs all increase the activity of serotonin, and constrict swollen blood vessels in the brain and scalp. They come in different forms, including tablets that are swallowed or that melt on the tongue, in nasal sprays, and by injection. There are no published studies on the best time of day to take these medications. People usually take them at the first indication that a headache is starting.

Pain Preventers

If you have severe headaches more than three times a month, your doctor may suggest that you take daily medications. These seldom stop headaches completely, but they usually reduce their frequency and severity. Many doctors view propranolol and other beta blockers, which relax blood vessels, as the treatment of choice, especially if stress plays a big role in triggering your headaches. Antidepressant drugs that change the way brain cells communicate and also reduce REM sleep help some headache sufferers, whether or not they also are depressed. If these medications don't help you, your doctor has a long list of other choices.

Timewise Tips

Keep a headache diary. (See page 273.)

Practice good sleep hygiene by getting enough sleep and getting up around the same time each day, including days off.

Eat meals at regular times. Don't skip meals.

Get outside every day. Regular exposure to daylight-intensity light may help prevent migraine attacks, some studies suggest. This is a curious finding, since many who suffer migraines find bright light disturbing, at least while their headaches are in progress. Bright light at other times, however, may elevate levels of serotonin in the brain, and protect against headaches.

Timewise Tips for Women with Migraines

If you have menstrual migraines:

If you take birth-control pills, talk to your doctor about changing the dose or brand. Ask about using the pills all month long, wearing an estrogen patch just before and while you are having your period, or using estrogen replacement therapy. Some women with disabling menstrual migraines that do not respond to other treatments benefit from using the drug bromocriptine.

If you have menopause-related migraines:

Talk to your doctor about starting hormone replacement therapy, or, if you already use it, changing the dose.

Headache Diary

Name _____

See a doctor promptly if a headache

- often wakes you up
- suddenly worsens
- lasts for more than a day
- follows a blow to the head
- includes convulsions or confusion

- includes weakness or loss of balance
- involves pain in the eye or ear
- accompanies a high fever and stiff neck
- starts or gets worse when you have sex

Make four or more photocopies of this page, and keep track of your headaches for a month or longer. Take this diary with you when you see your doctor.

Women: Date of Last Menstrual Period _____

Day/Date	Start Time	Stop Time	Awakened from sleep? Yes/No?	Warning Signs & Symptoms	Location of Head Pain	Severity Low High 1 2 3 4 5	Possible Triggers	Treatment Used

If you are pregnant:

Caution: Do not take any medication, even drugstore remedies, without talking to your doctor first. While some women have migraines more frequently in the first trimester, most women find that these headaches disappear while they are pregnant.

Timewise Tips If You Have Cluster Headaches

In a cluster period, avoid changes in your schedule, particularly in the time you sleep. Do not take afternoon naps, which often bring on this type of headache.

Avoid alcohol in a cluster period. A headache may start before you finish your first drink.

Anytime Tips

Exercise regularly. It's a great way to reduce tension in the muscles of the shoulders, neck, and scalp that might trigger tension headaches.

At work, take frequent breaks. Stand up and stretch if possible. Even sitting, you can turn your head, roll your shoulders, lift your arms over your head.

Pay attention to possible dietary triggers, and then avoid them.

If you smoke, stop. Smoking may trigger both migraine and cluster headaches.

Drink only in moderation. To ease a hangover headache, try honey, which helps the body burn alcohol faster, or caffeine, which helps dilated arteries tighten up again.

Learn tactics for stress reduction, such as relaxation techniques and biofeedback.

Talk to your doctor about medications so that you're ready the next time a headache strikes.

Study. Visit the Web sites of the National Institute of Neurological Disorders and Stroke (www.ninds.nih.gov) and the National Headache Foundation (www.headaches.org).

HEARTBURN

Heartburn, a burning sensation in the lower chest, peaks in the evening and at night. It occurs when a valve at the top of the stomach, designed to keep stomach contents from escaping, fails to stay shut. Stomach acid then backs up into the esophagus, the tube that conveys foods and liquids from your mouth to your stomach. While the stomach has a special lining to protect it from acid's caustic effects, the esophagus does not; that's why it hurts.

Your doctor may use the medical term for heartburn, *gastroesophageal reflux disease.*

Pain peaks in tandem with the daily rhythm of stomach acid secretion. Although the stomach secretes acid whenever you eat, it secretes two to three times more of it between 10 P.M. and 2 A.M. than at other times, even if you fast.[1] If the tissues lining your stomach are irritated or injured, this normal rise in stomach acid may trigger pain.

Since stomach acid helps digest food, the secretion of copious amounts late in the day may seem odd. But acid secreted when you eat gets neutralized by food. Acid secreted at night, several hours after day-active humans typically consume large meals, serves a secondary purpose: to destroy bacteria. It thus may help mop up the stomach, ridding it of any unwelcome residue from the day's meals. Our stomach acid secretion rhythm may be an evolutionary leftover, a tactic that enhanced survival when food safety was more dicey than it is now.

The pain of heartburn may spread sideways in the chest and upward into the neck, throat, jaw, and face. If severe, it may be confused with a heart attack. (Human nature being what it is, however, people more often dismiss the pain of a heart attack as mere indigestion.)

Heartburn also may include belching and regurgitation of a sour-tasting substance into the back of the throat. The pain warns of irritation to the delicate tissue of the esophagus, and is a symptom that should prompt a visit to your doctor. Sustained backup of stomach acid into the esophagus may cause ulcers and other injuries.

In one study, persons with heartburn experienced pain for fifteen minutes an hour on average, for several hours following their evening meal. If you often have heartburn while awake, you're likely to have it when you sleep, too. When you are awake, a few swallows will send the acid back down to the stomach. Saliva also acts as a natural antacid. But the recumbent posture of sleep makes it easier for acid to travel up into the throat. Moreover, people swallow ten times less often and produce less saliva while asleep than when awake.

To get rid of the acid, people often cough and choke in their sleep. The acid sometimes goes down the wrong way, entering the lungs instead of the stomach, worsening asthma or other chronic lung diseases.

Take Medication in the Evening for Nighttime Symptoms

Drugstore remedies may ease occasional heartburn, especially that occurring mainly after meals, but they don't last long enough to relieve nighttime heartburn. If you experience heartburn at night or at least two or three times a week, your doctor may suggest prescription medications that reduce acid secretion. Widely used drugs include ranitidine, cimetidine, famotidine, omeprazole, and lansoprazole.

If your symptoms occur chiefly or only at night, take medications that end in "-tidine" in the evening. These are members of a family called H_2-receptor antagonists. Studies show that taking a given dose of this type of medication only in the evening is much more effective than taking the same dose only in the morning. Dividing the medication into both a morning and an evening dose offers no advantage in terms of efficacy, and is less convenient than taking an evening dose alone.[2] Medications that end in "-prazole," known as proton-pump inhibitors, generally work best when taken once a day in the morning.

If your symptoms occur throughout the day, take your medication once a day before breakfast, or twice a day, with equal doses before breakfast and before your evening meal.[3]

Timewise Tips

If heartburn often bothers you:

Elevate the head of your bed, using six- to eight-inch blocks.

Eat your evening meal early, and don't snack after dinner. Avoid big meals, and spicy or fatty foods, carbonated drinks, or other foods or beverages that give you indigestion.

Sit up for two to three hours after meals; don't lie down on the couch to read or watch TV.

Don't exercise vigorously, or do chores that involve prolonged bending, soon after eating.

Keep a diary to record when you suffer heartburn, and when and what you ate. Take it with you when you see your doctor.

Anytime Tips

Wear loose clothing without tight waistbands or belts.

If overweight, shed some pounds.

Ask your doctor whether any of the medications you take may be contributing to your heartburn. These include both prescription drugs and remedies you buy in a drug store or health food store. Ask about prescription medications designed to relieve heartburn.

Study. Visit the Web site of the National Digestive Diseases Information Clearinghouse (www.niddk.nih.gov/health/digest/pubs/heartbrn/heartbrn.htm).

HEART DISEASE

Nearly every type of heart ailment, from heartbeat irregularities to heart attacks, displays daily, weekly, and annual biological rhythms.

Heart Attacks Peak in Morning

Heart attacks occur more often between 6 A.M. and noon than at other times of day. Records of calls for ambulances, times of emergency helicopter runs, and hospital admissions offer ample evidence. One study reviewed the times of 66,635 heart attacks: Mylan Cohen of Harvard Medical School and his colleagues analyzed results of more than thirty different studies published in medical journals between 1985 and 1996, all confirming this morning surge. The time pattern for more than 19,000 sudden deaths from heart disease proved strikingly similar.[1]

This vulnerable time is not clock time per se, but rather the first hours after waking. Scientists debated for many years whether heart attacks occurred more often in the morning, or if they were simply first noticed then. They knew that 20 to 25 percent of all heart attacks cause little or no pain, and are recognized only after additional problems occur. In such cases, they could only speculate about when the attacks had occurred.

Then, in 1985, Harvard Medical School researchers found that a specific enzyme, creatine kinase, shows up in an altered form in the blood about four hours after an injury to the heart muscle, allowing the onset time and even extent of a heart attack to be established. Using this heart-damage marker, James Muller and his colleagues studied over 700 patients, finding that their heart attacks began three times more often between 9 A.M. and 10 A.M., the peak time, than between 11 P.M. and midnight, the least frequent time.[2]

What Makes Mornings Risky?

Heart attacks are sudden events, like the closing of a dam in a mighty river. Men are more likely than women to show the so-called classic warning signs: pain may explode in the middle of the chest, and radiate to the neck, jaw, shoulder, arm (usually left arm), and back. A person in the grip of a heart attack may sweat profusely, feel dizzy, weak, and short of breath. In women, the first signs of a heart attack may be more subtle: nausea, vomiting, unexplained anxiety, palpitations, a feeling of pressure in the chest, or a cold sweat. Women, and even their doctors, sometimes do not recognize the importance of these often vague symptoms, delaying treatment. Feeling short of breath on awakening is a red flag for both sexes.

Just waking up can set this process in motion. This seemingly simple act proves to be a complex event. Most people awaken in REM sleep, or soon after it. Heart rate and breathing normally are more variable at this time.

Once you awaken, but before you even get out of bed, your heart beats faster, and blood pressure surges upward. These activities make the heart work harder, and increase the amount of oxygen the heart muscle needs by

50 percent.[3] The sudden demand for oxygen may make the heart beat irregularly, or even cause chest pain.[4]

Near your habitual time of awakening, the stress hormones adrenaline, vasopressin, and cortisol pour into your blood, readying you for the day's activities. Their cumulative effect is to narrow tiny arteries that supply blood to the heart muscles, restricting blood flow. At the same time, they speed up blood clotting and prompt a sudden increase in blood pressure.

The added force of blood surging through the heart may dislodge fat deposits clinging to artery walls, tearing tissue and causing bleeding. Blood cells called platelets are more "sticky" in the morning than later in the day. They clump together, forming clots at the site of the injury that may be large enough to block the arteries. Clot formation is most intense in the morning.

Sitting up, and then standing up, further increase your heart's workload. With age, blood vessels become less elastic. If your alarm clock's buzzer annoys you, the morning news distresses you, or your child appears at your side with a knot in her shoelace, your mental stress level also soars. The heart is exquisitely sensitive to such perturbations.

Morning heart attacks usually cause more heart-muscle damage than heart attacks at other times.[5] People are more likely to die from morning heart attacks, too, according to a study reviewing the times of some 20,000 sudden deaths caused by heart attacks.[6] Going back to bed won't change this picture. Patients confined to bed in hospitals and nursing homes still have more heart attacks in the morning.

Americans experience more than 1,100,000 new and recurrent heart attacks every year. Heart disease is the leading cause of death in the United States, killing 500,000 Americans annually. Few women develop heart disease before menopause, thanks to estrogen's protective effect. In women over age sixty, however, heart disease is the leading killer.

Angina (Chest Pain) Peaks in Morning

Angina pectoris, or pain in the chest, may produce a sensation of burning, pressure, or aching in the chest. It may be more discomforting than painful. The sensation often starts under the breastbone, and, as with a heart attack, sometimes spreads to the neck, jaw, shoulder, arm (usually left arm), and back. About 12 million Americans have angina.

Angina indicates that some muscles of the heart do not receive enough oxygenated blood. Trouble with either supply or demand may cause angina: too little blood may get through, or physical exercise or mental stress may require more blood than is available. Exertion and stress are the most common triggers for angina, but angina sometimes occurs when a person is resting. Angina attacks may even occur without causing pain. Indeed, an estimated 70 percent of angina attacks are "silent." Abnormalities in the heart's blood supply can be detected easily, however, because the electrical activity of the heart muscle shows characteristic changes. Continuous round-the-clock monitoring, using lightweight, portable, battery-powered monitors, provides a profile of the severity and times of even silent angina attacks.

For this procedure, small metal discs called electrodes will be pasted temporarily on your chest. Signals from your heart will be transmitted through the electrodes to wires connected to a small recorder and timer you wear on your waist or on a strap around your neck. After twenty-four or forty-eight hours, you'll return to the doctor's office, where the information will be downloaded to a computer. While wearing the monitor, you probably also will be asked to keep a diary to record any heart symptoms.

As with heart attacks, angina attacks associated with exertion or stress peak between 6 A.M. and noon, the first six hours of the daily activity period. Nearly three-quarters of angina attacks occur in these hours.[7] The duration of these types of angina attacks also exhibits profound circadian rhythmicity. A study at the University of Texas Medical Center in Houston found that angina attacks totaled only five seconds per hour on average between 2 A.M. and 4 A.M., their daily low, but 3.7 minutes per hour on average between 10 A.M. and 11 A.M., their daily high.

The angina that occurs when a person is at rest shows a different daily pattern. Attacks of this type of angina, called variant angina, occur thirty times more often between 2 A.M. and 4 A.M. than at other times of day.[8]

Caution: Chest pain has many causes, including indigestion and muscle strain. Women in their premenopausal years experience chest pain more often than men, although they seldom have underlying heart disease. Chest pain not caused by heart disease may be more frequent and more severe in both premenopausal women with high estrogen levels and postmenopausal women using estrogen replacement therapy than in women with lower estrogen levels. The Women's Ischemic Syndrome Evaluation study, a multicenter program funded by the National Institutes of Health that runs to 2001, is aiming to better understand the causes and consequences of chest pain in women.

Most episodes of chest pain do not reflect angina or heart attacks. Still, they are a message that something is wrong, and they deserve your attention.

Heart Attacks Jump on Mondays

This pattern suggests that small changes in daily routines may disrupt biological rhythms. Over the weekend, people often stay up late. They may miss sleep, or sleep much later than usual. They often consume more alcohol. A similar situation occurs after vacations, prompting an increase in what doctors call "holiday heart syndrome." One study found that twice as many episodes of life-threatening irregular heart rhythms occurred on Monday as on either Saturday or Sunday.[9]

Social factors may play a role here. Caught up in weekend activities, people may minimize chest pain. They may not be able to get in to see their usual doctor, or they may choose not to "bother" the doctor on a weekend.[10]

Heart Attacks Surge in Winter

Fatal heart attacks occur more often in winter than at other times of year. You may be tempted to blame cold weather activities that strain the heart, such as shoveling snow or breathing frigid air, but even areas where temperatures stay mild year-round show increased deaths in winter.[11] In one study, University of Southern California researchers analyzed death certificates for everyone who died of heart disease in Los Angeles for twelve years, more than 220,000 persons in all. They found 33 percent more deaths occurred in December and January than in June through September.[12] Heart attack deaths in the Southern Hemisphere peak in July, when it's winter there. What causes the winter peak remains a mystery, although annual rhythms in certain body functions, such as blood pressure and cholesterol levels, both higher in winter, along with complications of wintertime respiratory infections, may play a role. Changes in daylength may contribute to this rhythm, too. Nonbiological factors such as holiday overindulgence in food or alcohol and stress also may have an impact.

Is Morning Exercise Safe?

Morning exercise theoretically increases your risk of suffering a heart attack, as it further stresses the heart. But don't cancel your 7 A.M. bike ride or morning run. And don't use this information as an excuse to avoid exercise, either. One study looked at 221 persons with known heart disease, persons who had had heart attacks, heart surgery, or other cardiac conditions. All agreed to participate in a cardiac rehabilitation program.

Paul Murray and his colleagues at Wake Forest University divided the volunteers into two groups. Both groups exercised three days a week, one from 7:30 A.M. to 8:30 A.M., and the other for one hour sometime between 3 P.M. and 5 P.M. In more than 250,000 hours of exercise, only seven cardiac events occurred. That means that even in this at-risk group, the incidence of heart problems was extremely low. Time of day had no impact.[13]

If you have a healthy heart and work out regularly, your risk of having a heart attack while exercising presumably is even smaller. The benefits of regular exercise at any time of day far outshine the theoretical drawbacks. Indeed, a sedentary lifestyle virtually doubles your risk of having a heart attack. If you are a couch potato, particularly if you are overweight, and plan to start an exercise program, see your doctor for a heart health checkup first, and work out in the afternoon or early evening until you get in shape.

When Is Sex Safest?

Sexual activity, a rather special form of exercise, often prompts anxiety in persons who have had a heart attack. Until recently, doctors often told patients that strain on the heart in sex was the same as that of climbing a flight of stairs, and that if they could manage the latter, they could manage the former, too. But that was just a guess. In a recent study, Harvard Medical School researchers asked patients about sexual activity hour by hour in the twenty-four hours before their heart attacks occurred.

For a person who previously had a heart attack, the odds of suffering a nonfatal heart attack while having sex or in the two hours afterward are about two in a million. For someone not previously known to have heart disease, the risk is virtually identical, about one in a million, a difference too small to be of any practical significance, James Muller and his colleagues said. Given the low overall risk of heart attacks, the absolute hourly risk was extremely low.

The researchers interviewed 858 persons who were sexually active in the year before they had a heart attack. Seventy-nine of them reported sexual activity in the twenty-four hours before the attack, and twenty-seven in the two hours before it. The majority of these persons were men aged fifty to sixty-nine.[14]

The headline on an editorial accompanying a report on this study in the *Journal of the American Medical Association* suggested a collective sigh of relief: "Sexual Activity Triggering Myocardial Infarction [heart attack]: One Less Thing to Worry About."[15]

If you have had a heart attack, the best thing you can do to prevent another one is to exercise regularly, which will strengthen your heart's ability to handle extra effort. Among all the individuals in this study, the risk of having a heart attack soon after engaging in sex was highest in those who were sedentary, and lowest in those who habitually worked out.

The safest time to have sex if you've already had a heart attack thus appears to be . . . any time.

Chronotherapy Can Help *Prevent* Heart Disease

Hundreds of medications are available to regularize the heart rate, lower high blood pressure, open arteries in the heart, and reduce clotting. Few have been studied with respect to the best time to take them, although chronotherapy has made some important inroads.

Aspirin

Ask your doctor if you should take aspirin every day or every other day, either to reduce the odds that you will ever have a heart attack, or to prevent another one. Numerous studies show aspirin makes platelets less "sticky." It thus lowers or prevents the formation of clots in diseased blood vessels. Doctors and nurses volunteered for two large studies. Health professionals usually make good subjects, as they recognize the need to comply with the study regimen.

In one study, more than 22,000 male U.S. physicians took either one regular aspirin (325 milligrams) or a look-alike but inactive tablet every other day for eleven years on average. Those taking aspirin had 44 percent fewer first nonfatal heart attacks, and 60 percent fewer heart attacks in the first three hours after awakening, than those not taking aspirin.[16] In the other U.S. study, researchers kept tabs on nearly 88,000 female nurses, and found that women taking one to six aspirins a week had 25 percent fewer first nonfatal heart attacks and fewer morning heart attacks than those using less aspirin.[17] (See Strokes, page 354.)

These and other studies suggest that taking one "baby" aspirin (75 to 100 milligrams) per day or one regular aspirin (325 milligrams) every other day may help prevent a heart attack. For those taking the lower dose, additional twice-monthly doses of 325 milligrams, a booster dose, may further help prevent the formation of blood clots.

Aspirin clearly benefits people with known heart disease. Whether all healthy men and women should take aspirin regularly, when in life to start, and how much to take are still unresolved questions. These may be answered by research now in progress, such as the Women's Health Study, a trial evaluating a daily dose of 50 milligrams of aspirin in 40,000 U.S. female health care professionals. The American Heart Association stresses that aspirin is no substitute for a heart-healthy lifestyle that includes a low-saturated-fat diet, regular physical activity, and no cigarette smoking.

Talk to your own doctor before starting to take aspirin regularly. Aspirin may not be appropriate for you. Your doctor may advise against taking aspirin if you also are taking blood thinners, such as warfarin; other nonsteroidal anti-inflammatory drugs (NSAIDs); or acetaminophen (not a NSAID), as these drugs may interact with aspirin to increase digestive upsets, or if you have peptic ulcers, a bleeding disorder, or certain other chronic medical illnesses. If taking aspirin regularly, ask your doctor what to take for occasional headaches, muscle aches, and other minor pains. *If you do take aspirin, take it once a day at bedtime with a full glass of water to minimize stomach irritation.*

Controlled-Onset, Extended-Release Verapamil

Verapamil, a drug that lowers BP and reduces the heart's oxygen demand, now comes as a chronotherapy. Novel drug design allows users to take this

medication, Covera-HS, at bedtime. The medication is released
amounts tailored to the different day and night risk of angina
reduces attacks of angina, particularly in the morning, and, it's hoped,
will prevent heart attacks. (See High Blood Pressure, page 285.)

Cholesterol-Lowering "Statin" Medications

Cholesterol is a type of fat. Though cholesterol has a bad reputation, the
body needs certain types and amounts of it to build cells, make hormones,
and use as a source of energy. Most of the cholesterol you need is manufactured in your body by your liver at night. Eating cholesterol-laden foods, such
as red meat, rich cheeses, ice cream, and butter, introduces excess cholesterol
into your body. Some of it gets deposited on walls of blood vessels, narrowing
them, and increasing the likelihood that blood vessel blockages will develop.

Blood tests you get as part of a regular physical checkup tell your doctor
how much cholesterol is circulating in your body. The ideal total cholesterol
level for adults ranges between 140 and 200 milligrams per deciliter of blood.
For higher levels, doctors usually advise reducing dietary fat, and also may
prescribe cholesterol-lowering medications.

A family of drugs called "statins" are among those most commonly advised.
These drugs include fluvastatin, lovastatin, pravastatin, and simvastatin. They
typically are prescribed in single daily doses, and their effectiveness depends
on when you take them. In reviewing various statin drugs, the *Physicians'
Desk Reference*, the "bible" doctors consult for guidelines on medication use,
reports that these drugs are more effective when taken in the evening than
the same dose of the same drugs taken in the morning,[18] perhaps because the
body manufactures cholesterol at night.

Nitroglycerin Patches

These help prevent angina pectoris, pain in the chest caused by heart disease. Users wear these patches twelve to fourteen consecutive hours every day.
Wearing them longer may cause drug tolerance to develop, making the drug
less effective. Instructions do not specify a particular application time. These
drugs can be easily used in a chronotherapeutic manner, however. Persons
who have angina primarily in the morning, as well as those who have angina
overnight, may get the most benefit from the medication by applying the
patch at bedtime and taking it off around noon.

Chronotherapy Can Help *Treat* Heart Disease

If you think you may be having a heart attack, call 911 or another emergency
medical service. Immediately chew half a standard-sized aspirin to speed its
passage into your bloodstream, and wash it down with a glass of water. This act
helps avert severe damage to the heart muscle by clearing clots from tiny

blood vessels in the heart, allowing blood flow to resume. Lie down, and wait for help.

At the hospital, doctors aim to quickly restore blood flow through blocked arteries. Rapid treatment minimizes the death of heart muscles from lack of oxygen. Doctors often use a type of medication called tissue-type plasminogen activator (TPA) to dislodge clots. Studies show TPA dissolves clots better in persons who experience heart attacks between noon and midnight than in persons who have heart attacks between midnight and noon. Indeed, researchers found it worked best around 8 P.M. Knowing this fact may influence a doctor's choice of dosage or use of other medications in addition to this one at different hours. Such studies show doctors need to consider time of day in making medication decisions even in emergency situations.[19]

If you have chest pain from angina: Take this pain seriously since it warns that too little blood is getting through, and your heart is working too hard. See your doctor promptly for a complete evaluation, possibly including round-the-clock ambulatory monitoring.

Timewise Tips

Get out of bed slowly, particularly if you are forty-five or older. Sit at the edge of the bed for a minute before standing up. Try to minimize rushing and other stressful activities in the morning.

Keep your blood pressure in a normal range. See High Blood Pressure (page 285.)

Talk to your doctor about using verapamil chronotherapy if you have angina, about when to take statin medications, and when to wear nitroglycerin patches.

Exercise regularly. Three hours of brisk walking each week confers the same benefits as fifteen to twenty minutes of vigorous exercise every day. Both can cut your risk of a heart attack by 30 to 40 percent. If you are forty-five or older, see your doctor for a checkup before embarking on a strenuous exercise program. Exercise in the afternoon or evening until you get in shape.

Anytime Tips

If you smoke, stop. Just five cigarettes a day doubles your risk of heart disease.

Trim fat from your diet. If your cholesterol is high, talk to your doctor about good nutrition and cholesterol-lowering medications. If overweight, work on getting rid of extra pounds.

Use alcohol appropriately. One to two drinks a day, no more than twenty-four ounces of beer, eight ounces of wine, or two ounces of 100-proof whisky, may cut your risk of heart disease.

Keep stress in check. Stress boosts the heart rate and sends BP soaring.

Feelings of tension and frustration double the likelihood that too little blood will get to your heart, increasing your risk of having a heart attack.

Ask your doctor's advice about taking folic acid and vitamins B_6 and B_{12}. Persons who have a deficiency of these substances or who have elevated levels of homocysteine, a building block of protein in the body, may improve their heart health by modifying their diet or taking dietary supplements.

Study. Visit the Web sites of the National Heart, Lung and Blood Institute (www.nhlbi.nih.gov/nhlbi/nhlbi.htm) and the American Heart Association (www.americanheart.org).

HIGH BLOOD PRESSURE

The most common test performed in the doctor's office—a blood pressure reading—is just a snapshot of your blood pressure at a single time of day. It tells surprisingly little about your health. You wouldn't rely on one photo of yourself at the beach to explain what the ocean is like. Similarly, your doctor needs readings from different times of day and night to see the high tides and low tides in the ocean of blood circulating through your body.

Here's why: blood pressure normally is about 20 percent to 30 percent higher in waking hours than when you sleep, and higher in the afternoon than in the morning. Depending on when you see the doctor and have your blood pressure taken, your highs might be missed. Consistent high blood pressure boosts your risk of having a heart attack or stroke, losing your vision, and dying early.

Fortunately, you can prevent or lower your risk of such problems with a proper diet and other good health habits, and, when necessary, by also taking medications.

How Blood Pressure Works

Every time your heart beats, the walls of your arteries stretch. Between beats, the arteries relax. A blood pressure (BP) reading reflects the force of blood against artery walls at these two times.

BP must be high enough to push five quarts of blood through the roughly 60,000 miles of blood vessels in your body, shuttling oxygen and nutrients to every cell and taking waste matter away. If BP is too high, your heart has to work harder, and there's too much stress on vessels that carry blood, particularly the tiny ones in the heart, brain, eyes, kidneys, and other organs. These overstressed vessels may rupture and bleed, causing a heart attack or stroke. If BP is too low, cells don't get the oxygen and nutrients they need, and some wastes aren't removed.

Doctors use the terms "high BP" or "hypertension" to mean blood pressure that poses unacceptable health risks. Where to draw the line continues to be a matter of intense medical debate. Your age, weight, sex, race, and various health conditions, such as whether you are pregnant or have diabetes, determine the BP that is considered right for you.

3 in 10 Americans with High Blood Pressure Don't Know It

Only half of those who do know are getting treatment. Only one-quarter have normalized their BP. At the end of 1970s, surveys showed that only about half of those who had high BP knew this fact. By the 1990s massive public education efforts had improved this situation dramatically, using barbershops, grocery stores, churches, and other community organizations to spread the message. At the end of the century, however, Mayo Clinic specialists found evidence of backsliding, as AIDS, cancer, and other illnesses moved to the front burner of public awareness. More ominously, they noted that the number of deaths from strokes and heart attacks, which fell dramatically in the previous two decades, seemed to be leveling off, and even edging higher.[1]

The threat of high BP is real. The early identification and successful treatment of persons with high BP remains one of the nation's major public health goals. High BP affects men more often than women up until about age fifty-five, when the odds even out. Fifty million Americans have high BP. The disorder affects the elderly more than the young, and African Americans more than Caucasians. It is rare in children.[2]

Causes of High BP Still Unknown

Despite recognition of the dangers of high BP, the disorder's cause remains largely a mystery. In nine out of ten persons diagnosed with high BP, no medical cause can be found. Doctors term this type of high BP "essential" or "primary." Genetics presumably play a key role, as high BP often runs in families. Diabetes, kidney disease, sleep apnea, some hormonal disorders, complications of pregnancy, other medical conditions, and use of certain medications also may trigger high BP. This type of high BP is called "secondary."

Poor health habits increase your vulnerability. Not watching your weight, not exercising regularly, smoking, drinking excessively, and, in persons intolerant to salt, consuming excessively salty foods all contribute to high BP.

What the Numbers Mean

With each beat of your heart, BP briefly goes up. With each rest between beats, it briefly falls. A BP reading thus tells your high and low pressure at the time it is taken. The high, or systolic, pressure is written first, and the low, or diastolic pressure, next: 120/80 is one example.

To get these numbers, a cuff connected to a metering device must be wrapped around your arm. With a stethoscope held over the large artery of your arm, the doctor or nurse inflates the cuff. This temporarily cuts off the flow of blood in the artery, so no heartbeats can be heard. The doctor or nurse then slowly deflates the cuff. The first audible heart sound tells the pressure required to force blood past the inflated arm cuff. This is your systolic BP. The last audible sound reveals the pressure when your heart relaxes. This is your diastolic BP. Many physicians' offices, as well as drug stores, shopping malls, and fitness centers, now have devices that take BP readings automatically. You can buy a BP cuff and check your own BP at home.

BP readings commonly are followed by the abbreviation "mm Hg." This means "millimeters of mercury." The term is a carryover from the time when BP devices utilized a glass tube filled with mercury that offered a visible marker of how much BP rose or fell. Present-day devices often show these numbers on a dial or present them electronically.

BP goes up when you are active, falls when you are still, is higher when you stand than when you lie down, and higher when you talk than when you are silent. BP customarily is read while you are sitting up and relaxed, and at least thirty minutes after you consume caffeine or tobacco, since both caffeine and nicotine boost BP temporarily.

Stress also may elevate BP. Simply visiting the doctor has this effect on about one in four people of all ages, a condition doctors call *white coat hypertension*. Many persons who experience it relax after a few minutes, and their BP falls to its usual level. That's why a high reading usually prompts repeat readings in the course of a visit. Some persons don't settle down before the visit is over, however, and are mistakenly diagnosed as having high BP.[3] Worse, some then are subjected needlessly to expensive tests and even drug treatment for a condition that lasts only as long as they are in the doctor's office.

How Time of Day Alters BP

White coat hypertension highlights the inherent flaw of relying on one reading, or even several readings taken at about the same time. BP normally follows a roller-coaster path over the twenty-four-hour day.

To prepare your body to function best in waking hours, BP starts upward before you habitually wake up. Once you awaken, it surges abruptly. It climbs through the morning and afternoon, peaks in late afternoon or early evening, and then slides to its trough in sleep. Systolic BP ordinarily is about 25 to 30 mm Hg higher when you are awake than when you are asleep. Diastolic BP is about 15 to 20 mm Hg higher in the daytime.[4]

You may have heard that a blood pressure reading of 120/80 is "normal," but these numbers are just statistical averages. Moreover, they are just averages of readings taken in the daytime. A healthy person could have BP readings in what doctors view as a low, normal, and high range at different times of the day: 110/60 at 6 A.M., 130/85 at noon, 140/95 at 6 P.M., 120/70 at midnight, and 110/70 at 4 A.M., for example. The proper interpretation of any blood pressure reading requires knowledge of the time of day it was taken, and more important, its relation to other readings taken around the clock.

Current medical guidelines say BP in adults is "high" when systolic pressure consistently averages 140 mm Hg or higher, and diastolic pressure consistently averages 90 mm Hg or higher, as determined on three different visits to the clinic or doctor's office.[5] Since most clinics and doctors' offices are open only in the daytime, typically between 8:30 A.M. and 5 P.M., most diagnostic decisions currently are based on only daytime BP readings. That's not enough.

Monthly and Yearly Rhythms May Alter BP

Changes over the month and year generally aren't great, but they may be large enough to affect treatment in someone whose BP consistently is in the high range.

BP is a little higher in most women in the week or so before the start of a menstrual period than it is in mid-month, at the time of ovulation.[6] In women who use birth-control pills, both systolic and diastolic BP average about 4 to 5 mm Hg higher than in nonusers.[7]

Both systolic and diastolic BP vary slightly over the year in areas where temperature changes seasonally. Cold temperatures cause muscles of the small arteries to contract so as to retain heat in the body, and thus raise BP. This may aggravate underlying existing heart disease, and probably contributes to the higher death rate in cold weather. Heat relaxes these muscles and lowers BP. If you smoke, your BP is likely to be higher at all times than that of nonsmokers, and even more so in cold weather.[8]

Discover Your Daily Cycle

Determining whether BP gets too high and stays high for too long requires a round-the-clock study. It's good preventive medicine to check your own BP round-the-clock at least once a year for at least a day, and then several times a day for the next week. This is true even if you have no symptoms. Many people with high BP do not have symptoms until BP has caused serious damage. That's the reason doctors call high BP a silent killer.[9]

You can find reliable home BP measuring devices at pharmacies, department stores, and through catalogs for under $100. The most accurate devices include a cuff that wraps around your upper arm. Small, lightweight finger

Blood Pressure Diary

Name _____

See a doctor promptly if you

- have more than one daily reading of 140/90 or higher
- have frequent headaches, especially in the morning
- feel short of breath and lack stamina
- feel dizzy

- develop a chronic red face
- have frequent nose bleeds
- have fainting spells

Photocopy this page, and take your BP several times a day. Take measurements while sitting, after resting for five minutes, and at least thirty minutes after consuming caffeine or smoking. Take this diary with you when you see your doctor.

Women: Are you menstruating today? Y/N _____

Day/Date	Wake-up (Before Getting Out of Bed)	Before Breakfast	Before Lunch	Midday	Before Dinner	Bedtime	Mid-sleep (Set Alarm)
Sample Sun. 6/4/00	110/60	120/80	130/85	140/90	140/95	120/70	110/60

Medications used:

Name of medication _____ **Time taken** _____

Name of medication _____ **Time taken** _____

Name of medication _____ **Time taken** _____

and wrist BP monitors, though more convenient, are less trustworthy. Take the device you buy with you when you see your doctor to verify that the readings you get at home are comparable to those taken in the doctor's office. Use the diary on page 289 to keep track of your readings.

Taking your own BP and keeping a diary is a good start, but automated round-the-clock ambulatory monitoring will give your doctor a more comprehensive picture. For this procedure, you wear a BP cuff on your left arm while going about your usual activities. The cuff is connected to a small, lightweight, battery-powered device that makes it inflate roughly every fifteen to thirty minutes. The device stores your readings in a unit you wear at the waist or over the shoulder. When you take it back to the doctor's office, this information is downloaded into a computer. People typically wear these devices for twenty-four to forty-eight hours.

Some physicians and health maintenance organizations view ambulatory BP monitoring as too costly for general use. Others contend it pays for itself, by reducing unnecessary office visits, medical tests, and medications, including inappropriate treatment of persons who simply have white coat hypertension, possibly one-quarter of all those now thought to have mild to moderate high blood pressure.

Italian researchers, for example, found pregnant women with white coat hypertension are more likely to undergo cesarean delivery than are women whose BP remains normal. Such surgery carries higher health risks for mother and baby than a vaginal delivery. Using round-the-clock monitoring, Gianni Bellomo of Assisi Hospital and his colleagues found that nearly one-third of a group of 148 pregnant women who had high BP readings in the doctor's office in the last three months of their pregnancy simply had white coat hypertension. These women were just as healthy as women whose BP readings stayed in the normal range. Both groups of babies were equally healthy, too. Twenty-four-hour BP, the researchers concluded, is superior to office BP in predicting the outcome of pregnancy.[10]

White Coat Hypertension

◆ Betty, who is sixty-eight, had a BP of 157/103 mm Hg in the doctor's office. Her doctor tried to bash it down with medications, and indeed, kept increasing the doses because none worked. He then referred her to a specialist who saw that her BP stayed high, even after she sat in the waiting room for a while. The specialist fitted her with a twenty-four-hour monitoring device. Within an hour of leaving the specialist's office, Betty's BP had dropped to 123/85 mm Hg. Outside the doctor's office, Betty's BP was perfectly normal. She didn't need medications at all.

Few insurers in the United States currently include this worthwhile medical procedure as a part of their general health maintenance coverage. Medicare and Medicaid programs do not cover it either. Hence, people who wish to have it done usually must pay for it themselves.

As patients become more assertive about their health care needs, and further studies show how useful such monitoring can be, this situation may change. We're betting round-the-clock ambulatory monitoring eventually will become a standard part of a regular checkup for all adults, like the now-familiar measures of cholesterol in blood, sugar in urine, electrocardiograph monitoring of heart function, and Pap smears for women.

Daily BP Patterns Predict Health Risks

BP falls in sleep by 10 percent to 20 percent from its daytime average in most people: those with normal BP, as well as those with high BP. These persons are called *normal dippers.*

In some persons, however, BP doesn't fall, and even may jump higher than it does when they are awake.[11] They are called nondippers. African Americans are more likely to be nondippers than Caucasians. Other nondippers include persons who are intolerant of high-salt diets, many older persons, and those whose high BP stems from medical conditions such as sleep apnea, complications of pregnancy, and diseases of the central nervous or endocrine systems. Japanese researchers tracking more than 1,500 persons over age sixty found that nondippers were nearly three times more likely to die from a heart attack or stroke than normal dippers.[12]

In other persons, BP in sleep falls more than 20 percent from its daytime levels. These persons are *superdippers.*[13] A drop of this magnitude, which cannot be predicted from readings taken in the daytime, accelerates tissue damage, particularly in the eyes and heart. It may even trigger strokes.

In still other persons, BP rises too rapidly in the morning. Blood vessels weakened by age or disease are susceptible to damage in the same way that pipes can be in an older house. Just as a rush of water may dislodge bits of rust and cause leaks, *morning spurts* in BP may tear loose fatty deposits from the walls of small vessels of the heart and brain, causing bleeding. Clots form at the site of injury, perhaps creating a blockage. In the heart, a blockage may cause a heart attack, and in the brain, a stroke.

The bottom line: too little or too big a fall in BP in sleep, or too rapid a rise in BP in the morning, may have numerous adverse health consequences. Readings taken only in the doctor's office do not show these problems. The only way to identify them is to monitor BP round the clock and define its circadian rhythm.[14]

Chrono Success Stories: Preventing Blindness, Helping Babies

Preventing Blindness

Eye diseases that disrupt blood flow may cause sudden loss of vision. Three out of four persons with this problem discovered it themselves when they awakened from nighttime sleep or a daytime nap, a study of more than 500 episodes of sudden visual loss at the University of Iowa shows.

Eye specialist Sohan Hayreh and his colleagues monitored the patients' BP round-the-clock. The researchers found that sudden visual loss occurred more often in persons with high BP than in those with normal BP, and most often in those whose BP fell most precipitously when they slept.

The researchers made another important discovery: BP fell the most in persons who took certain BP medications in the evening. They advised patients to take these medications earlier in the day. As a result, the patients' BP fell less in sleep. This simple tactic probably spared many of them from further loss of vision.[15]

Boosting Odds of Having Healthy Babies

As many as one in seven pregnant women develop a condition called preeclampsia, usually late in pregnancy. Prominent symptoms include swelling of the face, hands, ankles, and feet, along with elevated BP. If not treated, preeclampsia may retard the baby's growth and lead to premature delivery. It even may progress to eclampsia, triggering seizures and coma that may be fatal to both baby and mother. The causes of these disorders aren't known.

By using twenty-four-hour monitoring, Spanish researchers found that BP rhythms predict which women are likely to run into trouble. In these women, BP may fail to dip normally in sleep. It also rises much higher than in healthy women, starting at about the fifth month of pregnancy.[16]

Could aspirin help? This drug has a high safety record in pregnancy, but initial studies in preeclampsia showed inconsistent results in preventing the disorder.[17] To see if timing mattered, Ramón Hermida of the University of Vigo and Diana Ayala of the University of Santiago recruited one hundred pregnant volunteers who had developed high BP and preeclampsia in earlier pregnancies, and assigned them randomly to take either 100 milligrams of aspirin or a look-alike but inactive pill at different times.

Women who took their aspirin in the morning were more likely to experience high BP in their pregnancy. Those who took it at bedtime had fewer BP problems. Most important, fewer women in the latter group developed preeclampsia or eclampsia.[18]

Caution: If you are pregnant, do not take aspirin or any other medications without first talking to your doctor. Keep track of your own BP by using the diary, page 289, and see your doctor regularly.

Medications for High BP: What Time Is Best?

As we discussed in chapter 14: "A Time to Heal," there is no scientific rationale for the times manufacturers recommend for taking most BP-lowering drugs.

Many of these medications come in a once-a-day tablet or pill. If you ask your doctor if it's okay to take your medication at any hour that suits you, you may be told that time doesn't matter, as long as you take your medication regularly. Many studies suggest this is not true.

In these studies, volunteers with high BP took a once-a-day BP-lowering medication either in the morning or the evening for several weeks, and then took the same dose of the same medication at the opposite time for an equal number of weeks. Some took the drug in the morning first, and then in the evening, while others did the reverse. Before and after several weeks of treatment, they wore twenty-four-hour ambulatory monitors to assess the effects of the different dosing times on their BP levels. Here's what researchers found:

Japanese investigators studied diltiazem, one of many widely used calcium channel blocking drugs that reduce high BP by relaxing muscles of the small arteries. When taken at 8 A.M., at the start of the daily activity period, diltiazem lowered BP more effectively at night than in the day. When taken at 7 P.M., it lowered BP more effectively in the day than at night. Since daytime is prime time for high BP, when this drug is taken may determine how much patients benefit from it.[19]

Australian researchers studied another type of commonly used medication, one of the family known as angiotensin converting enzyme, or ACE, inhibitors. These drugs lower BP by boosting the volume of urine the kidneys excrete and relaxing blood vessels. Their study participants took the ACE inhibitor perindopril in the morning for four weeks, and in the evening for four weeks. When taken at 9 A.M., the drug successfully lowered BP for twenty-four hours. When taken at 9 P.M., however, its BP-lowering effect lasted only twelve to fourteen hours. To achieve the same benefit, the researchers said, people would have to take twice as much of this drug in the evening as in the morning.[20]

Dozens of other studies show timing of medications also influences how low BP falls in sleep and how rapidly it spurts in the morning. The same drugs, in the same dose, may be helpful when taken in the morning but harmful when taken in the evening, or vice versa. Use this information to talk to your doctor about timing issues. Since there are many different types of drugs for high BP, and many different drugs in each category, ask your doctor to review any studies that may have been done on the best time to take the particular BP medication prescribed for you.

Using Chronobiology to Design Better Drugs

Growing evidence that tailoring a medication's delivery to body rhythms may make a drug both more effective and safe holds practical implications for drug design. The pharmaceutical industry has begun to take note.

The first chronotherapy for high BP was introduced in the United States by the pharmaceutical manufacturer Searle in 1996. It involves a novel way to deliver verapamil, a drug long known to be effective in lowering BP. This new medication comes in a tablet taken at bedtime. A coating on the tablet takes four to five hours to break down, exposing a membrane containing tiny openings. Fluid absorbed from the digestive tract expands chemicals in the tablet, pushing the verapamil through this membrane. The medication thus starts to go to work at the same time BP begins its daily rise. Most of the drug is released early in the day, when it is most needed, and less in the evening and overnight, when it is least needed.

This approach also acknowledges human nature: many people shower, dress, and have breakfast, and then take their medicine, perhaps an hour or more after they awaken. Because most blood pressure lowering drugs take a few hours to kick in, and few work with equal efficiency around the clock, people using conventional medications may be unprotected when they need the medication most.

In one study, William White of the University of Connecticut and his colleagues compared the new medication, called Covera-HS in the United States and Chronovera elsewhere, to another commonly used BP-lowering medication, nifedipine, which releases a constant amount of medication through the twenty-four-hour day. The researchers randomly assigned nearly 600 patients to take either one drug or the other for six weeks. Both medications worked equally well to lower BP in the daytime. But the nifedipine lowered BP nearly twice as much at night as the Covera-HS did. Markedly lowering BP could be risky for some people, particularly those aged sixty and over, since it induces a super-dipping BP pattern in sleep.

A long-term study, launched in 1996, will compare Covera-HS to now-standard BP medications in 16,600 persons with high BP at 660 medical centers in fifteen countries to see whether it reduces the likelihood of having a heart attack, or of dying from a heart attack and other heart diseases. Doctors need long-term results, or "outcome measures," to see whether the drug's effect on BP holds true significance for human health. Positive results in this very large study group likely would advance chronotherapy's march toward widespread acceptance by physicians. The first results are scheduled to be announced in 2002.

Other drug manufacturers already have adopted the chronotherapeutic approach. In 1999 Schwarz Pharma introduced Verelan-PM, also a controlled-onset extended-release capsule form of verapamil for high BP.

Initial studies show it also reduces abnormally high BP in the morning and afternoon.[21]

U.S. physicians write more prescriptions for medications to lower high BP than for any other single type of drug. The introduction of bedtime chronotherapies of high BP has had some unintended and unwelcome effects on medical practice. Some physicians have wrongly advised patients to take conventional once-a-day therapies at night. This practice may be dangerous. Most studies to date have assessed the safety of BP-lowering drugs taken in the morning. Until further studies are done, it's impossible to say which time is best.

Timewise Tips

Record your BP, using the Blood Pressure Diary on page 289. Take the diary with you when you see your doctor.

If your BP is high, and your doctor suggests that you take medication, ask about the new verapamil chronotherapies or other chronotherapies expected to be available soon.

Do not change the time you take any prescription medication without talking with your doctor. If no twenty-four-hour studies have been done on your particular drug, stick with the dosing time recommended by the drug's manufacturer, since premarketing studies showed that this time is acceptably safe.

Exercise regularly. Start your exercise program in the afternoon if you are out of shape. Exercise not only helps trim flab but improves blood circulation. It enlarges openings of arteries in the heart and adds new smaller vessels to handle increased blood flow when you exercise. Sedentary persons have a greater risk of developing high BP than those who engage in regular aerobic exercise.

Urge your insurer to pay for twenty-four-hour BP monitoring. It's your health that's at stake.

Anytime Tips

If overweight, shed some pounds. Six out of ten adults with high BP weigh at least 20 percent more than their ideal weight, based on standard charts. Losing 10 percent of body weight will reduce BP, possibly enough to eliminate the need for medication, or permit a lower dosage.

Eat plenty of fruits and vegetables. These foods contain fiber, potassium, magnesium, and calcium, all thought protective against high BP.

If you smoke, stop. Nicotine makes the heart beat faster and narrows arteries. A single cigarette raises BP for about thirty minutes. Stopping smoking will both reduce your BP and lower your risk of heart disease.

Reduce salt consumption. High salt consumption increases BP in about half of all persons with high BP, those with salt sensitivity. This problem is more common in African Americans, in persons who are overweight, have diabetes, or are over age sixty-five. Cutting back on prepared foods and fast foods is an important step; they are the source of 80 percent of the sodium in the typical American diet. There is no easy way to tell if you will benefit from salt reduction other than trying it, and seeing if it makes a difference. Lowering use of prepared foods and fast foods probably also will reduce fat and salt in your diet.

Use alcohol moderately. It's good news that one drink a day may help lower BP.

Explore stress management. Stress releases a cascade of hormones that make the heart beat faster and blood vessels constrict, elevating BP. Lifestyle modifications that reduce your daily stress level are likely to benefit BP. Many people find relaxation exercises, biofeedback, yoga, and similar tactics beneficial.

Study. Visit the Web sites of the National Heart, Lung and Blood Institute (www.nhlbi.nih.gov/nhlbi/nhlbi.htm) and the American Heart Association (www.americanheart.org).

MOOD DISORDERS

If you sleep longer and feel more sluggish in the winter yet also crave carbohydrates and eat more then, you've got plenty of company. One in six persons who live in temperate and higher latitudes suffers *winter blues.* As days lengthen in the spring, many of us cheerfully succumb to *spring fever,* a transient giddiness that makes us want to play hooky from school or call in sick at work.

Some of us feel more irritable for a week or so after the one-hour spring change to *daylight saving time,* and more cheerful after the fall change back to standard time. *Jet-lagged travelers* (see page 143), *shift workers* (see page 164), and persons with *sleep disorders* (see page 339) often report mood upsets tied to schedule changes. Many women experience *premenstrual syndrome* (see page 324), and some suffer depression at times of major shifts in reproductive hormones when pregnant, after childbirth, or at menopause.

These common experiences suggest that disruptions in biological clocks may be both cause and consequence of disturbed moods. Extensive research today focuses on exploring the contribution of such disruptions to severe mood disorders, a cluster of illnesses that often involve intense feelings of sadness and grief. In any year, about 7 percent of Americans, 17 million persons of all ages, experience mood disorders. Such problems rank among the top ten causes of disability worldwide, according to U.S. Surgeon General David Satcher's 1999 report on mental health.[1]

Some people suffer recurring depression in either winter or summer. They have *seasonal affective disorder*, aptly nicknamed "SAD." ("Affective" is the psychiatric term for "mood.")

In some mood disorders, including *major depression* and *bipolar disorder*, with its extreme ups and downs, people often sleep too little or too much, and their daily rhythms of hormone release and body temperature may undergo profound disruption. Episodes of these disorders, though possibly many years apart and once thought unconnected, today are recognized as additional beads on a string, recurrences of a chronic illness.

Treatment targeting body clocks can help persons with mood disorders maintain a more even keel and prevent or minimize future flare-ups, an important practical finding of recent research. This treatment may involve medications, timed exposure to daylight-intensity bright light, and changes in the timing or amount of sleep.

Seasonal Affective Disorder

Winter SAD

One in twenty to twenty-five adults experiences a true and recurring depression in winter. Twice as many women as men develop SAD, most starting between ages twenty and forty, but even young children may be affected. If you have SAD, you may sleep perhaps four hours longer than usual; lose interest in work, school, socializing, and other normal activities; eat more, and gain perhaps twenty pounds between October and March, when symptoms abate on their own. December, January, and February typically are the worst months.

In the spring, summer, and early fall, you probably feel fine. Creative persons with winter SAD often prove unusually productive in these seasons, psychiatrist Norman Rosenthal reports in his book, *Winter Blues*.[2] George Frideric Handel, known to be melancholic in winter, composed *The Messiah* in twenty-three days in the summer of 1741.

Think of Vincent van Gogh's painting *The Reaper*. It shows a robust young farmer striding across a fertile field, bathed in the summer sun's radiant light. "There's a certain Slant of light, Winter Afternoons," Emily Dickinson wrote, "That oppresses, like the Heft of Cathedral Tunes."

The frequency of winter SAD rises with distance from the equator, in tandem with the seasonal decline in hours of daylight. In the United States, winter SAD is ten times more common in New York than in Florida.[3] In Europe, people in Norway and Finland suffer from it more often than those in Italy and Spain.

Winter doldrums may underlie some so-called *holiday depressions*. Though many people find Christmas and the beginning of the new year stressful, these holidays seem to prompt less angst in the Southern Hemisphere, where seasons are reversed.

Folk names in many cultures testify to the strong link between winter and blue moods. U.S. residents often complain about *cabin fever*. Polar explorers have reported *Arctic hysteria*. Norwegians talk about *morketiden*, "the murky time." In Iceland, a single word, *skammdegistunglyndi*, describes the "heavy mood of the short days." Curiously, the incidence of SAD is lower in Iceland than in some other countries of comparable latitude, and even among descendants of Icelanders living elsewhere. Researchers suspect a genetic adaptation in Icelandic populations.[4]

Savvy Patient Kindles Light Therapy

Some 1,800 years ago, the Greek physician Galen likened winter "lethargicum" in some of his patients to hibernation in animals. In the spring of 1980, a New Jersey man with recurring winter depression learned from a news article that scientists at the National Institute of Mental Health (NIMH) had devised a way to measure melatonin in the blood. A research engineer, Herbert Kern thought melatonin might be a good biological marker for his seasonal mood changes, and contacted the researchers.

Kern came to the NIMH's Bethesda, Maryland, campus the following December when he was most depressed. Having found that exposure to light five to ten times brighter than ordinary room light could turn off melatonin secretion, a hint that light might affect other body rhythms as well,[5] Alfred Lewy, Norman Rosenthal, and their colleagues asked Kern to sit in front of a bank of fluorescent lights for three hours in both the morning and early evening. Their idea was to make spring come early. Within four days, Kern's mood improved so much that he was able to enjoy Christmas for the first time in years.[6]

A news report on this study swamped the research team with mail from others with winter depression, and studies of light therapy began at the NIMH and elsewhere. "Light therapy is one of the most successful and practical results of basic research in biological rhythms," according to Thomas Wehr, who directs NIMH biological rhythms research.[7]

Bright Light Now Treatment of Choice for Winter SAD

"Light is as effective as antidepressant medications are, perhaps more so," asserts Anna Wirz-Justice of the University of Basel in Switzerland.[8] She and other members of the Society for Light Treatment and Biological Rhythms, an international group of specialists in the field, have used light to relieve winter SAD in thousands of patients, and developed standards for treatment. About three in five persons with winter SAD who use light therapy get better, usually in just a few days. Antidepressant drugs, by contrast, often take three to four weeks to show similar benefits.

Over the years, the intensity of light used has gotten stronger, and the time required for treatment shorter. Although two hours' exposure to light with an intensity of 2,500 lux can relieve SAD, the now standard regimen calls for a thirty-minute daily exposure to light of 10,000 lux, the equivalent of sunlight about forty minutes after sunrise. Ordinary indoor lighting is about 300 to 500 lux. Sunlight at noon on a bright summer day may be 100,000 lux. Even on rainy or overcast days, natural daylight is brighter than conventional indoor lighting.

Studies show bright white light is more effective than dim light, and that bright light helps more people than red or green light and most other placebo treatments do. The efficacy of placebos is always a concern in psychiatry where even sham treatments help many patients, at least for a while. (The word "placebo" is Latin for "I shall please.")

Light devices, known as light boxes, are about the size of a briefcase, and now fit easily on a tabletop or portable stand. You can get treatment while having breakfast or watching television roughly three feet from the light box. Staring at the lights is not necessary; scanning them every minute or two is sufficient. Light boxes cost about $300, increasingly covered by medical insurance. The Society for Light Treatment and Biological Rhythms advises against trying to construct your own light box. Well-designed commercial units provide measured intensity light, filtered to remove ultraviolet wavelengths to protect your eyes.

Battery-operated light visors that resemble a baseball cap allow users to move about freely. Studies are in progress to explore delivery of light through computerized devices in the bedroom that can mimic exposure to a natural dawn or dusk at any latitude or time of year, and through light masks that would be worn while you sleep. The retina of the eye is most sensitive to early morning light, and enough light may come through closed eyelids to alter body rhythms. If found to be effective, the computerized devices would further boost the ease of getting light therapy.

The earlier in the day people get light therapy, the better they usually do. Morning light therapy helps most persons with SAD, although some benefit from light at midday or in the early evening. Lewy, now at Oregon Health Sciences University, and his colleagues found that morning light shifted secretion of the hormone melatonin in SAD patients to an earlier time, suggesting that these persons had an underlying disturbance of biological rhythms that light corrects.[9] How light works still is not known, but scientists suspect it boosts levels of brain chemicals that normalize moods, particularly serotonin.

Most persons with SAD need to use light therapy every day or most days throughout the fall and winter months. Some benefit from taking antidepressant medications as well. Taking melatonin in the midafternoon in tiny doses now available only in research studies also may augment light therapy. More work is needed to see if this treatment is practical.[10] Some people with SAD feel best if they use both light and antidepressant drugs year-round.

Some physicians have yet to open their eyes to the clear benefits of light therapy for SAD. They regard it, Wirz-Justice said, as "not molecular enough, a bit too Californian-alternative, a bit too media overexposed, merely a placebo response by mildly neurotic middle-aged women who don't like nasty drugs." On the other hand, SAD is included in the American Psychiatric Association's *Diagnostic and Statistical Manual of Mental Disorders*, and Canadian specialists have widely publicized their consensus guidelines on SAD treatment.[11] Light is easy to administer, Wirz-Justice notes, lacks major side effects, and is relatively inexpensive. "Whatever its mode of action," she asserts, "it demands inclusion in the antidepressant armamentarium now."

Summer SAD

Loss of appetite and weight, as well as insomnia, are primary symptoms of summer SAD. Linked to hot weather rather than long exposure to daylight, summer SAD is far less frequent than winter SAD, affecting perhaps only one in two hundred Americans. Little research has been conducted on summer SAD to date. Some small studies at the NIMH suggest persons with this disorder benefit from staying cool. Light treatment does not relieve symptoms.[12]

SAD Children

SAD may start early in life, prompting a child to complain about school or about "mean" teachers or parents. Grades in a child with SAD may fall in winter, and then improve in the spring. Though sometimes treated as a school phobia, SAD symptoms in children, as in adults, typically become most obvious in winter months, while school phobias usually erupt in the fall, soon after school opens.

Researchers in Finland found as many as 90 percent of nearly 1,500 seventh- and ninth-graders reported seasonal variations in their energy, mood, length of sleep, and social activity. Most boys and girls said they felt more lethargic and sad in the winter, and more energetic and happier in the spring and summer.[13]

Nearly half of 1,700 children in grades four through twelve reported at least one symptom of depression in winter, in a survey Brown University researchers conducted. Only 10 percent did so in the spring and fall.[14] About one in seven students attending a northern New England college reported SAD symptoms in another survey.[15] Children and teenagers with SAD respond well to light therapy.

Bulimia Nervosa

Persons with the eating disorder *bulimia nervosa* gorge themselves rapidly on large amounts of food, often twice or more a week, usually in the evening. Despite feelings of depression, guilt, and self-loathing, persons with this disorder often report feeling "out of control." Many then self-induce vomiting to avoid gaining weight, or abuse laxatives and diuretic drugs. Some exercise compulsively. Bulimia affects an estimated 1 percent to 3 percent of young women, most in their teens and twenties.

Bulimia may follow a seasonal course. About one-third of persons with it also have SAD, and binge and purge more often in winter, according to Raymond Lam of the University of British Columbia. They also report gaining more weight and sleeping longer in winter than persons with bulimia who don't have winter SAD. By contrast, persons with another eating disorder, *anorexia nervosa*, who literally starve themselves to stay thin, seldom show a seasonal pattern.

Persons with bulimia often seek help in January when they are most ill. This time of year follows a holiday season often associated with overeating in even healthy persons. The long winter nights also may foster binge eating and purging, both usually done indoors in evening hours. In a study of women with bulimia not selected on the basis of any seasonal patterns, Lam found 10,000 lux light therapy for thirty minutes in the early morning for two weeks cut bingeing and purging episodes by half. The women's depressed moods also improved. The women who showed seasonal patterns improved the most with light therapy.[16]

Regular meals throughout the day ordinarily help keep inner clocks in sync. The frequent and excessive evening eating in bulimia, Lam suggests, may disturb them. Light therapy may pull these rhythms back in line.

Major Depression

Most of us feel more cheerful a few hours after arising than we do at the start of the day. People with *major depression* often are profoundly gloomy and lethargic in the morning. Their moods may brighten over the day, and then sink again into despair by the next morning. This pattern, frequently combined with waking earlier than desired, often around 4 A.M. or 5 A.M., and inability to return to sleep, points to disordered biological rhythms in depression. Sleep cycles are disrupted, too: rapid eye movement sleep, or REM sleep, controlled by the same areas of the brain that govern emotions, often occurs too early in the night and contains many more eye movements than is normal.

Major depression, also called *clinical depression* to emphasize that it is a severe problem that needs treatment, differs from ordinary ups and downs in mood. It usually is more severe than SAD. Persons with major depression show loss of interest or pleasure in nearly all former activities, including sex. If you develop this disorder, you may experience changes in appetite or weight, loss of energy, feelings of worthlessness or guilt, and difficulty in thinking, concentrating, and making decisions. You also may dwell on thoughts of death or suicide. Some people focus on bodily symptoms, such as trouble sleeping and aches and pains, rather than feelings of sadness. Children and teenagers with major depression may be irritable rather than noticeably sad.

Over a lifetime, one in seven adults, twice as many women as men, will suffer at least one bout of depression that lasts two weeks or longer, and interferes with work and family life. Episodes of depression last about nine months on average if untreated. Most people return fully to normal functioning, but most also have recurring episodes that start within the next two years. Continuing difficulty with sleep often predicts recurrences.

Depression has many causes, including an inherited susceptibility to it and chance encounters with depressing experiences, such as death of loved ones, development of a serious illness, loss of a job, a divorce, or devastating events such as a house fire or hurricane. Depression affects up to half of those who have had heart attacks, and is more common in persons with some other chronic illnesses, including diabetes, cancer, and multiple sclerosis. It's also a side effect of some medications used for these and other illnesses. Lack of light exposure also may play a role.[17] Some evidence suggests rates of major depression, like those of SAD, rise with distance from the equator.

Suicides and admissions to mental hospitals for depression peak not in the darkest months but in the spring. One theory is that depressed people become more aware of symptoms as the seasons change, and may have just enough energy then to act on their darkest impulses. For some people, as T. S. Eliot noted, "April is the cruellest month."[18] The fall brings another, smaller, upturn in suicides and hospital admissions.[19]

Suicides are twice as common in persons over age sixty-five than in younger adults. While illness and bereavement rise with age, it's also true that older people spend more time indoors and report much lower exposure to daylight than younger persons. They also have more eye disorders that may reduce their light perception. Most people with depression today can gain relief from a variety of safe and effective treatments.

Medications Are Standard Treatment

The drugs most commonly prescribed today for major depression are known as selective serotonin reuptake inhibitors (SSRIs). These boost brain levels of serotonin, a chemical messenger important for normal moods. They also normalize the timing of daily rhythms of body temperature, the sleep/wake cycle, and some hormones, which usually occur too early in depression. Their benefits thus may rest, at least in part, on their ability to resynchronize a disorganized circadian timekeeping system.

SSRIs are popular because they work well, lifting moods in 70 percent of users, and have fewer side effects than most other antidepressants. They include fluoxetine (Prozac), sertraline (Zoloft), paroxetine (Paxil), citalopram (Celexa), and fluvoxamine (Luvox), all regarded as more alike than different. Some of these drugs have an alerting effect, often desirable in persons who are lethargic. But they also may cause insomnia at night. Hence, doctors often tell patients to take them once a day in the morning. By contrast, related newer antidepressants mirtazapine (Remeron) and nefazodone (Serzone) may be sedating, and often are given at night. All of these drugs may take three to four weeks to become fully effective. Many patients benefit from continuing to use them, as doctors now know that the same drugs that make people well can keep them well. Doctors sometimes prescribe these drugs along with other drugs to relieve anxiety or to improve sleep.

Drugs Often Used with Psychotherapy

Combining medications with talking therapy, or psychotherapy, may help people with depression more than either treatment used alone. Talking therapies generally focus either on exploring roots of the depression or on trying to rout feelings and behavior that cause a person difficulty or distress in coping with everyday life.

Persons with depression who feel most gloomy in the morning and whose mood improves in the afternoon possibly may benefit more from psychotherapy in the afternoon, too, as they may be more open and receptive to exploring feelings then. This notion has not been studied. Persons who are so severely depressed that they require hospitalization likely would participate in individual and group psychotherapy both mornings and afternoons.

Severely depressed persons also may benefit from electroconvulsive therapy, in which doctors induce a controlled seizure with a small electrical current. This treatment normalizes some daily rhythms, including body temperature, perhaps a factor in its ability to ease depression.[20]

Light Therapy May Benefit Major Depression

Light may lift moods in persons who are clinically depressed within one week, Daniel Kripke of the University of California at San Diego found, in research that predated the use of light for SAD.[21] In a review of studies of the efficacy of either light or drugs used alone, he found that light therapy reduced negative moods in persons with major depression by as much as 35 percent, as measured by a standard depression rating scale. Antidepressant medications yielded similar results.

Light and medications appear to work best for major depression when used together. Depressed patients can get speedy relief with light therapy,

Kripke said, while also starting on medications known to be helpful. Combined treatment thus may both ease distress sooner and lower treatment costs.[22]

"Wake-up" Therapy Offers Additional Help

Studies going back to the 1970s show that about six out of ten persons with depression deprived of all or part of a night's sleep get better, often dramatically so. Some one hundred studies involving more than 5,000 patients confirm this outcome. This is a curious finding, since persons with depression often complain they sleep poorly. Moreover, persons who are not depressed typically report their mood worsens when they miss sleep.

The timing of sleep deprivation may affect its success. Depressed persons deprived of sleep in the latter half of the night, that is, from about 3 A.M. on, often report feeling much better than those kept from sleeping earlier in the night. Persons whose mood varies considerably over the day and from day to day tend to do better than those whose mood changes relatively little.

These discoveries suggest that people with depression may be sleeping at the wrong biological time. The drastic curtailing of sleep somehow sets things right. The trouble with this treatment is that its benefits usually are short-lived. When allowed to nap the next day or to sleep the next night, most patients fall back into depression. Light therapy may help some to retain their improved moods.[23]

Shifting the timing of sleep, rather than cutting it short, however, has produced longer-lasting help. German researchers treated depressed persons who responded well to total sleep deprivation, asking them initially to go to bed at 5 P.M. and get up at midnight. On each subsequent day for the next week, they went to bed an hour later, until they reached the conventional sleep time of 11 P.M. to 6 A.M. Twenty of the thirty-three persons who followed this schedule maintained their improved moods, Mathias Berger and his colleagues at Freiburg University report.[24]

Doctors today may suggest that persons with depression try a night of total sleep deprivation. A positive result may give patients the confidence that they can get better, and encourage them to advance their sleep schedule by several hours temporarily. New studies suggest combining sleep deprivation with antidepressant medications or light therapy can both induce a rapid response and sustain it.

Bipolar Disorder

Persons with bipolar disease may experience highs, known as mania, alternating with either normal moods, or with depression. If you have this disorder, in your manic times, you may feel unusually elated, with a supercharged sense of self-esteem or grandiosity. (The word "mania" comes from a French word meaning crazed or frenzied.) You may function with little sleep and feel unusually productive. You may talk rapidly, feel thoughts racing, become distracted easily, and fidget a lot. Perhaps you also fly off the handle easily, if your grand schemes are thwarted.

Some people caught up in mania go on spending sprees, engage in sexual flings, quit their jobs, and make other impulsive decisions. In the throes of mania, actor Patty Duke reports in her book, *A Brilliant Madness,* she told Dick Cavett "and I do not know how many millions of other people that I was pregnant and that I was going to build an ark in the desert."[25] An estimated 1 percent of American adults have bipolar disorder. Both sexes are equally affected. The disorder may run in families.

Episodes may last for months, and often are seasonal. It's common to feel "up" in spring and summer and "down" in fall and winter, sometimes prompting persons with this disorder to be misdiagnosed as having SAD. If your moods swing up and down more than four times a year, you are a "rapid cycler." In some people, ups and downs follow a highly predictable pattern, more evidence implicating disturbed body rhythms. Some people experience "double-days" of forty-eight hours with little or no sleep when they switch from the lows of depression to the highs of mania. In some women, manic days occur most often near menstruation.

Rapid cyclers lead more disorganized daily lives than persons with normal moods, studies at the NIMH and the University of Pittsburgh Medical Center suggest. The bipolar patients vary more in when they get up, go to bed, have meals, and in their number of activities overall, Sharon Ashman and her colleagues found.[26]

Medications and Psychotherapy Are Standard Treatment

Lithium commonly is used to stabilize mania. Antiseizure medications also benefit some persons with bipolar disorder. These include carbamazepine (Tegretol, Atretol), and valproic acid (Depakene). The same antidepressants used for major depression also are used for bipolar disorder.

Psychotherapy aims to help persons with this disorder understand its chronic nature and the need to continue taking medication regularly. Electroconvulsive therapy, sleep deprivation, and light therapy benefit some patients. Families of persons with bipolar disorder need to be involved in treatment, so that they can watch for signs of impending crises and help their family member get appropriate care.

Pregnancy-Related Depression

Dramatic hormonal shifts may be the culprit in depression that surfaces both in pregnancy and following delivery. Treating depression in pregnancy is tricky, as a doctor must consider two patients, the mother and her baby.

Depressed women who stop using antidepressant medication early in pregnancy show a 50 percent relapse rate by the third trimester, according to an ongoing collaborative study at the medical schools of the University of California at Los Angeles, Harvard University, and Emory University. Women who continue to use these medications, fortunately, do not appear to have an increased risk for major malformations or higher rates of miscarriage, stillbirth, or prematurity.[27] Partial sleep deprivation[28] and morning light therapy[29] are alternative approaches. A small study suggests both may help.

About seven in ten new mothers suffer *baby blues.* Their mood swings, anxiety, and sadness typically appear within a few days of delivery, and resolve within a week without medication. About one in ten women develops a more severe *postpartum depression,* usually within a few weeks of delivery but sometimes months later. The diagnosis often is missed because new mothers feel ashamed to admit they are unhappy or simply attribute their poor mood to the inevitable lack of sleep; hospitals don't warn new mothers to watch for symptoms, and primary care physicians may focus on the child's physical health without assessing the mother-child interaction.

Mothers with postpartum depression talk less to their babies, display less affection, and are less responsive to infant cues than non-depressed mothers, according to Deirdre Ryan of the British Columbia Women's Hospital in Vancouver. At three months of age, their babies showed fewer positive facial expressions and more negative ones, and at six months, they had more problems with sleep and eating, and were more withdrawn than babies of healthy mothers. Group therapy benefits these women, she said, helping them overcome feelings of isolation.[30]

The presumed cause of postpartum depression is the sharp drop in estrogen that follows childbirth. Replacing this hormone may lift moods. In a British study, women with depression that began within three months of childbirth improved more when they used estrogen patches than women who used a placebo. Estrogen therapy may target the underlying cause of postpartum depression more directly than antidepressant medications, which also can provide effective relief.[31]

Breast-feeding may limit the choices of such medications, but it does not mean these drugs should not be used. Concerns about the use of antidepressants by nursing mothers, however, have prompted interest in nondrug therapy for postpartum depression. Sleep deprivation may be an answer, according to Barbara Parry of the University of California at San Diego. She found that sleep deprivation in the latter half of the night brought about improved moods within a day. Some women improved even more after a night of recovery sleep. Light therapy also may help.[32]

Timewise Tips

If you have winter blues:

Sleep in an east-facing room, if possible. Leave blinds or curtains open, and let the morning sun awaken you.

If you have trouble getting going in the morning, boost the lighting in your bedroom, bathroom, and kitchen.

If you must leave for work or school while it is still dark, spend time outdoors later, but as early in the day as you can.

Build sunlight exposure into your schedule by parking your car at the far end of the parking lot and walking to your office in the morning. Take a lunchtime or afternoon walk.

Anticipate an increased desire to snack, and have fruits and veggies readily available.

If you suspect you have winter SAD:

Ask your doctor for a referral to a specialist in this area. Other illnesses, including thyroid disorders and chronic viral infections, may mimic SAD. A specialist who prescribes light therapy for you also will monitor how well it works.

Talk to your doctor about the health of your eyes before starting light treatment. There is no evidence that light therapy causes eye damage or worsens existing disorders, but such dangers are at least a theoretical concern. If you have a disorder of the retina or optic nerve, glaucoma, or cataracts, you need to see your eye doctor regularly. Persons with illnesses that affect the retina, such as diabetes and lupus, and persons taking photosensitizing medications such as lithium, psoralen (used for some skin disorders), and even herbal treatments such as St.-John's-wort, also may need an eye exam.[33]

If you develop headaches, jittery feelings, insomnia, nausea, eye strain, or other symptoms while using light therapy, tell your doctor. Most side effects from light therapy are mild, according to Michael Terman of Columbia University, and will abate if you cut back on the duration of exposure.[34]

Take your vacation in the winter, in a sunny spot, if you can.

Maintain regular hours, particularly a regular morning wake-up time.

Study. Visit the Web site of the Society for Light Treatment and Biological Rhythms (www.sltbr.org). You'll find specialists in your community and light box manufacturers listed there. Join a support group, such as the National Organization for Seasonal Affective Disorder (www.nosad.org).

If you suspect you have summer SAD:

Stay inside in an air-conditioned environment as much as possible. Take cool showers, sip iced beverages, dress lightly.

If you think your child may have SAD:

Recognize that depressed children may act cranky or bored. They do not always appear despondent, tearful, or show other classic signs of depression.

Be alert to a drop in school performance, changes in sleep, social isolation, poor communication, sensitivity to rejection or failure, and frequent complaints of headaches, stomachaches, or other physical symptoms. In teenagers, drug or alcohol abuse, and aggressive or disruptive behaviors may be signs of depression.

Take seriously statements such as "I'd be better off dead," and try to address your child's feelings. The wave of school shootings that swept the U.S. in the 1990s provides a grim reminder that teenagers may yield to violent impulses toward themselves and others. Suicide is the second leading cause of death in the United States in persons aged 15 to 19 years.

Talk to your child's doctor about your concerns.

Study. Visit the Web site of the American Academy of Child and Adolescent Psychiatry (www.aacap.org).

If you have been diagnosed with bulimia:

Talk to your doctor about using light therapy, particularly if you note that your bingeing and purging worsens in winter.

Study. Visit the Web site of the American Psychiatric Association (www.psych.org).

If you have major depression:

Be sensitive to changes in your sleep patterns, particularly sustained insomnia. Sleep may grow progressively worse for several weeks before a full-fledged episode of depression, studies by Michael Perlis of the University of Rochester and his colleagues suggest.[35] Call your doctor, who may suggest medication or other treatment to prevent an acute episode.

If you take antidepressant drugs, and feel sleepy in the daytime, tell your doctor. Your medicine may be disturbing your sleep without your being aware of it. Changing the time or dose, or switching to another drug, may relieve this symptom. Some SSRIs trigger sleep-onset insomnia, and have been linked in a small number of cases to the development of the delayed sleep phase syndrome (see page 342.)[36]

Don't self-medicate with alternative remedies for depression without talking with your doctor first. Early studies suggest St.-John's-wort, widely used in Europe, may be helpful for mild depression and for SAD; an NIMH study to assess its efficacy is now in progress. (Recall that light-therapy users with eye disorders should avoid St.-John's-wort.) The value of many alternative remedies is still unproved. You may suffer needlessly by delaying proper care.

Study. Visit the Web sites of the National Institute of Mental Health (www.nimh.nih.gov/) and the Depression and Related Affective Disorders Association (www.med.jhu.edu/drada/).

If you have bipolar disorder:

Work hard to stick to a regular daily schedule for sleep, meals, work, exercise, even TV watching. Sleep loss may trigger a manic episode. Ask family members to let you know if you're becoming irritable or acting erratically, and to help you get treatment before the situation gets out of hand.

Study. Visit the Web site of the National Depressive and Manic-Depressive Association (www.ndmda.org).

If you are pregnant:

Know that occasional tearfulness, anxiety, and worries are normal. Talk about your feelings with your partner, doctor, and friends.

If you are a new mother:

Talk to your doctor. He or she can reassure you that baby blues are common and provide treatment if they last too long or deepen.

Join a support group in your community or online. Type "new mom" at any major search engine, and follow the links.

Study. Visit the Web sites of the American Academy of Family Practice (www.aafp.org/) and Postpartum Support International (www.iup.edu/an/postpartum/).

MULTIPLE SCLEROSIS

The film *Hilary and Jackie* chronicled the battle with multiple sclerosis (MS) of talented cellist Jacqueline du Pré. The film implied MS symptoms such as loss of coordination and bladder control always erupt without warning. In fact, many MS symptoms show rhythmic patterns across the day and, in women, across the menstrual cycle. These patterns allow persons with this illness some measure of control in planning their activities.

MS is a baffling disorder of the brain and spinal cord. For still unknown reasons, the body's immune system mistakenly turns on itself, attacking its myelin, the insulation on nerve fibers. The myelin wears away in patches, known as plaques. This damage leaves multiple scars, or sclerosis, that slow, garble, or stop transmission of nerve signals. Damage at multiple sites gives rise to a wide range of symptoms, including fatigue, weakness, poor coordination, blurred or double vision, tingling and other strange sensations in feet, legs, hands, or arms, and trouble walking.

Because the body normally works hard to repair itself, symptoms in the early stages of MS may come and go and range markedly in severity. In an estimated 40 percent of persons with MS, symptoms persist. They may worsen to include problems with bladder and bowel control, sexual dysfunction, slurred speech, trouble with balance and memory, depression, paralysis, and, in rare instances, early death. MS took the life of Jacqueline du Pré at age forty-two in 1987.

Symptoms usually first appear between ages twenty and forty. The illness is more common in persons who grew up in temperate climates, in the northern part of the United States, for example, than in warmer latitudes. It also is most common in persons with northern European ancestry. Early life exposure to an infectious agent thus may trigger MS in persons genetically prone to it.

If you have MS, you eventually may need a cane or crutches to aid in walking. You may require an electric scooter or a wheelchair. But even so, you probably have good days and bad days, and better times and worse times on any given day.

Daily Symptoms Often Tied to Body Temperature

Heat aggravates symptoms in many persons with MS by making damaged nerves even less efficient in transmitting signals. MS symptoms often prove least troubling in the morning, worsen in the late afternoon and early evening, and then lessen by bedtime, in tandem with the normal daily rise in body temperature from about 96° F near 4 A.M. to about 100° F around 7 P.M.[1]

A Day with MS

♦ "I try to do my errands in the morning, when I have more energy. One afternoon, in a department store, I felt as if I were walking through wet cement. I could barely move my feet. I was staggering, really. People must have thought I was drunk."

—Marla, age 37

"I can read the paper and watch TV just fine in the morning, but not in the afternoon. The six o'clock news is unpleasantly blurry. After about 8 P.M., I can watch TV again, read, and even work at my computer."

—Ron, age 42

Any activity that boosts body temperature, as well as hot, humid weather when sweating doesn't provide adequate body cooling, may aggravate symptoms, too.[2] Suffering a fever may have the same effect. Research in the 1950s showed that an increase of as little as .5° F above normal body temperature may make MS worse. This finding provided the basis for a short-lived diagnostic test, in which doctors placed persons suspected of having MS in a warm bath, and then in an ice bath, measuring their responses after each exposure. While heat-related symptoms fortunately are almost always reversible, doctors today use more reliable and sophisticated tests, such as magnetic resonance imaging.

The early studies affirmed, however, that cooling down may help relieve MS symptoms. Sudden exposure to cold weather, for reasons that are not clear, may worsen MS symptoms. Still, many persons with MS report they feel better in an air-conditioned environment. It is hard to lower body temperature and keep it down with cool air alone, however. The body's internal regulatory mechanisms are so efficient that body temperature soon returns to normal for the particular time of day.

Because water conducts temperature better than air, swimming or merely sitting in a cool pool or bathtub for thirty minutes or so can lower temperature for several hours. This finding prompted the design of cool suits and caps, not stylishly "cool," but literally so, adapted from technology devised to control body temperature in astronauts working in outer space.[3] Clothing and hats with pockets for ice or gel packs as well as battery-operated devices that circulate a cooling fluid already are on the market. A national multicenter trial to see if cooling therapy offers sustained benefits was in progress when this book went to press.[4]

Fatigue Disturbing but Invisible

Fatigue is virtually a universal complaint in MS. It is an invisible symptom, hard for those who suffer from it to explain it to their families, coworkers, and employers, and hard for doctors to assess. Fatigue severity is not correlated with the extent of a person's physical disability, nor with measures of MS detectable by magnetic resonance imaging.[5] Yet it causes considerable distress, as it sabotages performance of normal daily activities. If you have MS, tuning into your fatigue rhythms may help you to take advantage of your best times.

Researchers at the Rocky Mountain MS Center in Englewood, Colorado, have identified eight causes of fatigue. Some apply specifically to persons with MS and other neurological illnesses, and some may produce fatigue in anyone.[6] A person with MS may have several types of fatigue simultaneously. Possible causes of fatigue include:

MS itself. Many persons with MS say they experience an unusual and profound fatigue that differs from any sensation they experienced before becoming ill. "I feel like a sponge squeezed dry," "like being trapped in a giant spiderweb," or "like I am wearing heavy metal shoes" are typical complaints.

This overwhelming fatigue has a pronounced daily rhythm tied to the body temperature cycle.

Neuromuscular symptoms. After jogging for a few blocks, a young woman with MS started dragging her foot. A few blocks farther on, she could barely stand up. Damaged nerve fibers that can't cope with repetitive use cause this type of fatigue. While elevated body temperature may add to it, this problem may occur even while stretching gently in a cold pool. With rest, abilities return to their starting point.

Disability. Persons with MS expend more effort than other people on routine tasks, from pulling on socks to walking to the mailbox. Mobility aids, such as canes and walkers, and energy-saving strategies, such as sitting while preparing a meal, can be useful.

Deconditioning. It's the familiar "use it or lose it" refrain. If you feel weak and weary, it's hard to muster the energy to exercise. Unfortunately, a vicious circle may develop, and the less active you are, the greater your loss of muscle strength.

Depression. While it's understandable that persons with a chronic illness might feel depressed, persons with MS have higher rates of depression than persons with similar or even greater disabilities, such as spinal cord injuries causing paralysis. Depression may be both a reaction to the illness and a consequence of damage to nerve cells in some parts of the brain.[7] Antidepressant medications may improve mood; a bonus is that they also often ease MS pain.

Disturbed sleep. The need to urinate frequently, spasticity, pain, tingling, and other strange sensations may disrupt sleep. Some medications taken to combat daytime fatigue may cause insomnia at night. Persons with depression may sleep poorly; conversely, difficulty sleeping may upset a person's mood. Poor sleep habits, such as not keeping regular hours, can sabotage anyone's sleep. Research to date shows no specific sleep disorder in MS. That's good news, because it means medications of known efficacy for sleep disorders, and good sleep hygiene, may be helpful.

Poor diet. Snacking on sugary foods, not consuming enough carbohydrates, trying fad diets, and drinking too much alcohol may cause fatigue.

Exertion. Physical, mental, and emotional work may make anyone weary. This type of fatigue is normal, and improves after rest or sleep.

Attacks May Be Tied to Cyclic Hormones

Two-thirds to three-quarters of the 250,000 to 350,000 persons in the United States with MS are female. This fact suggests female sex hormones play an important role in the illness. In one study, nearly half of a group of sixty women with the relapsing-remitting form of MS said their symptoms predictably worsened just before or at the start of their periods, a pattern common to many illnesses. Estrogen levels are low at this time. (See page 123.) Many of the women without menstrual worsening were taking birth-control pills, which raised their estrogen levels. These findings suggest that low levels of estrogen make the immune system in women more reactive, and high levels dampen immune responses.[8]

More support for this theory comes from the observation that MS symptoms abate in the later stages of pregnancy, when the female hormone estriol, one type of estrogen, is prominent. The risk that the illness will flare rises in the six to nine months after childbirth, though fortunately not so severely as to prompt doctors to advise women with MS against pregnancy. Research studies showing estriol can inhibit or prevent MS-like disease in mice prompt interest in the possibility that it may help humans, too.[9]

In the first clinical trial of a pregnancy hormone in MS, Rhonda Voskuhl of the University of California at Los Angeles and her colleagues are giving estriol to twelve premenopausal nonpregnant women with MS. The researchers will track the status of the women's disease for six months before treatment, during treatment, and afterward. They hope to determine whether estriol provides any benefits, whether it is safe, and how much of it is needed to have an effect, setting the stage for a larger study. The pilot study is scheduled to be completed in 2000.[10]

At menopause, female sex hormones plunge, and many women report MS symptoms worsen. Symptoms such as hot flashes reflect problems with body temperature regulation, often an issue in MS flare-ups. In a British study, symptoms improved in three-quarters of a group of postmenopausal women with MS who used hormone replacement therapy (HRT).[11]

Sex hormones may play a role in MS in men, too. One study found that one-quarter of a group of men with MS had lower than normal levels of the male hormone testosterone. Some studies show that testosterone reduces the severity and incidence of an MS-like disease in mice. It is possible that it may have that effect on humans, too.[12]

Attacks May Vary Seasonally

The initial bout of MS, and later flare-ups of symptoms, according to several studies, occur 50 percent more often in the late spring and summer than in late fall or winter.[13] This pattern may be tied to environmental factors, such as changes in heat and humidity.

Variety of Medicines Requires Attention to Timing

To combat fatigue, physicians may prescribe stimulant medications. These work best when taken in the morning. When taken late in the day, they may disturb your nighttime sleep.

Fatigue Diary

Name _____

Make seven copies of this chart and fill them in for the coming week. Add columns for symptoms that trouble you most. Change times if you work at night. Take this diary with you when you see your doctor.

Day/Date _____

Time of Arising _____ A.M./P.M.

Bedtime _____ A.M./P.M.

Women: **Are you menstruating today? Y/N**

Time	Fatigue Severity Low High 1 2 3 4 5	Weakness Severity Low High 1 2 3 4 5	(Symptom) ————— Severity Low High 1 2 3 4 5	Possible Trigger	Length of Fatigue Episode	Treatment Used
8 A.M.						
10 A.M.						
NOON						
2 P.M.						
4 P.M.						
6 P.M.						
8 P.M.						
10 P.M.						
MIDNIGHT						

To calm acute flare-ups of MS, physicians may prescribe corticosteroid drugs, to be taken orally or given intravenously. These medications work best and cause the fewest side effects when given in the morning, in tandem with the body's normal peak production of cortisol.

To relieve stiffening of muscles, physicians may prescribe muscle relaxants. These drugs often cause sleepiness. If using them, don't drive until you see how they affect you. If you take them at bedtime, they may help you sleep better.

To reduce the frequency and severity of relapses, physicians may prescribe one of three drugs now approved in the United States for MS: Avonex, Betaseron, and Copaxone. The National Multiple Sclerosis Society recommends that people start taking one of these medications as soon as their diagnosis is confirmed. Patients inject these medications in the same way that some persons with diabetes give themselves insulin shots. The frequency of injections required for MS treatment ranges from once a day to once a week. No specific time is recommended for the injections, other than a consistent time. If you are using these medications, however, you may be able to avoid some associated short-lived symptoms, such as pain at the injection site or nausea, by giving yourself your shot at bedtime and escaping into sleep.

Timewise Tips

Chart daily, menstrual-cycle, and seasonal patterns in your MS, using the Fatigue Diary on page 314. Use this information to plan activities and rest periods.

Nap or schedule a rest period daily. Get enough sleep at night. Being overtired makes many MS symptoms worse. If you don't sleep well, talk to your doctor about possibly taking sleeping pills.

See whether changing the time you take medications makes your symptoms better or worse. Add your observations to your diary, and report them to your doctor.

Anytime Tips

Prioritize. Try to do your most important tasks first.

Avoid excessive heat and humidity. If your physician prescribes an air conditioner to ease your symptoms, its cost may be tax deductible. Ask your accountant.

See a physical therapist for tips on exercise, geared to all levels of disability, as well as information on ways to maximize energy and on mobility aids.

Exercise in a cool environment, such as a swimming pool or even the bathtub. You may feel weary after exercising, but you should see a gradual improvement in your endurance over time.

Get a flu shot annually. Having the flu would put you at higher risk of having a flare-up of MS.

Learn strategies of stress management and relaxation. Consider joining a sup-

)nline groups offer a special boon to persons who must operate
ice or who can't easily get to community meetings.

the Web site of the National Multiple Sclerosis Society
.w.nmss.org).

NOSEBLEEDS

Nosebleeds are four times as frequent at 8 A.M. as at 2 A.M., their least common time. There is another, smaller rise in nosebleeds at 8 P.M. Nosebleeds
also occur more than twice as often in January as in July.

These findings come from a study in Italy, where nosebleeds prompt
emergency-room visits more often than they do in most other countries. In
seven years 1,706 persons sought care for nosebleeds at the University of Fer-
rara, Italy, teaching hospital. Medical records for 1,340 of them included the
time the nosebleeds started.[1]

The morning rise in blood pressure that occurs around the time people
habitually awaken may contribute to this daily pattern. But nosebleeds prove
equally frequent in the morning in persons with and without high blood pressure. Thus, other body rhythms, even the action of chewing foods at breakfast, also may play a role. Seasonal differences in temperature and relative
humidity may be factors in the annual pattern.

Timewise Tips

If you have frequent nosebleeds, record the times they occur.

Keep a blood pressure diary. (See page 289.) Take both records with you when
you see your doctor.

Talk to your doctor about treatment to seal the bleeding blood vessel. If your nosebleeds typically occur at a particular time of day, schedule your appointment
at that time. This will boost the likelihood that the doctor can identify the
blood vessel causing your problem.

OSTEOPOROSIS

Your bone factory is busiest on the night shift. Bone remodeling, the ongoing
replacement of new bone for old bone, occurs mainly in sleep. Treatment
keyed to this time process may help slow bone loss in later years, perhaps
sparing millions of people pain, inconvenience, loss of function, and cost of
fractures.

Bone Up on Life Cycle Changes

In childhood and adolescence, new bone construction exceeds old bone demolition. Teenagers may grow six inches, sometimes even more, in a single year. For the next two decades, breakdown and buildup balance each other, and you replace 6 percent to 12 percent of the 206 bones in your skeleton every year. Starting about the fourth decade, bone loss outpaces new bone formation. Bones lose calcium, the mineral that makes them hard, faster than it can be replaced.

This process accelerates in women at menopause, with a drastic fall in production of the female sex hormone estrogen, which helps strengthen bones. For about three to seven years after menopause, bone loss speeds up. It then continues at a less rapid pace. Bone loss is more of a problem for women than men, as women's bones generally are smaller and lighter to start with. Short, thin men are more apt to have problems with bone thinning than are those built like linebackers.

Loss of bone density, if severe, may lead to osteoporosis, literally, "porous bones." This condition affects 10 million Americans, 80 percent of them women, mainly in their fifties and older. Porous bones, particularly those of the hip, wrist, and spine, break more easily than healthy bones. One in three women over age fifty will endure a fracture because of osteoporosis at some time. Americans suffer some 1.5 million fractures annually, at a cost to the nation of about $14 billion in medical expenses. Many experience continuing pain and limitations in ease of movement.

Why Old Bones Ain't Going to Rise Again

The disparity between bone loss and bone formation increases in later life. One study in postmenopausal women found that the blood level of deoxypyridinoline, a marker of bone loss, jumped by 62 percent at night; the women's blood level of osteocalcin, a chemical marker of bone formation, increased by only 5 percent at night.

Postmenopausal women prone to fractures excreted significantly more calcium in their urine at night than a comparable group not prone to fractures. This is a worrisome finding. Bone-building cells ordinarily pick up calcium that enters the bloodstream via food or medication, and use it to add strength to new bone. As much as 500 milligrams of calcium enters or leaves the adult skeleton every day.

The body also uses calcium to aid muscle contraction, transmission of nerve signals, and other functions. If blood calcium is low, the body takes the amount it needs for these other purposes by stealing it from existing bones, sapping their strength, particularly at night when people ordinarily do not consume calcium-containing foods or supplements.[1]

k?

g calcium intake increases bone mass in younger people, reduces bone loss in older people, and lowers the risk of suffering fractures. Milk, yogurt, spinach, and sardines and salmon with bones are among the many good food sources of this essential mineral. Indeed, calcium-rich foods are "the preferred source of calcium," according to a consensus statement on optimal calcium intake developed by the National Institutes of Health (NIH) and the National Academy of Sciences (NAS) in 1997.

The NAS guidelines for dietary reference intakes, or DRIs (formerly called recommended daily allowances, or RDAs), specify that both men and women aged nineteen and older need at least 1,000 milligrams of calcium a day. After age fifty-one, the DRI is 1,200 milligrams a day.

Most people don't get as much calcium as they need in their usual diet. Calcium supplements, however, are widely available and inexpensive. Many doctors advise taking 400 to 800 international units of vitamin D in addition to the supplements, to boost calcium's absorption.

What Is the Right Time to Take Calcium?

Since bone remodeling peaks at night, it might seem logical to make calcium available by taking calcium supplements at bedtime.

We asked leading experts in nutrition, endocrinology, and osteoporosis what time they recommended. They gave us these answers: "Morning." "Evening." "Both morning and evening." "Spread out through the day." "Any time." These opinions reflect the dearth of research that explores this question in a rigorous way.

In one study, researchers assessed markers of bone breakdown in eighteen women aged twenty to forty-seven, all premenopausal. The women then took 1,000 milligrams of calcium at either 8 A.M. or 11 P.M. for fourteen days. When they took calcium in the evening, their markers of bone breakdown fell by nearly 20 percent. When they took calcium in the morning, these markers stayed the same.[2]

Two other studies, however, failed to substantiate these findings. One found that taking calcium in the evening reduced bone loss only marginally,[3] while another found morning and evening doses of calcium had comparable effects.[4]

The timing issue is complicated further by the question of how much calcium you should take at one time. The NIH/NAS consensus statement says calcium supplements are absorbed best in individual doses of 500 mg or less. Higher doses, the expert panel noted, lead to higher amounts of calcium excreted in urine, and may increase the risk of kidney stones in some people. Higher doses also may trigger constipation in some people. Both bladder and bowel activity vary across the day, slowing down at night, and may alter the likelihood that such problems would occur.

In their book *Strong Women, Strong Bones*, Miriam Nelson and Sarah Wernick suggest spreading your calcium consumption, via both food and supplements, over the day. If most of your daily calcium intake comes from two supplements plus breakfast cereal with milk, they advise taking one supplement in the afternoon and the other in the evening.[5]

Whether you should take calcium supplements with food or between meals may depend on the type of calcium you take. The most common type of calcium supplement, *calcium carbonate*, is absorbed best when stomach acid is present. Take it with food, especially acidic foods, such as citrus juice or fruit.

Calcium citrate, however, is absorbed more easily on an empty stomach, that is, between meals. Doctors often recommend this form of calcium for persons taking medications that block stomach acid production, such as drugs used for heartburn or peptic ulcers, and for persons who produce little stomach acid, including many older adults and those who have had stomach surgery to reduce acid production.

The best time for you to take calcium also depends on other medications that you regularly take. Calcium may interfere with the absorption of an iron supplement, for example. Don't take both at the same time. Calcium also may inhibit absorption of tetracycline, and of aspirin and other medications containing salicylates. This is a lot to keep in mind. See Timewise Tips, page 320, for help in organizing your daily routine.

New Prescription Medicine May Slow Bone Loss

Women of menopausal age, and older, small-boned men, should get periodic bone-density scans. These are quick and painless imaging studies that provide a picture of your bone health and allow your doctor to compare you to healthy persons of the same height, weight, and age. If you develop significant bone loss, taking additional calcium will not be enough to halt this deterioration and reduce your risk of fractures. Many doctors recommend estrogen replacement therapy for women; research suggests it helps curb the risk of wrist and spine fractures by 50 percent and hip fractures by 25 percent. Women who cannot use hormone replacement therapy or choose not to may opt to use a selective estrogen receptor modulator, or SERM, a new type of drug that provides some of estrogen's benefits. Raloxifene (Evista) is one such drug. (See chapter 11: "Time for Sex.")

If your bone loss is severe enough to be classed as osteoporosis, your doctor may suggest taking a bisphosphonate drug to reduce bone loss and perhaps even build new bone. Two drugs of this type currently are available in the United States. The recommended dosing time for the widely used medication alendronate (Fossamax) is the morning.[6] There are no published studies examining its effects when it is taken at other times of day. There also are no published studies on the other bisphosphonate, etidronate (Didronel).

Timewise Tips

Ask your doctor to check your overnight urine for markers of bone breakdown and buildup. Empty your bladder before going to bed, making a note of the time. Collect all urine passed in the night, and the first voiding after you awaken in the morning, again noting the time.

Take alendronate (Fossamax) soon after awakening, sitting straight up, with a full glass of water, to avoid irritation to your esophagus. Wait thirty minutes before eating or taking other medications. This schedule may be incompatible with that for some other medications that need to be taken immediately on awakening, such as drugs to prevent high blood pressure. In this instance, ask your doctor to switch you to one of the blood pressure chronotherapies that are taken at night.

Tell your primary care doctor about all the medications you are taking, including those prescribed by specialists, and any herbal remedies or food supplements you regularly use. Make an hour-by-hour daytime schedule, and work out with your doctor the best time to take all of your medications to maximize their efficacy, reduce your risk of side effects, and lower the likelihood of drug interactions. Your pharmacist also can help you with these decisions.

Anytime Tips

Review your diet (many online programs will do this for you), and be sure you are getting an adequate amount of calcium via foods and supplements. Taking your calcium supplements at the same time every day will help ensure that you take them regularly. Keep supplements in your kitchen, bathroom, and purse so they're readily at hand when it's time to take them.

Walk briskly, run, dance, play tennis, lift weights. Regular weight-bearing exercise builds up bone mass early in life and maintains it later on.

Ask your doctor to order a bone scan to check the health of your bones, and discuss whether estrogen replacement therapy is appropriate.

Whatever your age, ask your doctor how best to decrease your risk of bone fractures. Your risk is higher if you

- are postmenopausal
- have small bones
- have a parent with osteoporosis
- are of Caucasian or Asian ancestry

- take certain medications, including thyroid hormone, corticosteroids, and drugs to prevent seizures
- smoke
- drink a great deal of alcohol
- had anorexia nervosa in early adulthood

Study. Visit the Web site of the National Osteoporosis Foundation (www.nof.org).

PEPTIC ULCERS

Peptic ulcers act up late at night for the same reason that heartburn intensifies then: the pain coincides with the daily peak in production of stomach acid between 10 P.M. and 2 A.M.[1] (See Heartburn, page 274.)

Peptic ulcers are craterlike sores that take their name from a key component of stomach acid, the enzyme pepsin. Peptic ulcers occur only in areas of the digestive tract bathed by stomach acid, that is, the lining of the stomach and the duodenum, the first part of the small intestine. The pain may last from several minutes to several hours. It rarely lasts until morning.

About 4 million American adults have peptic ulcers at any one time, and an estimated one in ten men and one in twenty-five women will suffer from them at least once in their lifetime. Older persons develop peptic ulcers more often than younger persons.

Appreciating why peptic ulcer pain worsens at night is new, but recognition of the disorder's pain pattern is not. In 1910 the prominent Irish surgeon B. Moynihan observed that peptic ulcer pain usually first surfaces about two hours after people eat their heaviest meal. As the illness progresses, he said, pain becomes noticeable about two hours after each meal. "It is a characteristic feature of pain," he wrote, "that it wakes the patient in the night. . . . Constantly the time of awakening is said to be 2 o'clock."[2]

Recent studies validate his observation. British researchers, for example, found that 88 percent of one hundred persons with duodenal ulcers they queried reported nighttime pain. Nearly half the patients said ulcer flare-ups caused pain as often as three or four nights a week. Stomach ulcer sufferers also reported bouts of nighttime pain, although somewhat less often than those with duodenal ulcers.[3]

Increased secretion of stomach acid at night ordinarily is beneficial. The acid helps cleanse the stomach after the day's meals. The lining of a healthy stomach and the duodenum normally provide adequate protection from irritation. When body rhythms are in tune, other nighttime bodily functions, such as the secretion of additional acid-buffering substances, help prevent injury.

Setting the Scene for Peptic Ulcers

Until the 1980s stress got most of the blame for peptic ulcers. Now, it's recognized that a chronic infection of the stomach lining by the bacterium *Helicobacter pylori* is the prime culprit in nearly all peptic ulcers. This bacterium, widely present in the world around us, may neutralize stomach acid or increase its secretion.[4] The mere presence of the bacterium in the stomach is not enough to cause peptic ulcers. About one-third of young adults and two-thirds of those over sixty-five are infected with this bacterium, but most have no symptoms.

Some people prove more resistant to *Helicobacter pylori* than others. This is where stress may play a contributory role, perhaps by disrupting normal ups and downs in the stomach's circadian rhythms. In animals with stomach ulcers, for example, rhythms that protect the stomach lining do not occur at the right time to balance daily acid production.[5] Upsets in circadian rhythms may explain why rotating shift workers and night-shift workers suffer peptic ulcers far more often than persons who work only on the day shift. Frequent changes in the hours of waking and sleep, and in mealtimes, prompt a continuing tug of war between factors that evoke ulcer disease and factors that resist it. (See chapter 13: "Clockwatching at Work.")

Even for those on the day shift, fast and irregular meals—the burger picked up at a drive-through restaurant and gulped on the road, the vending-machine sandwich downed at your desk—disrupt normal daily digestive patterns and increase your risk of peptic ulcers. Some substances add to this risk. Alcohol and caffeine, for example, are irritants. When consumed in large amounts, they erode the lining of the stomach and duodenum. Persons who smoke also are more apt to develop peptic ulcers, as smoking stimulates stomach acid production. Some persons have a higher inherited susceptibility to peptic ulcers than others.

Prolonged use of aspirin and other nonsteroidal anti-inflammatory medications, or NSAIDs, such as flurbiprofen and ibuprofen, for chronic pain cause perhaps 10 percent of peptic ulcers. (See Arthritis, page 207.)

Evening Dose of Acid-Suppressing Medicines Works Best

Treatment aims to relieve symptoms and heal the ulcer fast, keep the ulcer from recurring, and, if possible, avoid surgery. Treatment often involves a multifaceted approach, using several different types of drugs. People with peptic ulcers who take NSAIDs usually are told to stop doing so.

Antibiotics

If a *Helicobacter pylori* infection is the cause of your peptic ulcers, the usual treatment involves antibiotics, sometimes a combination of antibiotics, such as tetracycline and metronidazole, along with bismuth to coat the stomach. This approach has a greater than 90 percent success rate.[6] Antibiotics usually are taken three or four times a day, at roughly equal intervals, for a week or longer.

Antacids

Antacids neutralize stomach acid and may be useful for flare-ups, but they typically give only temporary and partial relief. Even if taken at bedtime, they seldom last long enough to suppress nighttime pain.

Acid-Suppressing Medicines

Several studies show ulcer healing is related directly to how well medications inhibit nighttime acid secretion.[7] Acid-suppressing medicines are much more effective than antacids, since they are more potent and their benefits last longer. When you take these drugs makes a huge difference in their ability to relieve pain and promote healing.

Widely used acid-suppressing medications, with names that end in "-tidine," including ranitidine and cimetidine, work best when taken in a single dose in the evening[8]—at dinnertime, not at bedtime. The dinnertime dose best inhibits acid secretion before it surges in late evening, as well as overnight, and on the following day.[9]

Since ulcers may act up throughout the day, you might think that it would help to take these medications in the morning as well as at night. Studies show that's not the case. Twice-a-day schedules for these drugs don't adequately suppress acid secretion at night.[10] New acid-suppressing medications called proton pump inhibitors, such as omeprazole and lansoprazole, appear to work effectively around the clock when taken in the morning.

Bleeding Ulcers Show Rhythmic Patterns

If peptic ulcers do not heal properly, they may destroy the lining of the stomach or intestine, causing it to rupture or perforate. This event produces sudden and severe abdominal pain. It is a medical emergency that can lead to extensive loss of blood and to shock.

Ulcer perforations occur two to three times more often in the afternoon and evening than at night. In a study of nearly 1,500 patients, Norwegian researchers found stomach ulcer perforations peaked between 11 A.M. and 1 P.M., but were uncommon between 2 A.M. and 8 A.M. Intestinal perforations were greatest between 2 P.M. and midnight and were least frequent between 5 A.M. and 10 A.M.[11]

Ulcer perforations also vary weekly and seasonally. They occur most often on Fridays and in winter.[12] While biologic rhythms likely contribute to these patterns, other factors undoubtedly also are involved, such as cyclic variations in environmental and emotional stressors, and varying use of tobacco and alcohol, both of which may aggravate ulcers. The virulence of the *Helicobacter pylori* bacterium also varies seasonally.[13]

Timewise Tips

If you often suffer indigestion and gnawing abdominal pain after meals and at night, see your doctor promptly. Ask your doctor to test you for the *Helicobacter pylori* bacterium.

If taking any medication for peptic ulcer disease, be sure you know the proper time to take it, and stick to your prescribed regimen.

If taking aspirin or other NSAIDs regularly for pain relief, tell your doctor if you experience digestive problems. Ask your doctor to time NSAID treatment to your particular symptom pattern. Also ask whether you should take your medication with food or milk to coat the interior of your stomach and help reduce further stomach irritation.

Anytime Tips

If peptic ulcers run in your family, adopt lifestyle habits to lower your risk. If you smoke, stop. Consume caffeine and alcohol in moderation.

Perform an annual self-test for hidden blood in your stool using a kit available from your doctor or at pharmacies. Peptic ulcers that cause little or no pain may still cause slow bleeding.

Study. Visit the Web site of the Centers for Disease Control and Prevention (http://www.cdc.gov/ncidod/dbmd/hpylori.htm).

PREMENSTRUAL SYNDROME AND PREMENSTRUAL DYSPHORIC DISORDER

Most women experience some discomforting symptoms in the four or five days before their periods start and for the first day or two of menstruation. These collectively are called *premenstrual syndrome,* or PMS.

Physical symptoms often include fluid retention with two or three pounds' weight gain, abdominal bloating, breast tenderness, joint or muscle pain, and poor sleep. Emotional symptoms often include feeling anxious, irritable, and sad, or having difficulty concentrating. Appetite-related symptoms include increased desire for food and cravings for sweet or salty foods. In many chronic illnesses described elsewhere in this chapter—asthma, migraines, diabetes, skin disorders, and others—menstruation triggers flare-ups.

Researchers have cataloged some 150 different symptoms of PMS. These vary in type and intensity from woman to woman, but tend to be fairly consistent for any one woman. Two thousand years ago, men thought menstruating women could sour wine and tarnish metal. In the twentieth century, a physician triggered an acrimonious debate by asserting women's "raging hormones" made them unfit for public office. Such attitudes and expectations may shape a woman's experience of menstruation. Nonetheless, most women adapt to what is normal for them, allow for variation from month to month, and seamlessly accommodate their lives to this predictable event. Relatively few seek a doctor's help, although some could benefit from treatments introduced in the 1990s.

Better understanding of the biological rhythms behind PMS debunks the fiction that PMS is merely "in the mind." The American Psychiatric Association (APA) forthrightly states that transient menstrually related mood changes "should not be considered a mental disorder."[1]

About one woman in twenty, however, finds that her menstrually related symptoms interfere markedly with her work and social life, and are temporarily disabling. These women may have a true psychiatric illness, called *premenstrual dysphoric disorder.*

What Causes PMS?

PMS "represents an abnormal response to normal hormonal changes," scientists at the National Institute of Mental Health (NIMH) reported in 1998. In the first study to demonstrate the long-suspected tie between the prime female sex hormones and PMS symptoms, Peter Schmidt and his colleagues assessed these hormones separately.

They made a surprising discovery: estrogen was as potent in triggering PMS symptoms as progesterone, long thought the prime culprit. Estrogen dominates the first half of the cycle, and progesterone the second. Both plunge when menstruation starts. (See chapter 11: "Time for Sex.")

The researchers recruited women with and without PMS via newspaper ads. The women all kept daily diaries for three months to verify that symptoms in those with PMS occurred only in conjunction with their periods. The women then received injections of either a drug that turned off secretion of sex hormones or an inactive saline solution. Ten of eighteen women with PMS improved when they got the drug. None of those with PMS who got the saline got better. The women who got better with the drug then participated in a further study, taking either estrogen or progesterone alone, and then both together in different months. In all instances, their PMS symptoms came back. The same hormone treatment had no effect on women without PMS.[2]

Yet all the women were very much alike. Both those with PMS and those without it had normal menstrual cycles, and normal hormone levels and activity. The women with PMS ordinarily had no symptoms in the first half of the month when their estrogen levels naturally were high.

Why, then, did estrogen alone make their PMS worse? Perhaps a sudden encounter with high amounts of estrogen may worsen symptoms, while the usual, gradual build up of estrogen in the body does not. Perhaps the hormone-suppressing drug itself altered estrogen's impact. Or perhaps the researchers, who knew which women were taking the drug, somehow influenced the women's response.[3] Doctors now need to look further at estrogen, never before thought to have negative effects on mood. They will try to find out what happens early in the month that fosters PMS later on. The NIMH study also showed that progesterone, still sometimes prescribed for PMS, is not a useful treatment.

There are no laboratory tests that reliably diagnose PMS. Keeping a diary (see end of this section) is the best way to show your doctor the pattern and severity of your symptoms.

What Is Premenstrual Dysphoric Disorder?

To be diagnosed with what the American Psychiatric Association calls premenstrual dysphoric disorder (PMDD), a woman must have experienced certain symptoms only in the week before her period started for most menstrual cycles in the past year. She must have had five or more symptoms that disappeared in the week after menstruation, including at least one of the first four on the following list:

- Feeling sad, hopeless, or self-deprecating
- Feeling tense, anxious, or "on edge"
- Having marked mood swings with tearfulness
- Having persistent irritability, anger, and increased interpersonal conflicts
- Having decreased interest in usual activities
- Having difficulty concentrating
- Feeling fatigued, lethargic, or lacking in energy
- Having marked changes in appetite, possibly including binge eating or food cravings
- Sleeping too much or too little
- Feeling overwhelmed or out of control
- Having physical symptoms such as breast tenderness, headaches, and bloating
- Having suicidal thoughts

Some psychiatrists already were leery about calling PMDD a mental disorder. The new research showing the biological underpinnings of this mix of emotional and physical symptoms heightens this debate. The APA's bible for clinicians, the *Diagnostic and Statistical Manual of Mental Disorders*, published in 1994, lists PMDD in an appendix of illnesses needing further study.[4] For the present, women probably benefit from having the disorder included in the manual. Medical insurance companies seldom provide reimbursement for care without an official diagnosis.

What Treatments Help Most?

New drug and nondrug treatments benefit an estimated 70 percent of women with severe PMS. These include:

Birth-control pills: Although most women with PMS have normal hormone levels, some may be unusually sensitive to hormonal shifts. Birth-control pills suppress ovulation, flattening out these swings. Many users report that PMS symptoms lessen. Women prone to depression, however, may find that the pills aggravate this disorder.

Drugs for specific symptoms: Numerous drugs target problems such as fluid retention, breast tenderness, headaches, and anxiety.

Drugs that boost levels of serotonin: In addition to inducing calmness, this brain chemical carries messages to and from the biological clock. A deficiency in serotonin may prompt the notorious cravings for sweets in PMS. Drugs that increase the supply of serotonin in the brain, known as selective serotonin reuptake inhibitors, ease PMS symptoms in about 70 percent of the women who use them. These drugs include fluoxetine (Prozac), sertraline (Zoloft), paroxetine (Paxil), citalopram (Celexa), and fluvoxamine (Luvox). Some women may need to take these medications every day, and others may benefit from taking them only in the two weeks before they menstruate.

Light therapy: This treatment may be helpful instead of, or in addition to, drugs. You might spend two hours in front of a bank of daylight-intensity lights either first thing in the morning or in the early evening. You do not have to stare at the light, just gaze at it every few minutes. Both morning and evening bright light, and evening exposure to dim red light, cut depressive symptoms by at least 50 percent in women with PMDD, a series of studies by Barbara Parry of the University of California at San Diego (UCSD) and her colleagues shows. Researchers are trying to determine when and how much light individual women need. Some women in the UCSD studies continued to benefit from light treatment eighteen months later, arguing against the possibility that light is simply a placebo. Placebo treatments typically don't work as well as active treatments, or hold up over time.[5]

Changing times or amount of sleep: Partial sleep deprivation, a useful treatment for persons with some other types of depression, may help those with PMDD, too. (See Mood Disorders, page 296.)

Drugs that eliminate menstrual cycling: Doctors reserve the drug leuprolide (Lupron) for women with severe PMDD who don't respond to other treatments. Leuprolide produces a chemical menopause.

Timewise Tips

Good health habits may prevent overall monthly discomfort. Certain tactics address specific PMS symptoms.

Keep a menstrual diary, and plan ahead. If you often get headaches on the first day of your period, for example, try not to schedule important business meetings then. Some women discover through diary-keeping that certain symptoms, such as stomach upsets or feelings of anxiety, are present throughout the month, and are simply more severe at menstruation. This information will help a doctor pursue the underlying causes of these symptoms.

Get enough sleep. Lack of sleep itself may upset your moods or trigger irritability. Three in four menstruating women report trouble sleeping just before or while having their periods, the National Sleep Foundation found in a 1998 survey. Taking longer than usual to fall asleep and waking more frequently topped the list of complaints.[6]

Exercise regularly. Exercise boosts both energy and mood, and may relieve menstrual cramps and backaches associated with PMS.

Eat complex carbohydrates. Whole grains, fruits, and vegetables may boost levels of the brain chemical serotonin and have a calming effect. They are high in fiber and help prevent constipation.

Avoid salty foods. These include fast-food meals, potato chips, packaged luncheon meats, and many other convenience foods. Salt makes you retain water, leading to weight gain, bloating, and ankle swelling.

Consume 1,000–1,200 milligrams of calcium a day. The minimum daily requirement for women aged nineteen to fifty is 1,000 milligrams. In a study of nearly 500 women with PMS, Susan Thys-Jacobs of St. Luke's–Roosevelt Hospital in New York City found that those who consumed 1,200 milligrams of calcium daily cut PMS symptoms by half within two to three months. About 30 percent of those taking a placebo improved. The difference between the two groups shows that calcium had a significant benefit.[7]

Cut down on caffeine. Doing so may curb irritability, insomnia, and stomach upsets. Coffee, tea, colas, chocolate, and many over-the-counter drugs such as pain relievers and cold remedies contain caffeine or related compounds.

Limit alcohol intake. Some women report alcohol makes them feel more "blue." Some report a decreased tolerance for alcohol premenstrually.

Avoid standing too long. Standing may intensify backaches and contribute to foot and ankle swelling. Don't sit still either. Build walking and stretching into your day.

Learn stress-reduction strategies, such as progressive muscle relaxation, yoga, or self-guided imagery.

Seek sexual release. Many women report orgasm reduces pelvic congestion, eases cramps, and improves mood.

Use pain-relieving drugs. Numerous medications you can buy without a pre-

Menstrual Cycle Diary

Name _____

Photocopy this page, and keep track of your cycles for several months. Circle dates when you have your period. List symptoms you experience, such as bloating, breast tenderness, headaches, food cravings, or stomach upsets, and mark the dates. If symptoms vary in intensity, rank them from 1 (mild) to 5 (severe). If you try a specific treatment, note what you did and if it helped on a separate page. Take your diaries with you when you see your doctor.

Date of Last Menstrual Period _____

Month _____

Symptoms	1	2	3	4	5	6	7	8	9	10	11	12	13	14	15	16	17	18	19	20	21	22	23	24	25	26	27	28	29	30	31

scription, such as acetaminophen, aspirin, and ibuprofen, ease muscle aches and pains, headaches, and similar symptoms. To minimize stomach irritation, avoid taking these drugs in the morning. Some PMS remedies also are available over the counter. Most have not been subjected to rigorous scientific study.

See your doctor if symptoms interfere with work or social life. Treatment will depend on your specific needs.

Study. Visit the Web sites of the American College of Obstetrics and Gynecology (www.obgyn.net/women/women.htm) and the American Medical Association, (http://www.ama-assn.org/women).

RESTLESS LEGS SYNDROME AND PERIODIC LEG MOVEMENTS

If you often experience creepy, crawly, prickly, itchy sensations in your legs, particularly in the evening while sitting or at night when you lie in bed, you may have restless legs syndrome (RLS). As many as one in fifteen Americans are thought to have this still little known disorder. RLS is a potent disrupter of both day and night, as it forces people to move vigorously, often necessitating walking around to gain relief. Persons with severe RLS sleep poorly, with many interruptions, and often get less than four hours' sleep a night.

"The Greatest Torture"

◆ More than three hundred years ago, a British physician, Thomas Willis, wrote a still-classic description of RLS.

"Wherefore to some, on being a-bed, they betake themselves to sleep, presently in the arms and legs, leaping and contractions of the tendons, and so great a restlessness and tossing of their members ensue that the diseased are no more able to sleep than if they were in the place of the greatest torture."[1]

Virginia Wilson, a Florida resident, watched movies and plays from the back of the theater because she couldn't sit still. She even played cards standing up. She and her husband had separate bedrooms.

For decades, Wilson saw different doctors without receiving help. Some doctors trivialized her complaints or attributed them to hysteria, stress, or depression. Wilson did not learn she had RLS until she saw a sleep specialist in 1986. She was then seventy-three.

The experiences prompted Wilson to start *The Night Walker Newsletter,* and led eventually to the founding of the RLS Foundation, a national organization that provides information and support to those with RLS. Wilson also wrote a book about RLS, *Sleep Thief.*[2]

Circadian Pattern May Be Key Diagnostic Clue

Symptoms usually erupt just before sleep, and either prevent sleep or interrupt it soon after it starts. They may widen in time to include the evening and the latter part of sleep. As the disorder worsens, they also may occur in the afternoon. While the circadian pattern may disappear in severe cases, most persons with RLS rarely have symptoms between 7 A.M. and 11 A.M.[3] "The morning is the best time of day to be awake," says one woman with RLS. "Unfortunately, it's also the only time I can sleep."

The day-night pattern of RLS parallels the body temperature rhythm. In one study, eight volunteers with RLS spent three days and nights in a sleep laboratory. They rated the severity of their own symptoms, while researchers monitored their body temperature. They slept, or tried to sleep, the first two study nights, and stayed awake on the third night. Whether they were asleep or awake, their symptoms worsened at night as body temperature fell, peaked at midnight, and improved in the morning as temperature rose. The sleep deprivation, however, made their symptoms act up even more than usual.[4]

RLS usually starts gradually. Symptoms may disappear for weeks or months, then resurge in waves several days a week or every day. Eventually, the creeping, crawling, tingling sensations become both more intense and more frequent, making it hard to sit still. Some persons say they try to avoid situations that unleash RLS symptoms, such as riding in a car or on a plane, and even going to the movies, markedly dampening the quality of their lives. Some say they spend their evenings pacing almost constantly, the habit that gives RLS its name.

Some persons develop creeping sensations in arms and other body parts as well. The symptoms are peculiar and often defy description. Some people report pain. Few report muscle cramps or numbness.

Periodic Limb Movements Add to Distress

Most persons with RLS also suffer from periodic limb movements in sleep, or PLMS. They flex their legs repeatedly while sleeping without realizing it. PLMS commonly occur every fifteen to forty seconds, hundreds of times a night. Episodes may last only a few minutes or virtually all night long. Often, their bed partners are the ones who identify the problem: they complain they get kicked out of bed. Some people even wear holes in their sheets with their leg movements. Those with severe RLS also may experience the same type of limb movements while awake. The severity of this disorder also follows a circadian pattern, with a peak around midnight and fewest symptoms around 9 A.M.[5]

Nearly everyone with RLS has PLMS, but the opposite is not true. Most persons with PLMS do not have RLS.[6] PLMS alone may affect one in three persons over age sixty. Their causes are many, and include the sleep disorder narcolepsy and kidney disorders.

Who Gets RLS?

RLS occurs in persons of all ages, from infancy onward. In childhood, it may be mistaken for growing pains (see page 259) or attention deficit hyperactivity disorder (ADHD); teachers say these kids can't sit still. Some children may have both RLS and ADHD. As many as one in four women experience RLS while pregnant, particularly in the last three months. It usually disappears after childbirth, but may reappear years later. It is most common later in life, and affects men and women equally. RLS and PLMS together may account for one in three cases of insomnia in patients over age sixty.

RLS may affect only one person in a family but it also appears to run in some families, and, in that situation, generally shows up earlier in life. It's more common in persons with kidney disorders and anemia. Persons with RLS sometimes have a deficiency of iron. Since low brain iron has been identified as a possible cause of this disorder, keeping body iron levels in the high normal range is an important part of treatment. Oral iron supplements may help. Folate and magnesium deficiency also may worsen RLS symptoms. Taking supplements to correct the specific deficiency may bring improvement. Caffeine, alcohol, and nicotine may aggravate RLS, making attacks more severe or more frequent.

Treatment Targets Daily Symptom Pattern

Treatment includes both self-help tactics, outlined in Timewise Tips below, and a variety of medications. When other illnesses appear to provoke or aggravate RLS, doctors treat them first.

The primary treatment for RLS includes drugs that alter the availability of the brain chemical dopamine. These include carbidopa/levodopa, pergolide, pramipexole, and others. These medications usually are taken an hour or two before bedtime. If your symptoms awaken you in the night, your doctor may prescribe a combination of controlled-release and short-acting tablets.

Sleeping pills and anticonvulsants also may be helpful. Painkilling medications with narcotics such as codeine may have specific uses, such as before a plane trip or long drive. Many persons with RLS report that a combination of medications works best. While finding the right mix may take experimentation, once achieved, it is likely to work well for many years. The same drugs and combinations of drugs may help persons with PLMS, whether or not they also have RLS.[7]

Some persons using drugs that affect dopamine experience a phenomenon known as *augmentation*: they may gain relief from RLS in sleep, but RLS symptoms start to show up in the afternoon, or even the morning, often with greater intensity. These complications demand a good working partnership between you and your doctor, and careful attention to the type and timing of your medications.

Timewise Tips

Use the Pain Diary on page 208, modifying the symptoms list as necessary. Note medications and tactics that ease or worsen symptoms. Take the diary with you when you see your doctor.

Seek flexible work hours with a late start time, so that you can sleep until 10 or 11 A.M., if possible. Research is in progress to see if timed exposure to sunlight-equivalent light in the morning will cause symptoms to occur earlier in the day, and enable persons with RLS to fall asleep earlier at night.

Get a pillow speaker or headphone, so you can listen to the radio or tapes as a distraction if you awaken at night.

Try to schedule car or plane trips for morning. Take along your most mentally engrossing "quiet" activity. Listen to recorded books or music on a portable tape player. On car trips, stop frequently to walk around. On plane trips, request an aisle seat at the back of the plane, where you may be able to stand and move about more easily.

Experiment with type and timing of exercise. Some persons with RLS like to use a stationary bike or a treadmill just before going to bed. Others find isometric exercises, such as standing with your back against a wall and your knees bent as if sitting in a chair, help fatigue muscles.

Anytime Tips

If obliged to sit in meetings frequently at work, wear a pager. When you need to get up, page yourself so you may leave without attracting notice.

Buy or build a standup desk so you can do paperwork in comfort.

Avoid caffeine, alcohol, and nicotine, as all may make RLS worse.

Wear flexible or slip-on shoes to make stretching easier.

Try hot or cold baths, hot or cold packs, whirlpool baths, rubbing your legs or other affected areas, and using vibratory or electrical stimulation on feet and toes at bedtime, all tactics some persons with RLS find helpful. Relaxation techniques such as biofeedback, meditation, or yoga also may ease symptoms.

Ask your doctor whether any medications you are taking for other illnesses are known to aggravate RLS. If so, other drugs may be available.

Study. Visit the Web site of the Restless Legs Syndrome Foundation (www.rls.org).

SKIN DISORDERS

Step up to any cosmetics counter and you'll hear salespersons extolling the virtues of day creams and night creams. Even persons unfamiliar with the term *circadian rhythms* recognize that the skin's appearance changes across the day.

The skin, the body's largest organ, displays in microcosm how biological rhythms govern body functions, alter the course of various diseases, and affect both the results of diagnostic tests and treatment.

The skin springs into action at night to repair cells damaged by daytime exposure to ultraviolet sunlight. Skin cells reproduce themselves thirty times faster at midnight, their peak proliferation time, than at noon, the low point on the cycle.[1] Glands that produce oil to make skin supple and flexible pump out twice as much at noon when we are active as they do between 2 and 4 A.M., when we typically sleep.[2] We sweat more in the late afternoon than earlier in the day. This rhythm runs in tandem with the daily rise in body temperature, and with the daily peak in muscle flexibility and coordination that favors late-afternoon exercise.[3]

All of these changes influence the skin's role as a gatekeeper, allowing or denying entrance to the body of various substances at different rates and times of day. Understanding skin rhythms and harnessing them is adding a new wrinkle to skin care and treatment.

Many Skin Disorders Follow Cyclic Patterns

The symptoms of many skin disorders follow daily, monthly, and annual patterns. If you have a skin disorder, paying attention to the pattern of your illness may help you to better cope with it.

Psoriasis

Skin cells normally reproduce themselves every twenty-eight to thirty days, another one of our monthly cycles. The body then sloughs off dead cells unnoticeably. In psoriasis, however, skin cells reproduce themselves as often as every three to four days, and accumulate in thickened, reddened patches, most commonly on the elbows, knees, and scalp. Rather than having an active period and a quiet period, skin-cell turnover in psoriasis occurs night and day.[4] In the outer skin layer, or epidermis, cell turnover is highest between 9 P.M. and 3 A.M., just as in people with healthy skin. But in the underlying layer of skin, or dermis, activity is higher in the morning than at night.[5] Inflammation also follows a daily pattern. It is highest at night and lowest in the morning,[6] suggesting a respectively greater and lesser need for anti-inflammatory creams at these times.

Atopic Dermatitis

Both children and adults with this allergic disorder develop a chronic, itchy inflammatory rash. The itching is most severe between 7 P.M. and 11 P.M., the time of peak production of histamine, a chemical that triggers itching and other allergic reactions, including overnight worsening of symptoms of asthma and hay fever.[7] The itching of atopic dermatitis also may disrupt sleep.

To ease itching, doctors often prescribe corticosteroid anti-inflammatory creams. They also may recommend taking sedating antihistamines by mouth to help reduce nighttime itching and keep it from interfering with sleep.

Skin Cancer

Animal studies show that the likelihood of developing some skin cancers depends on the time of initial exposure to tumor-causing chemicals. Animals exposed to toxic chemicals at times of day when they are active develop tumors more often than do those exposed in their rest period.[8] The same may be true for humans, another reminder of the critical need to minimize workplace contact with potential cancer-causing agents.

Skin Eruptions Mirror Menstrual Cycle

Women with acne, psoriasis, eczema, hives, and other skin disorders often report that their symptoms worsen in the days immediately preceding menstruation, when estrogen levels fall and progesterone levels rise. Some women report cycle-related changes in skin pigmentation, with premenstrual darkening of the skin surrounding the eyes and nipples. Women who take birth-control pills, which even out female hormone levels, sometimes report fewer skin problems.

The benefits of these drugs for acne has declined somewhat in recent years, some dermatologists say, following the reduction in the amount of estrogen the pills contain. The higher amount of estrogen in the early birth-control pills, however, was linked with an increased risk of developing blood clots and strokes. The oral contraceptive Ortho Tri-Cyclen, designed for women with moderate acne that does not respond to antiacne medications applied to the skin and for those as well who desire this method of contraception, received approval from the U.S. Food and Drug Administration in 1996.[9]

Rhythms Affect Diagnostic Test Accuracy

Allergy Tests

To identify the cause of skin rashes, runny noses, coughs, and other allergic symptoms, doctors may inject a small amount of one or more known common allergy triggers, or allergens, just under the skin of the upper arm or back. If you are allergic to a specific substance, you probably will develop a hive, a large red blotchy area with light-colored swelling in its center. The skin reacts two to three times more strongly in the late afternoon and evening. Try to schedule your appointment for skin-allergy tests as late in the day as possible. If you have such tests in the morning, the severity of your allergies and even the exact identification of your sensitivities may be less obvious.[10]

In women, the time of the menstrual cycle also influences test results. In women not using oral contraceptives, reactions are about 25 percent more pronounced at menstruation than in the middle of the month, at ovulation.[11] In the latter group, reactions show less variation across the cycle. The predictable menstrual worsening of symptoms here can be put to good use. You can see your doctor when your allergic sensitivities are most evident.

Tuberculosis Tests

Skin tests tell if you have ever been infected with tuberculosis (TB), a potentially fatal bacterial infection. If the test is positive, it still will take additional tests to determine if you have an active infection. Skin tests routinely are given to schoolchildren, military recruits, prisoners, and other persons coming together in large groups. For these tests, a small amount of a protein purified from killed TB bacteria is injected just beneath the skin of the forearm. If a small bump forms at this site in the next couple of days, the test is positive. Persons who have been exposed to TB show a nearly threefold greater reaction after getting the injection at 7 A.M. than they do after getting it at 10 P.M.[12] Morning tests, therefore, offer more reliable information.

TB has resurfaced as a major public health problem in recent years in tandem with the AIDS epidemic, as persons with suppressed immune systems are particularly susceptible to it. It is a leading cause of death worldwide. Coughing by infected persons expels TB bacteria from their lungs into the air, exposing other people to it.

Cosmetics Industry Embraces Body Rhythms

Ads claiming that cosmetics work in sync with body rhythms may be more than a marketing gimmick. Some are among a rapidly expanding group of products alleged to achieve druglike effects, such as the repair of sun damage and reversal of aging. Such products are popularly called *cosmeceuticals,* a term not officially recognized by the U.S. Food and Drug Administration (FDA), which regulates the manufacture and sale of cosmetics.[13]

Most studies of cosmetics are conducted by the manufacturers themselves. Few result in reports for scientific journals, as the findings are considered trade secrets. One published study conducted for Lancôme, however, compares two face creams, one with chemicals skin cells use for nighttime restorative processes, and a similar product lacking those substances. Two groups of twenty-four French women aged nineteen to fifty-five applied the creams for two to three weeks at a time, either soon after they awakened in the morning or just before they went to bed at night. Each woman rated the appearance of her own facial skin several times a day, using criteria such as "texture" and "brilliance of complexion." Nighttime use of the nighttime cream produced the highest ratings of improved skin appearance.[14]

Some Skin Creams Work Best in Afternoon

Skin Creams

Like cosmetics, medications applied to the skin may work better at some times of day than at others. Studies show many work best in the afternoon, when skin temperature is higher and skin may be more porous. Twice as much of the painkiller lidocaine, applied as a cream, is taken up by the skin at 4 P.M. as at 8 A.M., for example.[15] The same medication also relieves pain for twice as long when injected into the skin in the afternoon as it does when injected in the morning.[16]

Corticosteroid Creams

A widely used anti-inflammatory corticosteroid cream produced more extensive and prolonged shrinking of blood vessels, an indirect measure of its ability to reduce inflammation, when it was applied at 4 P.M. than at 9 A.M.[17]

Dermatologists generally tell patients to apply corticosteroid creams in the evening and at bedtime, both because the creams are absorbed better later in the day and because the creams may be messy, making people reluctant to wear them for daytime activity. Long-term use of large amounts of corticosteroid creams—applying them over half of the body surface, for example, as a doctor may tell a person with psoriasis or atopic dermatitis to do—is known to suppress the adrenal glands and reduce the body's normal morning release of the hormone cortisol. No studies to assess the effects of applying corticosteroid creams at different times of day on this important body rhythm, however, have been published in medical journals.

Skin Patches

Skin patches get drugs into the bloodstream directly. Medication taken orally must be absorbed by the intestine and processed by the liver before getting into the blood. Skin patches, round or square, roughly the size of a large postage stamp, release medication at a constant rate. Chronobiologically designed patches now under development will deliver more or less drug as needed at different times.

Patches now on the market include:

Nicotine patches. These aim to help people quit smoking by weaning them from cigarettes as a source of nicotine and cutting their nicotine intake. Users are told to leave the patch on for twenty-four hours, and then to apply a new patch. Instructions do not specify a particular application time, but some of the side effects associated with use of nicotine patches make morning the best time: these patches sometimes cause vivid dreams and sleep disruption. If that happens to you, try wearing your patch for sixteen hours, and then take it off at bedtime.

Pain-relieving patches. Patches that contain lidocaine are designed to relieve the often excruciating pain that accompanies shingles. This illness, a reactivation of a childhood infection with chicken pox, scars nerves in the skin and causes pain that may last for months or years. Lidocaine patches are large, about the size of a postcard. Patients may wear up to three at a time, for twelve hours, with a twelve-hour break before applying new ones.

Other pain-relieving patches contain fentanyl, a narcotic drug. These patches are used by persons with chronic pain, such as cancer pain, and are worn for seventy-two hours. Circadian rhythms in blood flow to the skin and medication absorption time may alter drug uptake, however, so they may not work equally well at all times. If you experience breakthrough pain while wearing a pain-relieving patch, note the time and tell your doctor, who may prescribe pain medicine to take orally at times when the patch does not provide adequate relief, or prescribe a different painkiller.

Other patches. Patches now in use deliver nitroglycerin to help prevent angina pectoris, pain in the chest caused by heart disease (see page 283); airway dilator medication to prevent nighttime asthma (see page 218); testosterone for men with low levels of this sex hormone (see page 140); and estrogen, or estrogen and progesterone together, for women going through menopause and afterward (see page 135). Using these patches as chronotherapies may improve their effectiveness and reduce unwanted side effects.

Timewise Tips

If using once-a-day steroid creams, apply them in the evening for best penetration. Use the lowest effective dose for the shortest possible time.

If itching from an allergy disrupts your sleep, tell your doctor. You may need a higher dose or different type of medication, or you may benefit from applying creams or taking pills at a different time.

Try to schedule allergy skin tests in the afternoon, and TB skin tests in the morning. Women, try to schedule allergy tests just before your menstrual period.

Get adequate sleep. The concept of "beauty sleep" has some validity. Fatigue produces dark circles under the eyes. Bags under the eyes in the morning, however, don't come from activity of the skin itself. They may reflect overnight fluid accumulation in fatty tissues. Nasal allergies and chronic sinus

infections also may produce "shiners." Taking an antihistamine or decongestant at bedtime may prevent this problem. Sleeping with two pillows or elevating the head of your bed on wooden blocks by a few inches also may help.

To reduce superficial wrinkles and combat skin dryness, take advantage of
heightened skin-cell activity at night. Dampen skin and apply heavier creams
designed for nighttime use. For chapped hands, dampen skin, apply creams,
and wear cotton gloves to bed.

If using skin patches to quit smoking, ease pain, or other purposes, note time-of-
day patterns in your symptoms. Tell your doctor, as you may need to change
the hours you wear the patches or the dose of medication, or use an additional or different medication.

Study. Visit the Web site of the American Academy of Dermatology
(www.aad.org).

SLEEP DISORDERS

Some people who complain of insomnia may have nothing wrong with their
sleep at all. It may be the timing of their sleep that is off, a mismatch between
their body clock and the world's clock.

Insomnia is a big umbrella. It covers trouble falling asleep or staying
asleep, or waking too early. The perception that sleep is not refreshing or
restorative is central, too, for insomnia is a disorder of the entire sleep/wake
cycle. It is a twenty-four-hour illness, not restricted only to the hours you
spend in bed. If you don't sleep well, you're likely to feel foggy, fuzzy, less
motivated, and less energetic while awake, too.

One in four adults worldwide reports trouble with sleep, and of these, one
in ten claims to have slept poorly most nights or every night for a month or
longer.[1] Insomnia is not a disorder in itself. It is a symptom of sixty discrete
disorders of sleep listed in the *International Classification of Sleep Disorders*, the
sleep field's chief diagnostic manual.[2]

Psychological problems, such as depression and anxiety (see page 296),
physical illnesses, such as restless legs syndrome and periodic leg movements
(see page 330), and conditions that produce pain cause three in four cases of
insomnia. But one in four poor sleepers may have a disorder of sleep timing.
These disorders cause persistent trouble sleeping when you want to or need
to, or at the right hours for your school, work, or social life.

Jet lag (see chapter 12) and shift work (see chapter 13) are the best-known
disrupters of sleep timing. Sleep habits that ignore the clock can sabotage
your sleep/wake cycle, prompting these common complaints:

- "I can't turn off my mind at bedtime."
- "I toss and turn all night."

Chaos in the biological clock itself can sabotage sleep, causing four distinctive circadian-rhythm sleep disorders that make people report:

- "I fall asleep too late."
- "I fall asleep too early."
- "I have frequent bouts of troubled sleep."
- "I sleep in snatches all day long."

If you have one of these problems, even if you have had it for many years, chronotherapies described here may help you sleep better. The first step is to identify your particular time pattern. Use the sleep/wake diary, page 353.

"I Can't Turn Off My Mind at Bedtime."

Poor sleep habits are a highly underappreciated cause of insomnia. Though we all like being able to stay up late whenever we feel like it, and to sleep in on days when we don't have to go to work, our bodies crave regularity. In youth and early adulthood, we take odd hours in stride. But in middle age and beyond, the body clock balks at accommodating to frequent schedule changes. A weekend schedule that differs vastly from that of the rest of the week may upset sleep and alertness for two or three days . . . and soon it's the weekend again. Sunday-night insomnia is a predictable consequence of late nights Friday and Saturday.

It's hard for most of us to acknowledge that we are architects of our own sleep misery. John Wiedman, who suffered from insomnia for more than ten years, tried many supposed insomnia cures, without success. He doubted that so simple a tactic as heeding the body's clock could make a difference, but grudgingly gave it a try. Wiedman's sleep improved dramatically within just a few weeks, he said, once he accepted responsibility for his own difficulties. In his book, *Desperately Seeking Snoozin'*, he tells readers, "You created the habits that are causing your insomnia, and you are going to get rid of those habits."[3]

Good sleepers can flout the rules, but people who have trouble sleeping often sleep better if they go to bed and get up at about the same time, give or take an hour or so, seven days a week. Keeping regular hours prompts body temperature to head downward before bedtime, fostering sleep. In people who have trouble falling asleep, temperature drops to its daily low more than two hours later than it does in good sleepers.[4] Wanting to go to sleep at a certain time isn't enough; you have to put your body in sleep mode.

People who have trouble falling asleep typically feel anxious. They search through their minds to identify all possible sources of stress. This feeling may be merely a function of being awake. "Anybody lying in bed in the dark awake is apt to worry," asserts Peter Hauri of the Mayo Clinic.

Some people, however, are champion worriers. They describe racing minds at bedtime, an endless parade of anxious thoughts. In sleep-laboratory studies, Canadian scientists found brains of such persons to be more revved up at bedtime and after sleep started than those of both normal sleepers and persons with psychiatric illnesses that disturb sleep. Worriers had more waking brain waves and fewer sleep brain waves in the drowsy period before sleep started, and they took nearly twice as long as the comparison groups to fall asleep.[5]

Some people, according to Hauri, are not great sleepers to begin with. Some are "sleep responders." They sleep poorly when under stress, just as others in similar circumstances lose their appetite or develop tension headaches. Perhaps your sleep problems started with an upsetting situation, such as having to stay awake many nights in a row to nurse an ill child, or with trouble at work.

For those susceptible to poor sleep, sleep problems may continue even after the crisis that triggered it resolves. At this juncture, sleep-scheduling problems often come to the fore. It's not surprising that natural born worriers fear vague but ominous consequences of not getting enough sleep. Some unwittingly throw their body clock further out of balance by going to bed several hours early in an attempt to make up for missed sleep. This is a mistake.

"I Toss and Turn All Night."

Someone with this type of insomnia may go to bed at 10 P.M. and get out of bed at 7 A.M., waking frequently and accruing only five or six hours' sleep. Sleep-laboratory studies show that numerous awakenings fuse in a sleeper's mind to create a convincing perception of not having slept at all. It is this experience that prompts the claim, "I didn't sleep a wink," while a bed partner often staunchly maintains that's not true.

Here is where chronotherapy can help. Insomniacs' dogged search for sleep prompted a seemingly paradoxical theory: to get more sleep, insomniacs should spend less time in bed. Reducing time in bed consolidates sleep, according to Arthur Spielman of the City College of New York. He and his colleagues devised a novel treatment known as *sleep restriction*.[6]

Insomniacs following this treatment start by limiting their time in bed to the number of hours they actually sleep, down to about five hours, the minimum time in bed most people find acceptable. Since most people have to get up at the same time each weekday for work, they must go to bed much later than usual. A five-hour sleeper with a 7 A.M. wake-up time, for instance, must go to bed at 2 A.M.

After a week on this regimen, and each week for the next four weeks, the five-hour sleepers add thirty minutes to the time they spend in bed. Six-hour sleepers add fifteen minutes. By the end of the month, most typically sleep solidly for seven hours a night, and find the quality of their sleep much improved. If trying this approach, plan in advance how you are going to spend the time after everyone else in your home has gone to sleep. Pick quiet activities, compelling enough to keep you awake, such as surfing the Internet, playing a video game, or doing needlework. It takes a hefty amount of willpower to stick with a sleep-restriction regimen, and to keep regular hours afterward.

"I Fall Asleep Too Late."

If you don't feel ready for sleep until 2 A.M. or even later, you may have a sleep clock that is out of sync with that of the rest of the world. Your schedule likely poses problems if you must get up to go to school or go to work at a job with a traditional daytime schedule.

Sleep experts call this problem *delayed sleep phase syndrome*, or DSPS.[7] Having a delayed phase means that your sleep occurs later than you wish or later than your lifestyle demands. If not forced to awaken early, persons with DSPS usually sleep quite well and get a normal amount of sleep. "When I have to get up early, I always feel sick, can barely function, and remain tired all day until evening when I get an energy burst right about the time I should be going to sleep," one woman with DSPS reports. Parents, teachers, and employers may view persons with DSPS as lazy, unmotivated, even mentally ill. One U.S. Marine faced a court-martial for his "failure to go" before doctors found he had DSPS. He was acquitted.[8]

The typical family doctor seldom diagnoses DSPS, but sleep experts say 5 percent to 10 percent of insomniacs suffer from it. Most persons with DSPS rank as extreme owls on the Owl/Lark Self-test (see page 43). They say they feel and function best in the evening and at night. Personality factors may come into play. Persons with DSPS often bridle at having to follow the world's rules. "In all of my professional life, people have complained because of my inability to get in by 9 A.M. This burns me up," said a message poster on an online list for self-described night owls.

Some people with DSPS report they were night owls as babies. Their late bedtimes and trouble getting up in the morning often set off family battles in adolescence, when the biological clock normally shifts to a later schedule. (See chapter 8: "The Growing Years.") The typical teenager prefers a 1 A.M. or 2 A.M. bedtime, but those with DSPS often do not go to bed until 4 A.M. or even later. Most teenagers are sleepy in morning classes. Those with DSPS may not even show up for school, or arrive quite late. They may sleep all day on weekends.

Fourteen-year-old Janet (not her real name) flunked the ninth grade. Her report cards, going back to early elementary school, noted she often slept in class. In the summer, she went to bed at 6 A.M. and slept until 2 P.M. or 3 P.M. Before school started in the fall, her mother brought her to a children's sleep specialist. Asked to go to bed at 11 P.M. for a sleep-laboratory study, Janet slept fitfully until 4 A.M., and then solidly until midafternoon. In waking hours, she was fully alert.

Janet's home life, the doctor discovered, lacked structure. "Mom essentially goes to bed and lets the kids run wild," Janet's doctor told colleagues, seeking their help in planning treatment. The resulting discussion, which unfolded in an online list for sleep specialists, shows how complex DSPS can be.

Consider exposure to sunlight, or sunlight-equivalent artificial light, from 7 A.M. to 8 A.M. on three successive days, suggested Peter Glusker of Stanford University. "This should advance her phase, so that she can go to bed at, say, 10 P.M., and get up at 7 A.M. But this change will not hold," he noted, "unless you can establish good sleep hygiene and habits thereafter, and make the home environment more supportive."

"Many of the underlying habits, patterns, and problems in this girl and her family probably have been entrenched for years," cautioned Ronald Dahl of the University of Pittsburgh. "It is extremely unlikely that any simple intervention, no matter how clever or chronotherapeutically sophisticated, will change things substantively.

"The first step," Dahl said, "is to assess the motivation of this girl and her family. What are the goals/consequences that are salient to them that can be used to motivate at least some changes in behavior? Does the girl really want to attend school and is she just not quite able to get things together because of the burden of the sleep problem? Or does she say that her late-night and weekend activities are more important to her than school, and that any treatment plan that excludes these is not an option to her? Is the family really motivated to improve things or are they in the clinic simply because the school is threatening to prosecute them for all the missed school?"

When patient and family agree to work on the problem, the best tactic for most youngsters with DSPS, Dahl said, is to shift their bedtime in three-hour blocks around the clock. This teenager would go to bed at 6 A.M. the first day, 9 A.M. the next day, noon the day after, and so on until her sleep time lines up with her desired schedule. Teenagers usually enjoy this experience, Dahl said, because they get to stay up later and later. They often don't need much parental input to accomplish it. Further, when they finally go to bed they feel sleepy, which encourages them to develop new positive sleep-onset habits.

The real challenge comes in locking onto this new schedule, including weekends. For families that work at this task, Dahl said, re-aligning sleep/wake schedules and getting the adolescent back to school can be an enormous and extremely rewarding achievement.

Janet's story has a happy ending. After counseling, Janet decided to give up late-night TV viewing. Although she must have weathered some difficult days, she managed to get to school on time and reset her sleep clock on her own. She started paying attention to her teachers and doing her homework, and she earned passing grades. A year later, she appeared to have settled comfortably into her new routine.

Janet is among the luckier ones. Many adults with DSPS say that once they started going to bed late, whether as teenagers or after working at night, they couldn't return to a normal schedule. Most report numerous unsuccessful attempts to fall asleep earlier, including going to bed at a conventional hour, taking sleeping pills, trying health food store remedies, and using relaxation techniques. To get up in the morning, they may need several alarm clocks, help from family or friends, and cold showers. Some adapt their night-owl lifestyle to their careers, working, for example, as bartenders, musicians, computer programmers, and emergency-room physicians and nurses.

Curiously, persons with DSPS do not keep moving around the clock. They manage somehow to grab onto certain time cues, such as school or work hours, or mealtimes, to keep themselves anchored in a twenty-four-hour world.

Sleep experts often advise them to get up at a conventional wake-up time every day, usually a terrible struggle for those with DSPS because they feel extremely sleepy. Those who can do it for a week or two may find that their sleepiness helps them to fall asleep earlier, closer to their desired time. Morning exposure to sunlight also may help realign the disordered day/night pattern.

Going to sleep three hours later every day until reaching an acceptable schedule may help adults as well as teenagers, but some adults have developed even worse schedule problems after trying it. Another tactic is to skip sleep entirely on a Friday night, stay up all day Saturday, and go to bed ninety minutes earlier than usual that night and for the next week, repeating this process the following weekend until reaching a desired bedtime.[9] Both of these regimens are hard to manage, and it is harder still to stick with the new routine. The challenge is like that faced by the dieter who loses forty pounds and then struggles not to regain the weight.

Many sleep centers today employ a combination of treatments. You might use bright-light exposure when you wake up in the morning, then take melatonin three hours before your current bedtime, and finally a sleeping pill at bedtime. You would need to set up a schedule for each activity, and then shift light, pills, bedtime, and wake time about fifteen minutes earlier every two to three days.[10] (See pages 349–52.)

"I Fall Asleep Too Early."

Some people are saddled with a clock that runs too early. Those with the *advanced sleep phase syndrome*, or ASPS, fall asleep and wake up much earlier than they wish. They may elect to go to bed as early as 6 P.M. After sleeping a normal amount of time, they may awaken at 2 A.M.

ASPS can be a social nightmare, causing people to miss dinner parties and prime-time TV in the evening, and to feel trapped and limited in what they can do in a household where everyone else is asleep when they get up. Turning on lights, or brewing coffee, for instance, is likely to disturb other sleepers in the middle of the night.

ASPS is an extreme version of the early to bed, early to rise lifestyle that Ben Franklin advocated. It occurs mainly in persons who are middle-aged and older, in contrast to DSPS, which affects mainly young adults. "The late age of onset of ASPS may account, in part, for the presumed rarity of the disorder," observes Scott Campbell of Weill Medical College of Cornell University.[11] But some studies suggest it actually affects one in one hundred adults. While older people normally go to bed and get up earlier than they did when they were younger, this tendency is much exaggerated in those with ASPS. Their circadian rhythm of body temperature also is displaced. Daily lows in temperature occur earlier than normal in persons who fall asleep and wake up too early, the flip side of the "too late" rhythm of DSPS.[12]

Like persons with DSPS, those with ASPS don't keep moving their sleep time around the clock. Even if they try to stay up later, exposure to morning light works against them. Seeing the sun come up prompts an internal alarm clock to wake the person early again the next day.

Treatment aims to push both bedtime and wake time later. If you have ASPS, spend time outdoors in the late afternoon. Consider using a device that provides sunlight-equivalent bright light, called a light box, in the early evening. Even improving home lighting may help. When you watch television in a darkened room, despite the apparent brightness of the TV screen, you don't get any more light than you would outdoors by moonlight. Leave room lamps on.

Dark cues are important, too. Room-darkening shades or drapes in your bedroom may help extend sleep. While trying to reset a too early clock, keep shades drawn until noon, and wear dark glasses if you go outside. It may help to take a thirty-minute nap in the early evening, and then to get up and stay active for another two or three hours. (For more on use of light, melatonin, and other tactics, see pages 350–52.)

"I Have Frequent Bouts of Troubled Sleep."

Most of us comfortably and automatically reset our longer than twenty-four-hour inner clocks to the world's schedule every day. But some people cannot manage this task. Instead, they follow their internal clock, much as if they were living in a cave or laboratory with no indicators of time.

Even if they use alarm clocks, work regular hours, eat meals at the same time each day, and have other stable habits, they still often report trouble with sleep and alertness. If they try to stick to a conventional schedule, attempting to sleep from 11 P.M. to 7 A.M., say, they likely feel wakeful at bedtime, sleep restlessly, and feel drowsy in waking hours for several weeks, until that brief period when their internal and external clocks once more jibe with their desired schedules. Think of it as near-permanent jet lag.

This problem, known as the *non-twenty-four-hour sleep/wake syndrome*, is rare in persons able to perceive light, but several surveys suggest it may affect eight out of ten persons who are totally blind.

As one example, some 83 percent of members of the largest national association of blind persons in France reported having at least one sleep problem. These included difficulty falling asleep, frequent awakenings, early awakenings, poor sleep quality, and shortened sleep duration. Blind persons were twice as likely as a comparison group of sighted persons to show variations in bedtimes, wake-up times, mealtimes, times of peak alertness, and other indicators of disordered circadian rhythms.[13]

This finding points up the critical role of light in governing body clocks in sighted persons, notes Robert Sack of Oregon Health Sciences University. A sleep diary kept for several months, noting good nights and bad nights, alert days and sleepy days, can reveal this pattern.

Patricia is blind, having lost her sight in a horrendous car crash in 1950 when she was only ten months old. She retained one eye, which, though damaged, enabled her to perceive some light while she was growing up, just enough to navigate doorways and steer clear of large objects. She developed glaucoma, however, and at age twenty-four, she lost all light perception. That is when her sleep troubles began.

"I had terrible bouts of insomnia," Patricia recalls. "It took me several years to figure out that these bouts were cyclical.

"The first sign is that I cannot get to sleep at a reasonable hour at night. Then I cannot sleep at all at night, although, if I did not have to go to work, I could sleep all morning. The cycle works its way around the clock, with sleep snatched in three- or four-hour naps in the day and two-hour naps at night. I begin to snap out of it when I can sleep from 9 P.M. to 2 or 3 A.M. I can always sleep if I am able to do it at the right time, the time my body wants to sleep.

"It is hard to go on with life without becoming a slave to this condition. Being blind is okay although something of an inconvenience," Patricia asserted. "Having a free-running sleep cycle can be awful."

Within the blind community, Patricia has found, sleep problems are little discussed. Many blind persons gloss over their difficulties, she said, although their partner or spouse may talk about the problem. "If you are trying to live a mainstream life," she said, "you try to minimize your differences." Many doctors who treat the nation's 150,000 totally blind persons are not familiar with this problem, either.

In 1993, at Sack's suggestion, Patricia began taking melatonin about ninety minutes before her desired bedtime, finding after several years that 15 milligrams works best for her. "I now sleep much better," Patricia reports. "I continue to have periods of insomnia, but they are milder and much more tolerable than they used to be. Now that I take melatonin, I can get some sleep every night, three hours at least, and often more. Before taking it, I frequently went several nights with no sleep. I'm more like a normal insomniac now. I continue to have a cycle of sleepiness, but it has become more subtle, as if my clock were running slower."

In further studies, Sack and his colleagues treated seven blind persons with patterns similar to Patricia's by giving them 10 milligrams of melatonin about an hour before their habitual bedtime for three to nine weeks. Even if they were at a point in their cycle in which they were alert at night (despite trying to sleep then), and sleepy in the daytime (despite trying to stay awake then), melatonin helped them sleep better at night. Additionally, once they regularly secreted their own melatonin at bedtime, a dose of only 0.5 to 1.0 milligrams proved sufficient to keep them on the desired schedule.[14]

Researchers are trying to find out how a very small number of blind persons—those who have neither conscious perception of light nor unconscious recognition of light as measured by sophisticated tests of eye and brain function—manage to stay in sync with their desired schedules. Elizabeth Klerman of Harvard Medical School has identified nine such persons. She has several theories about what may be going on. These persons may perceive some light that present tests can't detect, she suggests. Or it may be that the natural rhythms of their internal clocks run on a twenty-four-hour schedule. Perhaps alarm clocks and other nonlight time cues are enough to lock daily rhythms for some, particularly those with a near twenty-four-hour inner timekeeper. Finding the answers would help both blind and sighted persons with non-twenty-four-hour schedule problems.

"I Sleep in Snatches All Day Long."

If you've stayed in bed for a few days with the flu or a fever, you may have awakened and dozed in short bursts, taking little note of the time. Some people persistently have an *irregular sleep/wake pattern*, sleeping three or more times a day. They usually get some sleep between 2 A.M. and 6 A.M., but the rest may be at variable hours.

In healthy, usually young adults, this pattern may represent what Neil Kavey of Columbia University calls the "freelance writer's syndrome."[15] Writers, students, artists, and others who don't have work schedules that force them to go to bed around the same time each day may elect to sleep only when they feel like it. The problem comes when they have to change their sleep time to meet outside demands. Often they can't do it.

This problem is most common, however, in persons with chronic illnesses that limit mobility, or involve depression, dementia, or brain injury. Their pattern is similar to that of newborn babies, except babies get more sleep.

In one study, more than 200 nursing-home residents with dementia wore wrist-activity monitors to keep track of their daily behavior. The majority rarely slept for a full hour at a time. They rarely stayed awake for an entire hour either, Sonia Ancoli-Israel of the University of California at San Diego and her colleagues found.[16]

In addition to their poor sleep, persons with Alzheimer's disease, Parkinson's disease, or the effects of a stroke may experience confusion, disorientation, and agitated behavior. This constellation of symptoms sometimes is called *sundowning*, but Ancoli-Israel thinks that's a misnomer. The name comes from the perception by families and caregivers that disruptive behavior gets worse after the sun goes down. They feel this way, Ancoli-Israel suggests, because they are tired then themselves. When she and her colleagues observed and rated agitation in a large group of nursing-home residents with dementia every fifteen minutes for three days, they found it was worst around 1 P.M.

Disruptive behavior, particularly at night, however, is the chief factor families cite in their decision to institutionalize an older person.[17] Improving such behavior, therefore, might stave off some nursing-home admissions. In 1999, 13 percent of Americans were over age sixty-five. The first baby boomers will hit sixty-five in 2010, boosting this percentage dramatically. The nation's tab for long-term care already exceeds $43 billion. Nursing-home staff sometimes deal with agitated behavior by giving sedating drugs, which prompts families to complain that when they come to visit their relative seldom is awake.[18]

In nursing homes, patients often spend most of the day in bed, even eating meals there. They get virtually no exposure to bright light, only five minutes per day on average in one study Ancoli-Israel conducted. Her studies and those of other researchers suggest that providing two hours of exposure to daylight-intensity light in either the morning or the evening, or using melatonin, will both reduce agitation and improve sleep.[19]

Improving sleep in the nursing-home environment is a daunting task. A team of researchers at the University of California at Los Angeles worked closely with nursing-home staff to try to do just that. They suggested turning off unwatched television sets between 7 P.M. and 6 A.M. to curb noise, individualizing nighttime care of incontinent patients to minimize disruptions, and turning lights on and off fewer times. These tactics cut noise and light exposure substantially. But patients' sleep improved only slightly. Focusing on nighttime activities alone is not enough, the researchers concluded. Improving sleep requires better management of daytime activities, too.[20]

Caregivers can help minimize agitation by keeping the person awake and busy in the daytime, out of bed if possible, with outdoor activities that involve sunlight exposure, such as walking, if the person can manage it. Use of standard good sleep hygiene, such as avoiding caffeine, and creating bedtime rituals, such as listening to music, may benefit sleep. Leaving a night-light on helps keep the person from becoming confused if awakening in the night. It also may help prevent bumping into things, and possibly falling. For added safety, the person can wear an electronic wanderer monitor, available through medical supply centers.

Admission to a busy, noisy, brightly lighted intensive-care unit is a notable sleep-cycle disrupter. Patients often sleep poorly because of problems such as pain and trouble breathing. Procedures start early; meals may be served at times different from home mealtimes. To keep patients oriented to the correct time, many hospitals use large wall-mounted clocks visible from patient beds, old-fashioned round ones with large numbers and sweeping minute hands. Nurses greet patients by saying, "Good morning," or "Good afternoon," when they provide care. When possible, they dim lights at night. U.S. law requires that all hospital rooms constructed or remodeled after 1977 include a window or skylight. In rooms with windows, nurses open and close blinds or curtains at the proper times.

When Can Sleeping Pills Help?

Sleeping pills, by definition, are chronotherapies; you take them just before bedtime. They act at brain sites that generate sleep. Zaleplon (Sonata), a prescription sleeping pill first marketed in the United States in 1999, is designed specifically for trouble falling asleep. It has a half-life of only one hour, meaning it disappears from the body in about four hours. It's the first sleeping pill that can be taken after going to bed and discovering that you can't sleep, although you should not take it any later than four hours before you expect to get up. The most appropriate use for this medication is occasional stress, a time when you expect to have a hard time falling asleep, as may occur if you want to sleep on an overseas flight.

Zolpidem (Ambien), the nation's best-selling prescription sleeping pill in recent years, targets the same brain sites as zaleplon, and stays in the body a few hours longer, helping persons who have trouble both falling asleep and staying asleep. Though different in chemical structure, both of these drugs work much like benzodiazepines, a chemical family that includes a wide variety of effective medications to improve sleep, depression, anxiety, and related disorders.

About one in four Americans uses some chemical to help with sleep each year, according to Thomas Roth of the University of Michigan. Most use alcohol and over-the-counter sleep aids.[21] Only 4 percent use prescription sleeping pills. For short-term insomnia—that lasting less than two weeks—the benefits of the prescription drugs are clear, Roth said. Users fall asleep faster, sleep longer, wake less often, report better sleep quality, and feel less fatigued in the daytime.[22] Researchers believe these drugs rapidly lose their efficacy, although there are few studies showing what happens when people use them for more than two to three months.[23]

"The longer insomnia lasts, the weirder it gets," asserts William Dement of Stanford University. Different people may need vastly different treatment. Some develop an "insomnophobia." Fear of trouble sleeping dominates their lives. In such instances, taking a sleeping pill one or more nights a week, or perhaps just having pills in the medicine cabinet, may curb their anxiety.

The rule that doctors usually follow in prescribing sleeping pills is "the lowest effective dose for the shortest possible time," only seven days on average, and no more than two to three weeks. One concern is that pill users may experience daytime side effects such as drowsiness that interferes with driving. Frequent users also may become dependent upon the drugs, increasing the risk of side effects.

Numerous studies show that changing sleep behavior, following the rules described in Timewise Tips for Good Sleep, page 77, works much better than sleeping pills to improve sleep in the long term. Charles Morin of Laval University in Quebec and his colleagues analyzed fifty-nine studies involving more than 2,100 patients, finding that nondrug techniques produced reliable and durable benefits.[24] If you have a chronic problem with sleep timing, don't expect sleeping pills to solve it. What you need are good strategies to reset your clock.

Timewise Tips on Using Bright Light

Understanding how light shifts body rhythms offers practical help to persons with sleep/wake cycle disorders. The general principles are these: Exposure to sunlight or its artificial equivalent in the morning will make you more alert earlier. Light in late afternoon or early evening will make you more alert later.[25] If you think you have a circadian-rhythm sleep disorder, talk with your doctor or see a sleep specialist to be sure your self-diagnosis is correct and to discuss treatment options. The following tactics may then prove useful:

If you have trouble falling asleep and staying asleep, despite going to bed at a conventional time, get up at a regular time, say 7 A.M., and go outdoors as soon as possible for about thirty minutes. Don't wear sunglasses. Stay indoors in late afternoon. If you go outside then, wear the darkest glasses possible (dark goggles are ideal) to minimize your light exposure.

If you have delayed sleep phase syndrome, get up around 7 A.M., and go outside as soon as possible for about thirty minutes, in order to feel more alert in the morning. Even on cloudy days, outdoor light intensity far exceeds that of indoor light. Avoid napping, and avoid bright light from late afternoon on. The aim here is to make you feel sleepy closer to a conventional bedtime.

If you have advanced sleep phase syndrome, avoid sunlight in the morning (keep shades drawn), but go outside for about thirty minutes in late afternoon, or use a light box in early evening to stay up later. After a few days of this routine, you should start sleeping later, too.

If you are a sighted person with a non-twenty-four-hour sleep/wake schedule, you need to mobilize all possible time cues to help you live on a twenty-four-hour day: light (particularly in the morning), alarm clocks, mealtimes, regular exercise, and more. You also need a thorough checkup, possibly including a visit to a neurologist, to be sure there is no physical reason for your problem.

If you have an irregular sleep/wake pattern, make every effort to wake up at a consistent and conventional time each morning. If possible, go outside soon after waking up for about thirty minutes. If confined to bed, ask that bedroom shades be opened in the daytime and closed at night. Consider using a light box in the morning. Try to confine naps to the midafternoon, and don't nap for more than thirty minutes. At night, sleep in a dark room. *If you are the caretaker of someone with this problem,* adapt these guidelines as circumstances permit.

Timewise Tips on Using Melatonin

While light is a more potent rhythm-setter than melatonin, this hormone offers an additional aid to resetting internal clocks to conform with the world's light/dark cycle. Certainly, it is more convenient to pop a pill than it is to get light at certain times. Light and melatonin exert their peak impact on the clock about twelve hours apart: light proves most effective in resetting the clock in the early morning, and melatonin does so in the late afternoon. The two approaches, used together, may be more effective than either alone. The advice below pertains to those who sleep between about 11 P.M. and 7 A.M.—or would like to. Before starting melatonin, be sure your doctor has no objections. (For more on melatonin, see chapter 4: "How Your Body Clock Works.") Note that the times suggested here for taking melatonin pertain to each specific situation, and may differ from times used in studies reported earlier in this section. Also follow guidelines for light above.

If you have trouble falling asleep, start with a low dose of melatonin, 0.3 to 0.5 milligrams, about thirty minutes before bedtime. Irina Zhdanova and her colleagues at the Massachusetts Institute of Technology found in several studies that a low dose helped both healthy young adults and elderly insomniacs to fall asleep faster. It also helped older persons awaken less frequently, important because staying asleep is a bigger issue in late life than is difficulty falling asleep.[26] Contrary to a popular myth, however, melatonin does not necessarily fall as people get older. Jamie Zeitzer and Charles Czeisler of Harvard Medical School and their colleagues found that melatonin levels in healthy people aged sixty-five to eighty-one matched those of people aged eighteen to thirty.[27] Poor sleep stems from many causes other than a deficiency in melatonin.

If you have DSPS, your goal would be to move your natural melatonin onset and bedtime earlier. Determining your natural melatonin onset time presently requires an expensive laboratory test, so you need to experiment to see which time to take melatonin works best for you. The most logical times range from midafternoon to about an hour before your desired bedtime.

Caution: melatonin makes about one in ten people who take it in the daytime sleepy. Don't drive between the time you take it and your bedtime. Don't take it if you work in the evenings. Try it on a day you can stay at home. Start with 3 milligrams, the most widely available dose in health food stores and pharmacies, and take that dose for a week or so. In one study, 96.7 percent of sixty-one persons with DSPS who took 5 milligrams of melatonin at 10 P.M. every day for six weeks shifted the time they fell asleep from after 3 A.M. to around 11:30 P.M. on average. When they stopped taking it, however, 90 percent returned to their previous patterns, Yaron Dagan and his colleagues at Tel-Aviv University Medical School found. Persons with DSPS, this study suggests, may need to take melatonin indefinitely in the same way that persons with diabetes need to continue to take insulin.[28]

If you have ASPS, your goal would be to move your natural melatonin onset and bedtime later. If you awaken at 3 A.M. or 4 A.M., take 0.5 milligrams of melatonin then, and go back to bed. The idea is to trick your brain into thinking it's still time for sleep, just as you'd like.[29] Even if you don't sleep well at first, rest quietly in the dark until your desired wake-up time.

If you are a blind person with a non-twenty-four-hour sleep/wake cycle, try taking 3 milligrams of melatonin about an hour before bedtime. If after a week or so you still are having problems, try increasing the dose slightly. Once you feel in sync, try cutting back gradually.

If you have an irregular sleep/wake cycle, try taking 3 milligrams of melatonin about 9 P.M., the time melatonin secretion normally starts. If you are the caretaker of an elderly person with this problem, consult the person's doctor before giving melatonin.

Study. Visit the Web sites of the American Academy of Sleep Medicine (www.aasmnet.org), the Sleep Research Society (www.sleephomepages.org), the National Sleep Foundation (www.sleepfoundation.org), and the Society for Light Treatment and Biological Rhythms (www.sltbr.org).

Sleep/Wake Diary

Name _____

Make two copies of this chart. Record your schedule each day for the next two weeks. Each morning, rate the quality of your sleep on a scale of 0 (terrible) to 100 (terrific) in the column on the far right. On a scale of 0 (weary) to 100 (refreshed), rate how you feel about one hour after awakening. Take the diary with you when you see your doctor.

Start Day/Date _____   Women: Are you menstruating today? Y/N

M=normal meal	P=sleeping pill	Alc=alcohol	A=alarm	S=snack
D=other drug	X=exercise	N=nap	C=caffeinated drink	
↓ =in bed	I—I=asleep	...=awake	↑ =out of bed	

	P.M.						MIDNIGHT				A.M.								NOON				P.M.		
Day/Date	6	7	8	9	10	11	12	1	2	3	4	5	6	7	8	9	10	11	12	1	2	3	4	5	Sleep/Wake Quality
Sun., 6/18/00	...	...	...	...	...	S↓	—	—	—	—	S —	A —	M —	P A↑	L MX	E ...	...	...	...	M	...	C	...	...	90/80

STROKES

Like heart attacks, strokes of all types are more frequent in the morning than at other times of day. Heart attacks and strokes—now increasingly called *brain attacks*—have much in common. Merely waking up may set off both of these catastrophic events.

A review of the times of day of more than 12,000 strokes reported in thirty-one scientific studies affirmed the morning peak, particularly for *ischemic strokes*, which account for 80 percent of brain attacks. Ischemic strokes indicate a sustained blockage of an artery in the neck leading to the brain or in the brain itself. Transient ischemic attacks, or TIAs, which involve a brief interruption of blood flow within the brain, also peak in the morning. More than half of all ischemic events occurred between 6 A.M. and noon.

A third type of stroke, one involving bleeding from a ruptured blood vessel in the brain, is called a *hemorrhagic stroke*. More than one-third of hemorrhagic strokes occurred between 6 A.M. and noon. If the timing were random, only one-fourth of each type of stroke would occur in each six-hour segment of the day.[1]

Consequences of brain attacks often include partial or total loss of vision or hearing, dizziness, slurred speech, impaired thinking, weakness or paralysis of an arm or leg, loss of bladder and bowel control, and even death. Strokes are the leading cause of disability in adults and the third leading cause of death in the United States, following heart disease and cancer. Some 750,000 Americans suffer strokes annually, a figure likely to rise as baby boomers age. These facts fuel intensive efforts to find better ways to prevent strokes and to treat them.

What Makes Mornings Risky?

The normal sudden morning rise in blood pressure (BP) makes blood surge through all blood vessels in the body. The force of blood may be enough to rip fatty deposits from blood vessel walls. In the tiny blood vessels of the heart and brain, these deposits may be large enough to form a blockage. Additionally, blood vessels weakened by age or disease, like old pipes, may burst when BP suddenly rises in the morning. Also, the increased stickiness of blood cells in the morning may cause clots to form in the brain, as well as in the heart.

Get Treatment Promptly If You Suspect a Stroke

If you think you may be having a stroke, or suspect one in someone else, call 911 or another emergency medical service right away. Some treatments, including tissue-type plasminogen activator, or TPA for short, a clot-dissolving medication, must be started within three hours of the onset of stroke symptoms to be effective. Prompt care can reduce further damage or death of brain cells. The National Stroke Association offers this reminder: "Time is brain."[2]

Ask your doctor if you should take aspirin. This drug may benefit persons at high risk of stroke, but it also increases the risk of bleeding and thus is not appropriate for everyone. When doctors suggest aspirin for stroke prevention, the usual dose is one "baby" aspirin (75 to 100 milligrams) per day or one regular aspirin (325 milligrams) every other day. To minimize stomach irritation, take aspirin in the evening with a full glass of water.

Timewise Tips

Check your BP regularly at home, and record it in the diary on page 289. Take the diary with you when you see your doctor.

Ask your doctor if the new BP medications, designed to work in synchrony with body rhythms, could benefit you. (See page 294.) If your BP is high, work with your doctor to get it under control and keep it there.

Follow Timewise Tips for heart disease, page 284.

Anytime Tips

If you experience brief episodes of slurred speech, lapses in awareness, blurring of vision, sudden weakness, or any other symptom you find strange, tell your doctor as soon as possible. Though TIAs seem minor at the time, people who have them are ten times more likely to experience a major stroke later.

Watch your temper. Anger boosts the heart rate and sends BP soaring. Men prone to outbursts of anger have twice the risk of having a stroke as men who keep their tempers under control.

If you smoke, stop. This is especially important if you are a woman who has ever used birth-control pills. Smoking plus use of this medication increases your risk of blood clots. Smoking makes you four times more likely to have a stroke. The older you get, the higher your risk.

Study. Visit the Web sites of the American Stroke Association (www.stroke-association.org) and the National Stroke Association (www.stroke.org).

SUDDEN INFANT DEATH SYNDROME

Sudden infant death syndrome (SIDS), also called crib death, is the sudden and unexplained death of a presumably healthy baby in its first year of life. About eight out of ten SIDS deaths occur while the baby is thought to be asleep. Most deaths occur in the small hours of the night.[1] "I didn't notice anything unusual when I put the baby to bed. When I returned a few hours later, the baby was dead," stunned parents typically report.

SIDS deaths peak in winter months, most likely because of the seasonal increase in infectious viruses that cause trouble breathing. In 1997, the latest year for which statistics were available when this book was written, three thousand babies died of SIDS in the United States. One-third more SIDS deaths occurred in January, the peak month, than in July, when the fewest babies died.[2]

Time-of-day and time-of-year links are helping researchers to target potential causes of this much studied, but still baffling, tragic disorder. One likely scenario is that some babies are born more susceptible than others, and that some triggering factor, such as heat, cold, or viruses, tips the balance. We review here some plausible theories derived from studies of body rhythms.

What Makes Early Morning Hours Risky?

Two-thirds of the babies who die of SIDS are between two and four months of age, and 90 percent are under six months old. Only 1 percent are older than one year.[3] Between about two and four months of age, infants lose antibodies they acquired in the womb that protect them from infectious agents early in life. They also start to secrete cortisol in a more adult pattern, in a morning burst, and their nighttime cortisol levels drop dramatically. In older children and adults, lowered levels of cortisol at night increase susceptibility to inflammatory responses, triggering asthma attacks near dawn, for example. Until infants' cortisol rhythm becomes established, they also may experience an increased susceptibility to infectious agents.

"If the switch to the circadian rhythm pattern (of cortisol) occurs in an infant when maternal antibodies are still present or after they have developed their own active immunity, the infant could neutralise common viruses, toxins or bacteria," suggests A. E. Gordon of the University of Edinburgh. "However, if this switch occurs in an infant when antibody levels are low," he reported, "this could be a window of vulnerability during which infants are at an increased risk of death."[4]

The daily rhythm of body temperature also evolves in the first months of life. Since overheating is thought to contribute to some SIDS deaths, researchers are exploring the tie between temperature control and breathing. New Zealand researchers found that temperature varies more in sleep in young infants than it does later in life.[5]

Some babies who die of SIDS may have a subtle heart disorder, making them more vulnerable to sleep-related irregularities in heart activity. Italian researchers recorded heart activity on the third or fourth day of life in 34,442 newborns, and then followed these babies for one year. In this time, thirty-four of the children died, twenty-four of them from SIDS. The researchers found that the SIDS babies had a specific heart defect. It would be premature to perform electrocardiograms routinely on all newborns. More research is needed to validate this finding and determine the appropriate treatment.[6]

Sleep itself is another active area of study. Some scientists believe SIDS involves a deficiency in arousability, an important defense mechanism. If breathing stops during sleep, the oxygen-depleted brain ordinarily prods the sleeper to restart it. SIDS babies, according to parents' later reports, often were harder to awaken and moved less often than healthy babies.

"Back to Sleep" Campaign Lowers SIDS Deaths

Some researchers postulate that babies who sleep on their tummies may rebreathe their own expired gas, causing a possibly fatal buildup of carbon dioxide and a decrease of oxygen in their blood. Suffocation is even more likely if babies sleep on soft mattresses, comforters, or water beds.

In 1992 the American Academy of Pediatrics recommended that parents place infants on their back or side to sleep.[7] In 1994 this organization, in collaboration with other health groups and the federal government, launched a national "Back to Sleep" campaign. At the same time, health authorities also urged changes in other practices thought to increase the risk of SIDS. They advised women not to smoke while pregnant, to breast-feed, to protect the newborn baby from exposure to tobacco smoke, to put the baby to sleep on a firm surface without pillows, and to avoid letting babies get too warm.

In 1992 about 70 percent of American mothers placed newborns on their tummies to sleep, according to a large national survey.[8] By 1997 only 21 percent did. The prevalence of breast-feeding did not change substantially in this time, but about one-quarter fewer women reported that they smoked cigarettes while pregnant. The SIDS rate fell by a remarkable 42 percent from 1992 to 1997, according to preliminary data from the National Center for Health Statistics.[9] Still, African-American and Native-American babies remain more than twice as likely to die of SIDS as Caucasian babies, pointing to a need for continued and targeted public health education efforts. The national goal is to have fewer than 10 percent of U.S. babies sleeping on their stomachs.

Other countries around the world adopted back to sleep campaigns, some ahead of the United States. In many with less diverse populations than in this country, results are even more impressive. In England, where three in four babies sleep faceup, SIDS rates are 70 percent lower than they were when the educational campaign started. In Hong Kong, where babies almost always sleep on their backs, SIDS rarely occurs.

Although some parents and doctors initially expressed concern that babies might choke on spit-up or vomit more often if sleeping on their backs, researchers showed the opposite is true. When babies sleep tummy-down, they swallow less frequently, about twenty-one times per minute, compared to thirty-two swallows per minute when they sleep on their backs. They also take fewer breaths. These findings come from an Australian study in which researchers, with parents' consent, gave a tiny amount of water to ten healthy one-month-old babies while they were sleeping in either the tummy-down or face-up position, and assessed their responses. The findings suggest that normal airway protective mechanisms work less well even in healthy babies when they sleep tummy-down. A baby with a cold and postnasal drip probably would have even more trouble breathing in that position.[10]

In the first four months of life, the high risk time for SIDS, babies almost always stay in the same position in which they are put down. They don't start turning over in sleep until they also do that while awake, usually around six months of age. While babies who sleep on their backs may develop motor skills more slowly than those who sleep tummy-down, studies show they catch up by eighteen months of age. Back-sleeping babies also may experience some flattening of the back of the head, but this, too, corrects itself. Parents can minimize it by alternating placing the baby's head to the left or right each time they put the baby to sleep.

How Risky Is Bedsharing?

Breast-fed babies have a lower risk of SIDS. Around the world, most breast-feeding mothers keep their babies next to them through the night. Yet some health groups that advocate breast-feeding disagree on the relative benefits and risks of bedsharing. The idea that babies should sleep alone is a Western one that surfaced only 150 to 200 years ago. Even in the United States, contrary to popular belief, bedsharing is not rare. Two studies found that 19 percent of whites, 59 percent of African Americans, and 26 percent of Hispanics in New York City and Cleveland reported frequent all-night or part-night bedsharing.

Some studies suggest that bedsharing may prevent long episodes of very deep sleep. Vulnerable infants theoretically may have trouble arousing from a prolonged pause in breathing or a drop in body temperature that may occur at this time.

Thirty-five mother-infant pairs volunteered for a study that Sarah Mosko, Christopher Richard, and their colleagues conducted at the University of California Irvine Medical Center. Twenty mother-infant pairs shared a bed most nights, while fifteen did not. All the mothers were Latina, because bedsharing is an accepted practice in this ethnic group. All were breast-feeding, in good health, and had had uncomplicated pregnancies, labors, and deliveries. All had chosen their sleeping practice for reasons other than infant temperament, that is, not because their babies were "fussy." The infants were eleven to fifteen weeks old at the time of the study, the age when SIDS most often occurs. All the infants were healthy and developing normally.

All mother-infant pairs spent three nights in the sleep laboratory. On the first night, they followed their home sleeping arrangement, and on the second and third nights they either shared the bed or slept alone, in random order. When sleeping alone, the infants slept in a standard crib in a room adjacent to that of their mothers, with the door between them ajar. Mothers and babies went to bed and got up at their usual times. Researchers monitored sleep stages, muscle movements, and breathing.

On the bedsharing night, all of the infants experienced less very deep sleep, considered a positive outcome in babies this age. The total amount of time spent in rapid eye movement or REM sleep—a time when breathing becomes more variable—was about the same in both conditions.[11]

In a second study, the same research group found that bedsharing also minimized face-down sleeping by the baby. Mothers and babies slept very close together, often less than eight inches apart, and maintained a high degree of mutual orientation, suggesting an awareness of each other's presence. This finding argues against the belief that bedsharing carries an inherent risk of overlying and accidental suffocation.[12]

Nonetheless, researchers at the U.S. Consumer Product Safety Commission warned in 1999 that adult beds are not safe places for children under age two to sleep. Suad Nakamura and her colleagues reviewed national data on deaths of children younger than two years in standard adult beds, daybeds, and water beds from 1990 through 1997.

They found 515 deaths, 121 of which allegedly resulted from overlying of the child by another person and 394 from entrapment in the bed structure. Most of the deaths, they said, appeared to have resulted from suffocation or strangulation, caused, for instance, by entrapment of the child's head between the mattress and a wall adjoining the bed, or between the mattress and headboard. The most common cause of the seventy-nine water bed–related deaths was airway obstruction. These infants were found facedown.

This study attracted a lot of national publicity, but some pediatric sleep experts felt the commission's recommendation was not justified by the data it reported. Not all the deaths were from SIDS; entrapment of a child's head is a known cause of death. Clearly, far more babies die alone in their cribs than die in their parents' bed. Nearly 34,000 babies died of SIDS in the United States, most in their own beds, in the years covered by the commission's study. The American Academy of Pediatrics cautions against routine cosleeping in a family bed in its *Guide to Your Child's Sleep*.[13]

Whether or not to sleep with your baby is a decision only you can make. Wherever the baby sleeps, you need to provide a firm sleeping surface and safe environment, and to place the baby on its back. For further guidance, talk to your child's doctor.

Specter of Child Abuse Complicates SIDS Investigations

SIDS, by definition, has no discernible cause. The great majority of infants who die suddenly may have still unrecognized heart, lung, or nervous system defects, or other illnesses, possibly genetic in origin. Many parents in their grief wonder if there was something they could have or should have done or noticed. Support and reassurance from family, friends, and doctors that they did nothing wrong may help the healing process.

It would be an error, however, to view the SIDS story as solely a medical one. Ghastly as it is to contemplate, some infant deaths result from child abuse. A book published in 1997, *The Death of Innocents: A True Story of Murder, Medicine, and High Stakes Science,* brought this issue to public awareness. Science writers Richard Firstman and Jamie Talan described in meticulous detail the deaths of five children in one family in the 1960s, and the trial and conviction of the children's mother for murder three decades later.[14]

A physician who treated the children, Alfred Steinschneider, had blamed the infants' deaths on SIDS. In an article published in 1972 in the prestigious journal *Pediatrics,* he suggested that a sleep-related breathing disorder, sleep apnea, was at fault, that SIDS could run in families, and that it could be prevented.[15] His report spawned a multimillion-dollar industry in infant apnea monitors used in the home by anxious parents.

Firstman and Talan's book prompted *Pediatrics* to renounce its publication of the 1972 Steinschneider article. "Some physicians still believe SIDS runs in families," Jerold Lucey, the editor of *Pediatrics,* wrote. "It doesn't— murder does."[16]

Deaths of infants at the hands of their caretakers probably is far more common than now is believed, authorities say. An extensive study conducted by *The Washington Post* in 1998 concluded that at least one child in the Washington, D.C., area died each week as a result of abuse or neglect, far more than were identified by official police counts or court cases.[17]

The American Academy of Pediatrics recommends an autopsy, an extensive battery of tests, and a detailed investigation that includes a visit to the scene at which a child was found dead before ruling that SIDS was the likely cause.

Timewise Tips

Put your baby to sleep on his or her back on a firm surface. Remind babysitters, too.

Remove fluffy blankets, comforters, stuffed toys, and pillows while the baby sleeps.

Keep room temperature at a level that feels comfortable when you are wearing a short-sleeved shirt. Put the baby in a sleeper suit, or use a light blanket that reaches no farther than the shoulders.

Anytime Tips

Breast-feed, if possible.
  Do not expose your baby to secondhand smoke.
  For more information on SIDS, see "Back to Sleep" (www.nih.gov/nichd).

TOOTHACHE

Toothaches erupt twice as often between 3 A.M. and 8 A.M. as they do between 3 P.M. and 8 P.M., their least frequent start time.[1] This rhythm may be tied to the body's secretion of a key inflammation-fighting hormone, cortisol, which is virtually absent at night. Cortisol secretion occurs in a burst about the time you usually awaken. The way your body responds to pain, and the efficacy of drugs to block that pain, also varies over the day. Here are some key findings of dental-pain studies in heroic volunteers:

Tooth Nerve Sensitivity Highest at Night

In one study, researchers applied an electric current to volunteers' teeth every three hours around the clock. It took 25 percent less current to induce pain at night than in the afternoon. In another study, the same researchers touched volunteers' teeth with a frozen cotton ball at different times. The subjects felt the pain 30 percent sooner at night than in the afternoon.[2]

Local Anesthetics Last Longest in the Afternoon

Marie Anne Reinberg, a French dentist, scheduled appointments hourly between 7 A.M. and 7 P.M. for persons who needed a cavity filled in an upper front tooth. She injected the same amount of lidocaine, a widely used dental anesthetic, into the gum above the tooth, and then started a stopwatch. After drilling the tooth to remove the decay, and with the patient's consent, she left the cavity temporarily unfilled.

Applying a cold stimulus to the tooth, she found that lidocaine relieved pain almost three times longer between 1 P.M. and 3 P.M. than between 7 A.M. and 9 A.M. The anesthetic lasted thirty-two minutes in the afternoon but only twelve minutes in the morning.[3] Similar studies by other scientists, assessing other painkilling medications in persons undergoing root canal surgery, tooth extraction, gum surgery, or other painful procedures, show comparable results.

Post-Surgical Pain Is Worst Near Dawn

The times people choose on their own to take painkillers after dental surgery also reveal daily pain rhythms. In one study, 714 people who had undergone oral surgery noted when they took aspirin and a similar medication, indomethacin, for the next few days. On the day of surgery, most people took pain relievers in the afternoon and evening. But in the following three days, they took such drugs far more often between 4 A.M. and 6 A.M. than they did in the afternoon. These findings suggest that pain arising from dental surgery is more intense at night, or that pain-relieving medications are less effective then. With healing, the patients stopped waking up needing to take pain relievers, and took them at bedtime instead.[4]

Aspirin Works Better for Dental Pain in the Morning

Aspirin and indomethacin appear to relieve dental pain better in the early-morning hours and in the afternoon than they do at night. This finding comes from studies in which researchers applied a cold stimulus to teeth after patients took one of these medications at different times. In these studies, the pain relievers offered little benefit when taken at midnight.[5] Dental pain, fortunately, usually is short lived. Although aspirin and related drugs may be more effective for this type of pain in the early morning, they also cause more stomach irritation when taken at this time. If you must use these drugs in the morning, ask your doctor if you should take them with food.

Timewise Tips

If you are having extensive dental work requiring a local anesthetic:

Ask for a midafternoon appointment if pain relief is your prime concern.

Ask for a morning appointment if you want to minimize numbing of the lips that may interfere with talking or eating later in the day.

Ask your dentist to prescribe a long-lasting pain reliever to get you through the night after having a wisdom tooth extracted, or undergoing a similar procedure.

Study. Visit the Web site of the American Dental Association (www.ada.org).

URINARY DISORDERS

From about ages five to fifty, our bodies produce up to 75 percent less urine at night than in the daytime. A healthy bladder holds this amount comfortably for about six to eight hours. This synchrony of time and function lets sleep proceed undisturbed. As we grow older, the peaks and valleys of this daily rhythm flatten, and we need to urinate more frequently both day and night.

If you awaken at night, you may get up to use the bathroom. Awakenings are not invariably triggered by the need to urinate, however. Airplane noise or a bedpartner's movement may have disturbed your sleep. A true need to urinate prompts awakenings mainly in older adults and in young children.

In both instances, various physical causes play key contributory roles. Parents of children who wet their beds fervently beg the doctor to "do something." Older persons often view nighttime urination, or *nocturia,* as an inevitable infirmity of age, and few seek medical help. For both the young and the old, however, medical treatment may bring substantial relief.

Bedwetting Usually Stops by Age Five

By four to six months of age, most babies show a clear circadian pattern in urine formation. They soak their diapers more thoroughly and more often in the daytime. Most start to stay dry for two- to three-hour periods around their second birthday and start to show interest in the potty chair at that time. Most learn to control urination and bowel movements in the daytime by their third birthday. But one in three normal, healthy four-year-olds continues to wet at night.

Pediatricians regard bedwetting as a problem only when it persists after age five. Most children who continue to wet their beds after this age never reached the stage of continuous dry nights. Doctors call this type of bedwetting *primary enuresis.* One in ten six-year-olds continues to wet the bed.

More boys than girls have continuing difficulty with bedwetting. The problem often runs in families and may simply reflect a maturational delay. If your child has it, ask your parents how old you were when you stopped wetting. The answer may reassure you that your child eventually will outgrow it, too.

Bedwetting usually occurs in the first three hours of sleep when sleep is soundest. Older children sometimes report that they dreamed they were in the bathroom. Sleep laboratory studies show, however, that wetting nearly always occurs in nondreaming sleep. Such "dreams" likely reflect the mind's quick attempt to account for wet pajamas. A child who offers this explanation is *not* telling a lie.

What Causes Bedwetting in Children?

The circadian rhythm of a hormone that controls urine production, arginine vasopressin, often is out of sync in children with primary enuresis. High levels of this hormone keep urine production down, while low levels boost it.

Although the body normally produces twice as much of this hormone at night as in the daytime, some children make too little of it.[1]

A child who has stayed dry for three to six months or longer sometimes starts wetting the bed again after an illness or a psychological stress such as the birth of a sibling or a move. Doctors call this type of bedwetting *secondary enuresis*. An estimated 10 to 30 percent of children who continue to wet the bed after age six have this problem.

Some children who continue to wet have a smaller than average-sized bladder, or a more active bladder than other children. Some have difficulty arousing from sleep, which makes them less aware of the need to urinate when the bladder is full.

Childhood-onset diabetes may trigger night-wetting: a child who develops diabetes may be excessively thirsty and drink large quantities of liquids in the daytime. (See Diabetes, page 245). The sleep-related breathing disorder, sleep apnea, is another possible culprit. Interruptions in the flow of oxygen to the brain trigger arousals, and the awakening sometimes prompts wetting. In this instance, children often snore loudly. Seizures may cause night-wetting and may occur at night even in children not known to have seizures in the daytime. (See Epilepsy, page 250).[2]

Psychological Distress Is Common

Older children who wet their beds often try to hide wet pajamas and bedclothes from parents. They fear sleeping over at a friend's house or going away to summer camp, depriving them of the social skills such experiences provide. An adolescent with this problem would be taunted in a college dorm. Perhaps one in a hundred eighteen-year-olds continues to wet the bed, at least occasionally. Young men sometimes are discharged from military service for this reason.

Timewise Tips for Parents

Take comfort in knowing that nearly all children who wet their beds well into childhood do outgrow the problem. Treatment typically involves both behavioral tactics and medications, so you'll need to coordinate your efforts with those of your child's doctor.

Don't worry about restricting fluids in the evening, unless your child is drinking huge amounts.

Arouse your child at your bedtime and walk him or her to the bathroom. Children usually fall back asleep rapidly.

Give an older child who wets the responsibility for washing himself, and changing his own pajamas and bedclothes. Leave a nightlight on and supplies by the bathroom hamper. Reward dry nights with a star chart and dry weeks with grown-up treats, such as going to a movie.

Consider use of a bed-wetting alarm. Such devices may involve buzzers worn on the wrist or shoulder and connected by wires to moisture sensors attached to pajamas. Others involve moisture-sensitive pads placed under the sheets, also connected to an alarm. Some devices turn on bedside lights. Urination activates the alarm and awakens the child. With repeated experience, about 70 percent of children using such alarms learn to recognize the sensation of a full bladder and to awaken before urination starts. Studies suggest success can be achieved within about six weeks.[3] These devices typically cost less than $50 and are widely available through catalogs.

Work on bladder training in the daytime, too. Encourage your child to drink freely, and then to try to hold urine as long as possible. Practicing stopping and starting also teaches better control.

Talk to the doctor about using medications such as imipramine and desmopressin (DDAVP). Imipramine decreases bladder excitability. Desmopressin is a synthetic version of the hormone that controls the daily rhythm of urine production. Taken at bedtime in a nasal aerosol spray or a tablet, desmopressin acts as a chronotherapy of primary nighttime enuresis by reducing the volume of urine formed in sleep.[4] Swedish researchers who gave desmopressin for two three-month courses to teenagers with persistent bed-wetting found that about a third were cured when treatment stopped, and most of the others continued to improve afterward. Four in five stayed dry seven years later, a higher cure rate than would have been expected to occur spontaneously.[5]

Study. Visit the Web sites of the American Academy of Family Practice (www.familydoctor.org), and the American Academy of Pediatrics (www.aap.org).

Age and Illness Chief Factors in Adult Nocturia

By age sixty, people produce about half their daily urine volume at night.[6] The circadian rhythm of arginine vasopressin changes with age. Older persons secrete less of this hormone at night than younger adults do.[7]

Half of all healthy sixty-year-old men and women awaken at least once a night to use the bathroom. As age progresses, this necessity becomes even more common. Nocturia understandably compromises sleep quality and may contribute to daytime fatigue. It also contributes to nighttime falls: sleepy people walking barefoot across dimly lighted rooms are apt to stumble.[8] People sixty and over also may take medications designed to help them stay asleep and thus are even more groggy when they get out of bed at night. Older persons urinate more frequently in the daytime as well.[9]

Illnesses that make muscles too weak or too active or that interfere with nerve signals unfortunately also become more common as people grow older. Congestive heart failure, diabetes, sleep apnea, kidney disorders, multiple sclerosis, strokes, recurrent urinary tract infections, and dementia are among the many conditions that increase the likelihood of needing to urinate at night. Enlargement of the prostate gland in older men puts added pressure on the bladder, contributing to nocturia.[10] Men who feel the urge to urinate frequently at night, particularly if they then have trouble doing it, should report this symptom to the doctor. While usually caused only by an enlarged prostate, these symptoms also occur in prostate cancer.

An estimated seventeen million Americans, largely women, report needing to urinate more than eight times a day, and waking to urinate two or more times a night, every night. The most common daytime complaint is that urine leaks when they exercise, cough, sneeze, laugh, or lift heavy objects, a condition doctors call *stress incontinence*. In premenopausal women, this problem may worsen a few days before menstruation when levels of estrogen fall. Some adults report they cannot hold urine long enough to get to the bathroom; this is *urge incontinence*.[11] Least common is a frequent or constant dribble of urine from a full bladder, or *overflow incontinence*. These problems require medical treatment. They are not a normal part of the aging process.

Concern about possible incontinence makes some women reluctant to go to stores, museums, or places where they aren't sure of the rest room availability. It's also fostered a big market in incontinence pads worn to minimize the likelihood of public embarrassment.

Bedwetting may be a lifelong condition. Dutch researchers surveyed more than 13,000 adults aged eighteen to sixty-four living in a community. One in every two hundred persons reported having wet their bed at least once in the previous month. Few had talked about the problem with their doctors, and most regarded it as untreatable. It did complicate their lives, however, limiting personal relationships as well as careers, since these people hesitated to travel for work or vacations.[12]

A U.S. survey of nearly 4,000 persons over age sixty-five found accidental wetting even more common. About three in one hundred women and one in one hundred men reported this problem. These people had higher rates of depression than other adults.[13] Incontinence is a key factor in the decision to admit a person to a nursing home.

Behavioral Treatment and Medications Can Help

Two hundred older women with urge incontinence or urge plus stress incontinence volunteered for a study at the University of Alabama at Birmingham. All reported about sixteen episodes of incontinence per week. Karen Burgio and her colleagues taught one-third of the women skills and strategies to prevent incontinence and gave one-third a medication commonly used for this problem, oxybutynin. The others did not receive treatment and served as a control group. The behavioral tactics included a biofeedback session to help the women identify and learn to control pelvic muscles. The women were told not to rush to the toilet when they felt an urge, but rather to sit down if possible, relax their bodies, contract pelvic muscles repeatedly to cut urgency, and then to walk to the toilet at a normal pace. They practiced these skills daily. After eight weeks, those in the behavioral group averaged three accidents per week, and those receiving the medication, six accidents. Those in the behavioral group also reported higher satisfaction with their treatment; nearly all said they would continue to work on their new skills.[14]

Biofeedback training requires a skilled instructor, and behavioral tactics require practice. Some people prefer the speed and convenience of medications. Desmopressin is the drug of choice for nocturia. Taken at bedtime, it reduces the amount of urine produced at night. The drugs of choice for urge incontinence are oxybutynin (Ditropan) and tolterodine (Detrol). Vaginal estrogen creams can aid postmenopausal women.

For men with moderate prostate enlargement, medications such as terazosin (Hytrin) and doxazosin (Cardura), both taken once a day at bedtime, cut the frequency of nighttime urination. Finasteride (Proscar) shrinks the prostate gland by lowering blood levels of the male sex hormone testosterone. Though effective in curbing urinary frequency, these drugs have a side effect that makes some men reluctant to use them: they sometimes cause erectile dysfunction.

Timewise Tips for Adults

Record your daily urinary pattern for two consecutive days using the diary on page 369. Take the diary with you when you see your doctor.

Limit fluids only after dinner. Eight glasses of water a day are recommended for most adults. Avoiding fluids may not only lead to dehydration but also slow down the digestive system and cause constipation.

Avoid coffee, tea, colas, and other caffeine-containing drinks, as well as alcohol, which are diuretics. Also avoid highly acidic and spicy foods, which irritate the bladder and increase its contractions.

Practice the "urge strategies" described above. Try to hold urine as long as possible, ideally for four hours between voidings. This tactic helps strengthen the muscles used in urinary control and may decrease nighttime awakenings.

Women should practice Kegel exercises to strengthen muscles in the pelvic floor that weaken after childbirth and after menopause when estrogen levels decline. Locate these muscles by stopping your urine flow midstream. To do the exercises, contract and relax these muscles rapidly ten times, rest for ten seconds, and contract and hold for ten seconds or longer. Repeat often during the day, while waiting at a stop sign, watching TV, every time you think of it. If you experience leakage while exercising, wear a tampon or a device called a pessary; both press against vaginal walls and compress the urine passageway, or urethra.

Consider the side effects of all medicines you take, even those you buy without a prescription. Decongestants and nonprescription sleep remedies, for example, may increase both difficulty urinating and leakage.

Talk to your doctor. You may have an underlying medical problem that contributes to night urination. Treating that problem may improve both conditions. Your doctor may suggest biofeedback training; prescribe medications that increase the contractability of the muscle that opens and closes the urethra, or relax the bladder; or suggest that you have injections of collagen to add bulk to the muscle that opens and closes the urethra. This procedure can be performed in the doctor's office. Surgery to restore muscle support sometimes is advised. The American Urological Association says that treatment can cure or improve 80 percent of cases of incontinence.[15]

Study. Visit the Web sites of the American Urological Association (www.drylife.org); Netwellness, a joint information project of the University of Cincinnati, Ohio State University, and Case Western University (www.netwellness.org); and the National Institute on Aging (www.nih.gov/nia/health/agepages/urinary.htm).

Urination Diary

Name_____

See a doctor if you

- urinate more than once a night
- urinate more than eight times a day
- experience incontinence

- have pain or burning when you urinate
- have trouble starting urination or stopping midstream
- have blood in your urine

Make copies of this chart and fill them in for at least two consecutive days. Use a disposable cup marked in ounces to measure urine excreted in the two hours following each time listed below. Take this diary with you when you see your doctor.

Day/Date_____

Time of Arising_____ A.M./P.M.

Bedtime_____ A.M./P.M.

Women: Are you menstruating today? Y/N

Time	Episode of Urination or Incontinence	Volume of Urine Voided	Fluid Consumed (Type and Amount)	Exercise, Coughing, or Other Trigger	Medications (Name and Dose)
8 A.M.					
10 A.M.					
NOON					
2 P.M.					
4 P.M.					
6 P.M.					
8 P.M.					
10 P.M.					
MIDNIGHT					
2 A.M.					
4 A.M.					
6 A.M.					

Better Health in the
Twenty-first Century

Practitioners of chronomedicine, circa 2000 and beyond, will routinely ask you how your symptoms wax and wane over the day, the month, and even the year. Your chronorecord will be a standard part of your medical history, helping to identify illnesses in their earliest, most treatable stages.

Your doctor will schedule tests at optimal biological times, and interpret test results in relation to time-of-day norms. More doctors' offices and outpatient treatment centers will offer appointments in the evening and at night.

You may wear or have implanted under your skin a microsensor that continuously monitors your heart rate, blood pressure, body temperature, hormonal rhythms, and other bodily functions relevant to your specific health needs. You'll use a special scanning device to collect this information, something like a bar-code reader now used in stores, sending data via the phone to your doctor's office for analysis.

In the future, you also will take a more active role in your own health care than most people do today. You will chart rhythms of disease activity at home, and conduct self-tests of various bodily functions. A study at the University of Illinois at Chicago Medical Center shows persons with long-standing high blood pressure gain better control when they take their own readings. The participants measured their blood pressure at home with an easy-to-use electronic device as often as three times a day: when they got up in the morning but before they took their medication, a few hours after the medication kicked in, and in the evening. The monitoring device contained a computer modem, enabling them to send results to a secure site on the Internet over phone lines.

At the medical center, clinical nurse specialist Mary Bondmass reviewed the results as they arrived. She considered each patient's daily pattern and what it showed about how well treatment was working. In collaboration with the person's doctor, she then adjusted medications as necessary. She also suggested ways to improve diet or make other modest lifestyle changes. Within a month, patients achieved blood pressure control that had eluded them for the previous year, despite using medications. They kept their blood pressure down for the remaining two months of the study. About one in ten patients, thought for many years by their doctors to have high blood pressure, proved to have only white coat hypertension. When they took their own readings at home, their blood pressure was normal.[1]

Computers Foster Chronotherapy

In the future, doctors will make greater use of computers to determine the best timing and dose of medications for you. They will integrate the health information you collect with their understanding of your illness and the rhythms that govern it and a vast database of the world's scientific literature. In so doing, they will weigh differences over the day in how the body responds to various drugs, takes them up into tissues, breaks them down, and excretes them. They will apply this information to your specific circumstances.

You won't face the hassle of complicated dosing schedules that require you to take pills, liquids, shots, or use inhalers several times a day. Chronobiologically designed medicines will be more widely available. Pharmaceutical manufacturers will make greater use of new biomaterials to provide drugs in the right amount at the right time, targeting only the active disease sites in the body. You will be able to take a pill in the morning that will start to work later in the day when you need the medication most. You will be able to take a pill on Monday that lasts for the whole week, with more of the drug being released at some times and less at others, in tandem with daily rhythms in disease activity and side effects. Some medications will work over the menstrual cycle or even around the year in this fashion.

If you have diabetes, asthma, heart disease, or other chronic illnesses, you may wear a small computerized device resembling a wristwatch that dispenses your medication, checks its blood level, and doles out the exact amount you need every minute of the day. A person with diabetes will be able to count on having insulin automatically available just before mealtimes and while exercising. A person with asthma will be protected from middle-of-the-night airway narrowing, and a person with heart disease, from a too rapid rise in early-morning blood pressure. Delivery systems for hormones will mimic the body's natural secretion patterns, providing the hormones in preprogrammed pulses. Growth hormone, for example, will be released in the early part of sleep, and cortisol before a person's usual wake-up time. These advances will enable persons with chronic illnesses to live healthier, longer, and blissfully more ordinary lives.

Everyone Will "Think Chrono"

In everyday life, in health as well as sickness, we all will be better attuned to our body rhythms. We will take advantage of our best times to be more productive at work, learn more in school, get the most out of exercise, and enjoy our leisure more fully. We will assess a prospective mate's morning and evening preferences and consider how it meshes with our own chronotype. We will be more sensitive to chronotypes in choosing jobs, and in rearing our children and structuring family life.

We will pay more attention to lighting in schools, homes, workplaces, and hospitals, using bright lights at the right times to boost alertness and mood, help us adapt faster after jet travel and job-schedule changes, and keep daily rhythms in synchrony. We will accommodate, not fight, our body's demand for sufficient sleep. In so doing, we will discover that we feel better, work better, view the world with greater optimism, and enjoy a higher and overall more satisfying quality of life.

We Need More Chrono Education

These advances are not the stuff of science fiction. Many are feasible, or nearly so, today. Their implementation, however, requires changes at every level of education, from the earliest grades through medical updates for health practitioners. It also requires continuing communication via the news media with the general public.

Innovative efforts already are in progress. *Online Hamsters* teaches the latest findings about how body clocks work to future doctors and patients, now in their early teens. This program invites middle school students to solve "the mystery of sleepy adolescents" by observing live-action hamsters in a chronobiology research laboratory at the University of Virginia over the Internet (www.cbt.virginia.edu/olh). Students can download results as they are generated. They learn how to formulate hypotheses and conduct long-term science experiments to answer their own questions, studies they could not conduct in a typical classroom. This feature is a special boon to schools that lack comprehensive science labs. The studies involve observation only, no surgery, although students do learn that surgery may be part of research, and why. *Online Hamsters* was developed by the Center for Biological Timing of the University of Virginia, with funding from the National Science Foundation.

Crash in Bed, Instead aims to teach high school students about the dangers of driving while sleepy, and the benefits of getting sufficient sleep. Designed for use in driver education, biology, science, and health classes, this program is a project of the American Academy of Sleep Medicine, a national organization of sleep professionals (www.aasmnet.org/).

Unintentional dozing is common in both high school and college students. While most teachers frown on napping in class, psychologist Scott Doran elevated it to the curriculum. His summer class on circadian rhythms and sleep at the University of Oregon met in the afternoon Monday through Friday for eight weeks. After Doran's ninety-minute lecture, the students trooped to a quiet adjacent carpeted room, spread out blankets and pillows, and rested for twenty minutes. While not all managed to sleep every day, most came away with new appreciation for daily rhythms of alertness and sleepiness, said Doran, now at the University of Pennsylvania.[2] In the future, students will learn this lesson earlier. They will monitor and chart their rhythms in health and disease from childhood on.

Chronobiology and chronotherapy do not need to be shoehorned as separate courses into the already tightly packed medical-school curriculum. Every aspect of the body from the cellular level to the whole person has its chronobiological component. Good teachers can integrate this information easily into their current lectures, showing students the ubiquity of biological time across all fields of biology and medicine.

The professors simply need to let go of their long-entrenched belief that the body strives for homeostasis, for internal constancy. They need to acknowledge instead that the body strives for predictability. The "chrono" aspect of our biology enables us to anticipate changes in the outside world, such as daylight and environmental temperature, and changes in our interior world, including our schedules of activity, meals, and sleep, over the day, month, and year, for our entire lives. Members of the American Association of Medical Chronobiology and Chronotherapeutics, established in 1999, will try to raise their colleagues' awareness of body time with lectures, symposia, and scientific publications.

Medical practice, circa 2000, will soon be known as the "bad old days."

Notes

Chapter 1: It's about TIME

1. Smolensky, M.H. Knowledge and attitudes of American physicians and public about medical chronobiology and chronotherapeutics. Findings of two 1996 Gallup surveys. *Chronobiology International.* 1998;15:377–394.

2. 1999–2000 APPMA National Pet Owners Survey. Greenwich, Conn.: American Pet Products Manufacturers' Association. 1999.

3. Bertman, S. *The Human Cost of Speed.* Westport, Conn.: Praeger Publishing. 1998.

4. Moore, J.G., et al. Day and night aspirin-induced gastric mucosal damage and protection by ranitidine in man. *Chronobiology International.* 1987;4:111–116.

5. Mormont, C., et al. Mechanisms of circadian rhythms in the toxicity and efficacy of anticancer drugs: relevance for the development of new analogues. In Lemmer, B. ed., *Chronopharmacology.* New York: Marcel Dekker. 1989:395–437.

6. Hagen, A.A., and Hrushesky, W.J.M. Menstrual timing of breast cancer surgery. *American Journal of Surgery.* 1998;104:245–261.

7. Quoted in Porter, R. *The Greatest Benefit to Mankind.* London: HarperCollins. 1997:14.

8. Hippocrates. *On Endemic Diseases (Air, Waters and Places).* Vol. 5. Mattock, J.N., and Lyons, M.C., eds. Cambridge: Heffer & Sons. 1969.

9. Binkley, S. *Biological Clocks: Your Owner's Manual.* Amsterdam: Harwood Academic Publishers. 1997.

10. Burton, R. *The Anatomy of Melancholy.* Vol 1. New York: Dutton. 1961. Originally published in 1621.

Chapter 2: Your Body Is a Time Machine

1. Moore-Ede, M.C. Physiology of the circadian timing system: predictive versus reactive homeostasis. *American Journal of Physiology.* 1986;250(5Pt 2):R737–752.

2. Births, marriages, divorces, and deaths: Provisional Data for 1998. *National Vital Statistics Reports.* 1999;47(21):2.

3. Weber, G.W. Height depends on month of birth. *Nature.* 1998;39:754–755.

4. Mortensen, P.B., et al. Effects of family history and place and season of birth on the risk of schizophrenia. *New England Journal of Medicine.* 1999;340:603–608. Andreasen, N. Understanding the causes of schizophrenia. *New England Journal of Medicine.* 1999;340:646–647.

5. Smolensky, M.H., et al. The chronopharmacology of methlyprednisolone: clinical implications of animal studies with special emphasis upon moderation of growth inhibition by timing to circadian rhythms. In Smolensky, M.H., et al., eds., *Recent Advances in the Chronobiology of Allergy and Immunology.* Oxford, England: Pergamon Press. 1979:137–171.

6. Arendt, J. Biological rhythms: the science of chronobiology. *Journal of the Royal College of Physicians of London.* 1998;32:27–35.

7. Harter, J., et al. Studies on an intermittent corticosteroid dosage regimen. *New England Journal of Medicine.* 1963;296:591–595.

8. Shock, N., et al. *Normal Human Aging.* Baltimore: U.S. Department of Health and Human Services, National Institute on Aging. NIH publication 84-2450, 1984.

Chapter 3: The Discovery of Inner Clocks

1. Hahn, R. *The Anatomy of a Scientific Institution: The Paris Academy of Sciences, 1666–1803.* Berkeley: University of California Press. 1979:87.

2. De Mairan, Jean Jacques Dortous. *Observation Botanique.* Paris: Proceedings of the Royal Academy of Sciences. 1729:35. Translation by Nidra Pollar, October 1998.

3. Hine, E.M. Dortous de Mairan and eighteenth century "systems theory." *Gesnerus.* 1995;52:54–65.

4. Aschoff, J. Bicentennial Anniversary of Christoph Wilhelm Hufeland's *Die Kunst das menschliche Leben zu verlängern* (The Art of Prolonging Human Life). *Journal of Biological Rhythms.* 1998;13:4–8.

5. Duhamel, H.L. *La Physique des Arbres.* Paris: H.L. Guerin and L.F. Delatour, 1798;2:158, cited in Ward, R.R. *The Living Clocks.* New York: Mentor (New American Library). 1971:54–55.

6. De Candolle, A.P. *Physiologie Végétale.* Paris: Béchet jeune. 1832:859. Cited in Ward, R.R. *The Living Clocks.* New York: Mentor (New American Library). 1971:57–58.

7. Darwin, C., and Darwin, F. *The Power of Movement in Plants.* Unabridged replication of the 1881 edition. New York: Plenum Publishing. 1966.

Chapter 4: How Your Body Clock Works

1. Richter, C.P. Sleep and activity: their relation to the 24-hour clock. In *Sleep and Altered States of Consciousness.* Association for Research in Nervous and Mental Disease. Baltimore: Williams & Wilkins. 1967:45:8–29.

2. Stephan, F.K., and Zucker, I. Circadian rhythms in drinking behavior and locomotor activity of rats are eliminated by hypothalamic lesions. *Proceedings of the National Academy of Sciences (USA).* 1972;69:1583–1586.

3. Moore, R.Y., and Eichler, V.B. Loss of circadian adrenal-corticosterone rhythm following suprachiasmatic lesions in the rat. *Brain Research.* 1972;42:201–206.

4. Ralph, M., and Menaker, M. A mutation of the circadian system in golden hamsters. *Science.* 1988;241:1225–1227.

5. Ralph, M., et al. Transplanted suprachiasmatic nucleus determines circadian period. *Science.* 1990;247:975–978.

6. Wever R. *The Circadian System of Man. Results of Experiments under Temporal Isolation.* New York: Springer Verlag. 1979:151.

7. Czeisler, C.A., et al. Entrainment of human circadian rhythms by light-dark cycles: a reassessment. *Photochemistry and Photobiology.* 1981;34:239–247.

8. Lewy, A., et al. Light suppresses melatonin secretion in humans. *Science.* 1980;210:1267–1269.

9. Boivin, D.B., and Czeisler, C.A. Resetting of circadian melatonin and cortisol rhythms in humans by ordinary room light. *Neuroreport.* 1998;9:779–782.

10. Shaddock, J. Florence Nightingale's *Notes on Nursing* as a survival memoir. *Literature and Medicine.* 1995;14:23–35.

11. Beauchemin, K.M., and Hays, P. Dying in the dark: sunshine, gender and outcomes in myocardial infarction. *Journal of the Royal Society of Medicine.* 1998;91:352–354.

12. Beauchemin, K.M., and Hays, P. Sunny hospital rooms expedite recovery from severe and refractory depressions. *Journal of Affective Disorders.* 1996;40:49–51.

13. Espiritu, R.C., et al. Low illumination experienced by San Diego adults: association with atypical depressive symptoms. *Biological Psychiatry.* 1994;35:403–407.

14. Koehler, Wilfried. Cited in Lamberg, L. Dawn's early light to twilight's last gleaming . . . *Journal of the American Medical Association.* 1998;280:1556–1558.

15. Klerman, E.B., et al. Simulations of light effects on the human circadian pacemaker: implications for assessment of intrinsic period. *American Journal of Physiology.* 1996;270:R271–R282.

16. Campbell, S., and Murphy, P. Extraocular circadian phototransduction in humans. *Science.* 1998;279:396–399.

17. Turek, F. Melatonin: pathway from obscure molecule to international fame. *Perspectives in Biology and Medicine.* 1997;41(1):9–19.

18. Kayser, C. Le rhythme nycthéméral des mouvements d'energie. *La Revue Scientifique.* 1952;90:173–188; cited in Reinberg, A., and Smolensky, M., eds., *Biological Rhythms and Medicine.* New York: Springer Verlag. 1983:4–5.

19. Sothern, R.B. Circadian and circannual characteristics of blood pressure self-measured for 25 years by a clinically-healthy man. *Chronobiologia.* 1994;21(1&2):7–20.

20. Rabatin, J.S., et al. Circadian rhythms in blood and self-measured variables of ten children 9 to 14 years of age. In Halberg, F., et al., eds., *Chronobiology.* Proceedings XIII, International Society of Chronobiology. Milan: II Ponte. 1981:373–385.

21. Binkley, S. Wrist activity in a woman: daily, weekly, menstrual, lunar, annual cycles? *Physiology and Behavior.* 1992;52:411–412.

Chapter 5: Are You a Lark, an Owl, or a Hummingbird?

1. Steele, M., et al. Morningness-eveningness preferences of emergency medicine residents are skewed toward eveningness. *Academic Emergency Medicine.* 1997;4:699–705.

2. Scott Adams's personal communications to Lynne Lamberg. August 13, 1995, and June 15, 1999.

3. Katzenberg, D., et al. A Clock polymorphism associated with human diurnal preference. *Sleep.* 1998;21:569–576.

4. Bloomberg, M., with Winkler, M. *Bloomberg by Bloomberg.* New York: John Wiley. 1997:29–30.

5. Walters, B. The mind of Bill Gates. *ABC 20/20.* January 30, 1998.

6. Hafner, K. *Where Wizards Stay Up Late.* New York: Touchstone. 1998.

7. Duff, C. Pick up on this: just don't answer, let freedom ring. *Wall Street Journal.* January 14, 1998. A1,14.

8. Miller, Henry. Cited in Mack, K., and Skjei, E. *Overcoming Writing Blocks.* Los Angeles: J.P. Tarcher. 1979:56.

9. Pat McNees's personal communication to Lynne Lamberg. November 14, 1997.

10. G. Howard's personal communication to Lynne Lamberg. May 13, 1999.

11. Van Dongen, H. Inter-and intra-individual differences in circadian phase. Leiden University Department of Physiology. Leiden, The Netherlands. 1998.

12. Hall, E.F., et al. Interval between waketime and circadian phase differs between morning and evening types. *Sleep Research.* 1997;26:716.

13. Howard, G. Ibid.

14. Schur, C. *Birds of a Different Feather: Early Birds and Night Owls Talk about Their Characteristic Behaviors.* Saskatoon, Canada: Schur Goode Associates. 1994.

15. Larson, J., et al. Morning and night couples: the effect of wake and sleep patterns on marital adjustment. *Journal of Marital and Family Therapy.* 1991;17:53–65.

16. Lange, A., et al. Sleep/wake patterns of partners. *Perceptual and Motor Skills.* 1998;86:1141–1142.

17. Jones, C., et al. Familial advanced sleep-phase syndrome: a short-period circadian rhythm variant in humans. *Nature Medicine.* 1999;5:1062–1065.

18. Gale, G., and Martyn, C. Larks and owls, and health, wealth, and wisdom. *British Medical Journal.* 1998;317:1675–1677.

19. Martin, J. Morning is no excuse for rudeness. *The Sun* (Baltimore). February 15, 1998:5K.

Chapter 6: Your Mind at Work

1. Van Dongen, H., and Dinges, D. Circadian rhythms in fatigue, alertness and performance. In Kryger, M.H., et al., eds. *Principles and Practice of Sleep Medicine.* Third edition. Philadelphia: W.B. Saunders. 2000.

2. Monk, T.H., and Carrier, J. Speed of mental processing in the middle of the night. *Sleep.* 1997;20:399–401.

3. Monk, T.H. Circadian rhythms in subjective activation, mood, and performance efficiency. In Kryger, M.H., et al., eds., *Principles and Practice of Sleep Medicine.* Second edition. Philadelphia: W.B. Saunders. 1994:321–330.

4. Folkard, S., et al. Time of day effects in school children's immediate and delayed recall of meaningful material. *British Journal of Psychology.* 1977;68:45–50.

5. Folkard, S. Time of day and level of processing. *Memory and Cognition.* 1979;7:247–252.

6. Carrier, J., and Monk, T.H. Effects of sleep and circadian rhythms on performance. In Turek, F. and Zee, P., eds., *Regulation of Sleep and Circadian Rhythms.* New York: Marcel Dekker. 1999:527–556.

7. Leirer, V.O., et al. Time of day and naturalistic prospective memory. *Experimental Aging Research.* 1994;20:127–134.

8. Monk, T.H., and Folkard, S. Concealed inefficiency of late-night study. *Nature.* 1978;273:296–297.

9. Zammit, G., et al. Postprandial sleep in healthy men. *Sleep.* 1995;18:229–231.

10. David Dinges spoke with Lynne Lamberg June 23, 1999.

11. Mitler, M., et al. Catastrophes, sleep, and public policy: consensus report. *Sleep.* 1988;11:100–109.

12. Broughton, R. Chronobiological aspects and models of sleep and napping. In Dinges, D., and Broughton, R., eds., *Sleep and Alertness: Chronobiological, Behavioral, and Medical Aspects of Napping.* New York: Raven Press. 1989:71–98.

13. Garza, A. Mexican workers lose afternoon break. Mexico City: Associated Press. *ABC-NEWS.com.* March 19, 1999.

14. Anthony, C. and W. *The Art of Napping at Work.* Burdett, N.Y.: Larson Publications. 1999.

15. Kerkhof, G. The 24-hour variation of mood differs between morning- and evening-type individuals. *Perceptual and Motor Skills.* 1998;86:264–266.

16. Boivin, D., et al. Complex interaction of the sleep-wake cycle in circadian phase modulates mood in healthy subjects. *Archives of General Psychiatry.* 1997;54:145–152.

17. Thayer, R. *The Origin of Everyday Moods: Managing Energy, Tension and Stress.* New York: Oxford University Press. 1996.

Chapter 7: A Good Night's Sleep

1. Shakespeare, W. *King Henry IV,* Part II. Act III, Scene 1, line 5:1597–1598.

2. Shakespeare, W. *Macbeth.* Act II, Scene 2, line 36.

3. Dinges, D., et al. Cumulative sleepiness, mood disturbance, and psychomotor vigilance performance decrements during a week of sleep restricted to 4–5 hours per night. *Sleep.* 1997;20:267–277.

4. Spiegel, K., et al. Impact of sleep debt on metabolic and endocrine function. *Lancet.* 1999;354:1435–1439.

5. Kreuger, J.M., and Majde, J.A. Microbial products and cytokines in sleep and fever regulation. *Critical Reviews in Immunology.* 1994;14:355–379.

6. Brown, R., et al. Suppression of immunity to influenza virus infection in the respiratory tract following sleep disturbance. *Regional Immunology.* 1989;2:321–325.

7. Wehr, T.A. The impact of changes in nightlength (scotoperiod) on human sleep. In Turek, F.W., and Zee, P.C., eds., *Regulation of Sleep and Circadian Rhythms.* New York: Marcel Dekker. 1999:263–285.

8. Maimonides. *Misheneh Torah.* Sefer Hamada. Hilchoth De'oth. Ch. IV., No. 4:1180. Translation by Arthur Lesley, Baltimore Hebrew University, Baltimore, Md.

9. Kripke, D.F., et al. Short and long sleep and sleeping pills. Is increased mortality associated? *Archives of General Psychiatry.* 1979;36:103–116.

10. Ancoli-Israel, S. Sleep problems in older adults: putting myths to bed. *Geriatrics.* 1997;52:20–29.

11. *1999 Omnibus Sleep in America Poll.* Washington, D.C.: National Sleep Foundation. 1999.

12. Jeffrey, N.A. Sleep: the new status symbol. *Wall Street Journal.* April 2, 1999:W1, W12.

13. Felsenthal, E., and Stevens, A. The year 2000: now what? *Wall Street Journal.* December 31, 1999; W1, W8.

14. Bliwise, D. Historical change in the report of daytime fatigue. *Sleep.* 1996;6:462–464.

15. *1999 Omnibus Sleep in America Poll.* Ibid.

16. Johnson, E.O. *1998 Women and Sleep Poll.* Washington, D.C.: National Sleep Foundation. 1998:11.

17. Dement, W., and Vaughan, C. *The Promise of Sleep.* New York: Delacorte Press. 1999.

18. Roehrs, T., et al. Sleep extension in sleepy and alert normals. *Sleep.* 1989;12:449–457.

19. Institute for Traffic Safety Management and Research. *New York State Task Force on Drowsy Driving Status Report.* Albany, N.Y.: New York State Governor's Traffic Safety Committee. May 1996.

20. Edgar, D., et al. Effect of SCN lesions on sleep in squirrel monkeys: evidence for opponent processes in sleep-wake regulation. *Journal of Neuroscience.* 1993;13:1065–1079.

21. Lavie, P. Ultrashort sleep-waking schedule. III. "Gates" and "forbidden zones" for sleep. *Electroencephalography and Clinical Neurophysiology.* 1986;63:414–425.

22. Bruck, D., and Pisani, D.L. The effects of sleep inertia on decision-making performance. *Journal of Sleep Research.* 1999;8:95–103.

23. Wehr, T.A. A "clock for all seasons" in the human brain. In Buijs, R.M., et al., eds., *Progress in Brain Research.* Vol. 111. Amsterdam: Elsevier. 1996:319–340.

24. Moorcroft, W., et al. Subjective and objective confirmation of the ability to self-awaken at a self-predetermined time without using external means. *Sleep.* 1997;20:40–45.

25. Dement, W., and Vaughan, C. Ibid.

26. Rechtschaffen, A. The control of sleep. In Hunt, W.A., ed., *Human Behavior and Its Control.* Cambridge, Mass.: Schenkman Publ. Co. 1971:75–92.

27. Bliwise, D.L. How lack of sleep can make you fat. *New York Times* (letter). August 3, 1994.

28. Rechtschaffen, A. Current perspectives on the function of sleep. *Perspectives in Biology and Medicine.* 1998;41:359–390.

29. Kräuchi, K., et al. Warm feet promote the rapid onset of sleep. *Nature.* 1999;401:36–37.

30. Dorsey, C.M., et al. Core body temperature and sleep of older female insomniacs before and after passive body heating. *Sleep.* 1999;22:891–898.

31. Stevenson, R.L. My first book. In *Treasure Island.* New York: Penguin. 1999.

Chapter 8: The Growing Years

1. Freudigman, K., and Thoman, E.B. Ultradian and diurnal cyclicity in the sleep states of newborn infants during the first two postnatal days. *Early Human Development.* 1994;38:67–80. Sada, A., et al. Newborns' sleep-wake patterns: the role of maternal, delivery and infant factors. *Early Human Development.* 1996;44:113–126.

2. Harkness, S. Quoted in Brown, N. The lullaby's too late. *Research/Penn State.* September 1995:10.

3. McGraw, K., et al. The development of circadian rhythms in a human infant. *Sleep.* 1999;22:303–310.

4. Mann, N.P., et al. Effect of night and day on preterm infants in a newborn nursery: randomised trial. *British Medical Journal.* 1986;293:1265–1267.

5. Quinn, G.E., et al. Myopia and ambient lighting at night. *Nature.* 1999;399:113–114. Zadnik, K., et al. Vision: Myopia and ambient night-time lighting (Brief communication). *Nature.* 2000;404:143–144. Gwiazda, J., et al. Vision: Myopia and ambient night-time lighting (Brief communication). *Nature.* 2000;404:144. Stone, R.A., et al. Vision: Myopia and ambient night-time lighting (Reply). *Nature.* 2000;404:144.

6. Daws, D. *Through the Night: Helping Parents and Sleepless Infants.* New York: Basic Books. 1993.

7. Weissbluth, M. Naps in children: 6 months–7 years. *Sleep.* 1995;18:82–87.

8. Mindell, J. *Sleeping through the Night: How Infants, Toddlers, and Their Parents Can Get a Good Night's Sleep.* New York: HarperCollins. 1997.

9. Ferber, R. *Solve Your Child's Sleep Problems.* New York: Simon & Schuster. 1985.

10. Richard Ferber spoke with Lynne Lamberg in March 1998.

11. Owens, J., et al. Television-viewing habits and sleep disturbance in school children. *Pediatrics* 1999;104:E27.

12. Foulkes, D. *Children's Dreaming and the Development of Consciousness.* Cambridge, Mass.: Harvard University Press. 1999.

13. Carskadon, M.A., et al. Pubertal changes in daytime sleepiness. *Sleep.* 1980;2:453–460.

14. Wolfson, A.R., and Carskadon, M.A. Sleep schedules and daytime functioning in adolescents. *Child Development.* 1998;69:875–887.

15. Carskadon, M. When worlds collide. Adolescent need for sleep versus societal demands. *Phi Delta Kappan.* January 1999:348–353.

16. Dahl, R. The consequences of insufficient sleep for adolescents. *Phi Delta Kappan.* January 1999:354–359.

17. Wahlstrom, K. The prickly politics of school starting times. *Phi Delta Kappan.* January 1999:345–347; Kyla Wahlstrom spoke with Lynne Lamberg in December 1999.

18. Kubow, P.K., et al. Starting time and school life. *Phi Delta Kappan.* January 1999:366–371.

19. Mary Carskadon spoke with Lynne Lamberg March 20, 1998.

Chapter 9: Fitness by the Clock

1. Edgar, D., and Dement, W. Regularly scheduled voluntary exercise synchronizes the mouse circadian clock. *American Journal of Physiology.* 1991;261(4 Pt 2):R928–933.

2. Winget, C.M., et al. Chronobiology of physical performance and sports medicine. In Touitou, Y., and Haus, E., eds., *Biologic Rhythms in Clinical and Laboratory Medicine.* Heidelberg: Springer-Verlag. 1992:230–241.

3. Smith, R. A comparison of peak performance, competition and training times in elite athletes. *Sleep Research.* 1996;25:574.

4. Reilly, T., Atkinson, G., and Waterhouse, J. *Biological Rhythms and Exercise.* Oxford: Oxford University Press. 1997.

5. Winget, C., et al. Circadian rhythms and athletic performance. *Medicine and Science in Sports and Exercise.* 1985;17:498–516.

6. Conroy, R.T.W.L., and O'Brien, M. Diurnal variation in athletic performance. *Journal of Physiology.* 1974;236:51P.

7. Hildebrandt, G., et al. Circadian variation of isometric strength training in man. In Morgan, E., ed., *Chronobiology and Chronomedicine.* Frankfurt: Peter Lang. 1990;2:322–329.

8. Burt Strug, M.D., Personal communication on November 19, 1999.

9. Reilly, T., Atkinson, G., and Waterhouse, J. Ibid.

10. Smith, R., et al. Circadian rhythms and enhanced athletic performance in the National Football League. *Sleep.* 1997;20(5):362–365.

11. Steenland, K., and Deddens, J. Effects of travel and rest on performance of professional basketball players. *Sleep.* 1997;20(5):366–369.

12. Recht, L.D., et al. Baseball teams bested by jet lag. *Nature* (letter). 1995;377:583.

13. Youngstedt, S.D., et al. Is sleep disturbed by vigorous late-night exercise? *Medicine and Science in Sports & Exercise.* 1999;31:864–869.

14. Kobayashi, T., et al. Effects of the late evening exercise on sleep onset process. *Sleep Research Online.* 1999;2(Suppl. 1):233.

15. Guilleminault, C., et al. Nondrug treatment trials in psychophysiologic insomnia. *Annals of Internal Medicine.* 1995;155:838–844.

16. King, A.C., et al. Moderate-intensity exercise and self-rated quality of sleep in older adults: a randomized controlled trial. *Journal of the American Medical Association.* 1997;277:32–37.

17. Eastman, C.I., et al. Phase-shifting human circadian rhythms with exercise during the night shift. *Physiological Behavior.* 1995;58:1287–1291.

18. Huguet, G., et al. Morning versus afternoon gymnastic time and diurnal and seasonal changes in psychophysiological variables of school children. *Chronobiology International.* 1997;14:371–384.

Chapter 10: Time to Eat

1. Aschoff, J., et al. Meal timing in humans without time cues. *Journal of Biological Rhythms.* 1986;1:151–162.

2. Cugini, P., et al. Chronobiometric identification of disorders of hunger sensation in essential obesity: therapeutic effects of dexfenfluramine. *Metabolism: Clinical and Experimental.* 1995;44(2 Suppl. 2):50–56.

3. Monk, T.H., et al. Differences over the life span in daily life-style regularity. *Chronobiology International.* 1997;14:295–306.

4. Finch, G.M., et al. Appetite changes under free-living conditions during Ramadan fasting. *Appetite.* 1998;31:159–170.

5. Ze, A. Daily practices, study performance and health during the Ramadan fast. *Journal of the Royal Society of Health.* 1997;117:231–235.

6. Iraki, L., et al. Ramadan diet restrictions modify the circadian time structure in humans. A study on plasma gastrin, insulin, glucose, and calcium and on gastric pH. *Journal of Clinical Endocrinology & Metabolism.* 1997; 82:1261–1273.

7. Habbal, R., et al. Variations of blood pressure during the month of Ramadan. *Archives des Maladies du Coeur et des Vasseaux.* 1998;91:995–998.

8. Waterhouse, J., et al. Chronobiology and meal times: internal and external factors. *British Journal of Nutrition.* 1997;77(Suppl. 1):S29–S38.

9. Schenck, C., et al. Sleep-related eating disorders: polysomnographic correlates of a heterogeneous syndrome distinct from daytime eating disorders. *Sleep.* 1991;14:419–431.

10. Waterhouse, D. *Why Women Need Chocolate: How to Get the Body You Want by Eating the Foods You Crave.* New York: Hyperion. 1995.

11. Lee, I.M., and Paffenbarger, R.S. Life is sweet: candy consumption and longevity. *British Medical Journal.* 1998; 317:1683–1684.

12. Spring, B., et al. Carbohydrates, protein, and performance. In Marriott, B., ed., *Food Components to Enhance Performance.* Washington, D.C.: National Academy Press. 1994:321–350.

13. Goo, R.H., et al. Circadian variation in gastric emptying of meals in man. *Gastroenterology.* 1987;93:513–518.

14. De Castro, J.M. Circadian rhythm of the spontaneous meal pattern, macronutrient intake, and mood of humans. *Physiology and Behavior.* 1987;40:437–446.

15. Mejean, L., et al. Chronobiology, nutrition, and diabetes. In Touitou, Y., and Haus, E., eds., *Biologic Rhythms in Clinical and Laboratory Medicine.* Berlin: Springer-Verlag. 1992:375–385.

16. Reinberg, A. Chronobiology and nutrition. In Reinberg, A., and Smolensky, M.H., *Biological Rhythms and Medicine.* New York: Springer Verlag. 1983:265–300.

17. Young, L.R., and Nestle, M. Portion sizes in dietary assessment: issues and policy implications. *Nutritional Reviews.* 1995;53:149–158.

18. Gortmaker, S.L., et al. Inactivity, diet, and the fattening of America. *Journal of the American Dietary Association.* 1990;90:1247–1252.

19. Robinson, T.N., et al. Reducing children's television viewing to prevent obesity: a randomized controlled trial. *Journal of the American Medical Association.* 1999;282:1561–1567.

20. Halberg, F., et al. Chronobiology and metabolism in the broader context of timely intervention and timed treatment. *Diabetes Research Today.* Meeting of the Minkowski Prize Winners. Symposia Medica Hoechst 12 (Capri). Stuttgart: F.K. Schattauer-Verlag. 1976:45–95.

21. Graeber, R.C., et al. *Human Eating Behavior: Preferences, Consumption Patterns, and Biorhythms.* Technical Report: TR-78-022. Natick, Mass.: U.S. Army Natick Research and Development Command. 1978.

22. Halberg, F. Some aspects of the chronobiology of nutrition: more work is needed on "when to eat." *Journal of Nutrition.* 1989;119:333–343.

23. Halberg, F., et al. From biological rhythms to chronomes relevant for nutrition. In Marriott, B., ed., *Not Eating Enough.* Washington, D.C.: National Academy Press. 1995:361–372.

24. Bellisle, F. Obesity and food intake in children: evidence for a role of metabolic and/or behavioral daily rhythms. *Appetite.* 1988;11:111–118.

25. Fricker, J. Circadian rhythm of energy intake and corpulence status in adults. *International Journal of Obesity.* 1990; 14:387–393.

26. Hill, S.W., and McCutcheon, N.B. Contributions of obesity, gender, hunger, food preference, and body size to bite size, bite speed, and rate of eating. *Appetite.* 1984;5:73–83.

27. Marmonier, C., et al. Metabolic and behavioral consequences of a snack consumed in a satiety state. *American Journal of Clinical Nutrition.* 1999;70:854–866.

28. Winter, A., and Winter, R. *Smart Food: Diet and Nutrition for Maximum Brain Power.* New York: St. Martin's Griffin. 1999:209.

29. Romon, M., et al. Circadian variation in diet-induced thermogenesis. *American Journal of Clinical Nutrition.* 1993;57:476–480.

30. Pendergrast, M. *Uncommon Grounds: The History of Coffee and How It Transformed Our World.* New York: Basic Books. 1999:6.

31. Bonnet, M.H., and Arand, D.L. Impact of naps and caffeine on extended nocturnal performance. *Physiology and Behavior.* 1994;56:103–109.

32. Horne, J., and Reyner, L. Vehicle accidents related to sleep: a review. *Occupational and Environmental Medicine.* 1999;56:289–294.

33. Institute of Medicine. *Caffeine Formulations for the Sustainment of Mental Task Performance during Military Operations.* Washington, D.C.: National Academy Press. 2000, in press.

34. Braun, S. *Buzz: The Science and Lore of Alcohol and Caffeine.* New York: Oxford University Press. 1996:38–39.

35. Arfken, C.L. Temporal pattern of alcohol consumption in the United States. *Alcoholism: Clinical and Experimental Research.* 1988;12:137–142.

36. Roehrs, T., et al. Sleep extension, enhanced alertness and the sedating effects of ethanol. *Pharmacology Biochemistry & Behavior.* 1989;34:321–324.

37. When (and how) to take your vitamin and mineral supplements. *Tufts University Health & Nutrition Letter.* March 1999:4–5.

Chapter 11: Time for Sex

1. Reinberg, A., and Lagoguey, M. Circadian and circannual rhythms in sexual activity and plasma hormones (FSH, LH, testosterone) of five human males. *Archives of Sexual Behavior.* 1978;7(1):13–30.

2. Leonard, L., and Ross, M.W. The last sexual encounter: the contextualization of sexual risk behavior. *International Journal of STD and AIDS.* 1997;8:643–645.

3. Palmer, J.D., et al. Diurnal and weekly, but no lunar rhythms in human copulation. *Human Biology.* 1982;54:111–121. Udry, J.R., and Morris, N.M. Frequency of intercourse by day of the week. *Journal of Sex Research.* 1970;6:229–234.

4. Adams, D.B., et al. Rise in female-initiated sexual activities at ovulation and its suppression by oral contraceptives. *New England Journal of Medicine.* 1978;299:1145–1150.

5. Cavanagh, J.R. Rhythm of sexual desire in women. *Medical Aspects of Human Sexuality.* 1969;3:29–39.

6. Harvey, S.M. Female sexual behavior: fluctuations during the menstrual cycle. *Journal of Psychosomatic Research.* 1987;31:101–110. Stanislaw, H., and Rice, F.J. Correlation between sexual desire and menstrual cycle characteristics. *Archives of Sexual Behavior.* 1988;17:499–508. Dennerstein, L., et al. The relationship between the menstrual cycle and female sexual interest in women with PMS and volunteers. *Psychoneuroendocrinology.* 1994;19:291–304. Udry, J.R., and Morris, N.M. Distribution of coitus in the menstrual cycle. *Nature.* 1968;220:593–596.

7. http://www.uneet.com/. Accessed December 21, 1999.

8. Angier, N. *Woman: An Intimate Geography.* New York: Houghton Mifflin. 1999:199.

9. Reinberg, A., and Lagoguey, M. Ibid.

10. Smals, A.G.H., et al. Circannual cycle in plasma testosterone levels in man. *Journal of Clinical Endocrinology and Metabolism.* 1976;42:979–982.

11. Reilly, K., and Binkley, S. The menstrual rhythm. *Psychoneuroendocrinology.* 1981;6:181–184.

12. Hood, K.E., as cited in Golub, S. *Periods: From Menarche to Menopause.* Newbury Park, Calif.: Sage Publications. 1992:99.

13. Golub, S. *Periods: From Menarche to Menopause.* Newbury Park, Calif.: Sage Publications. 1992:100.

14. Baines, C.J., and Dayan, R. A tangled web: factors likely to affect the efficacy of screening mammography. *Journal of the National Cancer Institute.* 1999;91:833–838.

15. Wright, T.C., et al. HPV DNA testing of self-collected vaginal samples compared with cytologic screening to detect cervical cancer. *Journal of the American Medical Association.* 1999;283: 81–86.

16. Attila Lörincz spoke with Lynne Lamberg on January 31, 2000.

17. Golub, S. Ibid.:64–65.

18. Golub, S. Ibid.:69;117–119.

19. American Psychiatric Association. *Diagnostic and Statistical Manual of Mental Disorders.* Fourth Edition. Washington, D.C.: American Psychiatric Association. 1994:715–718.

20. Case, A., and Reid, R. Effects of the menstrual cycle on medical disorders. *Archives of Internal Medicine.* 1998;158:1405–1412.

21. Roenneberg, T., and Aschoff, J. Annual rhythm of human reproduction: II. Environmental correlations. *Journal of Biological Rhythms.* 1990;5:217–239.

22. Albright, D., et al. Seasonal characteristics of and age of menarche. *Chronobiology International.* 1990;7:251–258.

23. Dewan. E.M. On the possibility of a perfect rhythm method of birth control by periodic light stimulation. *American Journal of Obstetrics and Gynecology.* 1967;99:1016–1018. Dewan E.M., et al. Effect of photic stimulation on the human menstrual cycle. *Photochemistry and Photobiology.* 1978;27:581–585.

24. Lacey, L. *Lunaception: a Feminine Odyssey into Fertility and Conception.* New York: Coward, McCann & Geoghegan. 1975.

25. Lin, M., et al. Night light alters menstrual cycles. *Psychiatry Research.* 1990;33:135–138.

26. Rex, K.M., et al. Nocturnal light effects on menstrual cycle length. *Journal of Alternative and Complementary Medicine.* 1997;3:387–390.

27. Kripke, D.F. Light regulation of the menstrual cycle. In Wetterberg, L., ed., *Light and Biological Rhythms in Man.* Oxford: Pergamon Press. 1993:305–312.

28. McClintock, M.K. Menstrual synchrony and suppression. *Nature.* 1971;229:244–245.

29. Weller, A., and Weller, L. Menstrual synchrony under optimal conditions: Bedouin families. *Journal of Comparative Psychology.* 1997;111:143–151.

30. Weller, L., et al. Menstrual synchrony in a sample of working women. *Psychoneuroendocrinology.* 1999;24:449–459.

31. Weller, L., et al. Human menstrual synchrony in families and among close friends: examining the importance of mutual exposure. *Journal of Comparative Psychology.* 1999;113:261–268.

32. Weller, A., and Weller, L. Prolonged and very intensive contact may not be conductive to menstrual synchrony. *Psychoneuroendocrinology.* 1998;23:19–32.

33. Stern, K., and McClintock, M.K. Regulation of ovulation by human pheromones. *Nature.* 1998;392:177–179.

34. McClintock, M.K. Whither menstrual synchrony? *Annual Review of Sex Research.* 1998;9:77–95.

35. Wilcox, A.J., et al. Timing of sexual intercourse in relation to ovulation. *New England Journal of Medicine.* 1995;333:1517–1521.

36. Driver, H., and Baker, F. Menstrual factors in sleep. *Sleep Medicine Reviews.* 1998;2:213–229.

37. Askling, J., et al. Sickness in pregnancy and sex of child (letter). *Lancet.* 1999;354:2053.

38. Perry, D.F., et al. Are women carrying "basketballs" really having boys? Testing pregnancy folklore. *Birth.* 1999;26:172–177.

39. Trentacoste, S.V., et al. Sleep/wake disruptions in the final weeks of pregnancy. *Sleep Research.* 1998;21:276.

40. Lee, K.A., et al. Parity and sleep patterns during and after pregnancy. *Obstetrics and Gynecology.* 2000;95:14–18.

41. Lee, K.A. Alterations in sleep during pregnancy and postpartum: a review of 30 years of research. *Sleep Medicine Reviews.* 1998;2:231–242.

42. Smolensky, M.H., et al. Chronobiology of the life sequence. In Itoh, S., Ogata, K., and Yoshimura, H., eds., *Advances in Climatic Physiology*. Tokyo: Igaku Shoin. 1972:281–318.

43. Trends in the attendant, place, and timing of births, and in the use of obstetric interventions: United States, 1989–97. *National Vital Statistics Reports*. 1999;47(27):1–16.

44. Caton, D., and Wheatley, P. Nativity and the moon: do birthrates depend on the phase of the moon? Tucson: American Astronomical Society meeting. 1995.

45. Utian, W.H., and Boggs, P.P. The North American Menopause Society 1998 Menopause Survey. Part 1: Postmenopausal women's perceptions about menopause and midlife. *Menopause*. 1999;6:122–128.

46. Albright, D., et al. Circadian rhythms in hot flashes in natural and surgically-induced menopause. *Chronobiology International*. 1989;6:279–284.

47. Woodward, S., et al. Ambient temperature effects on sleep and mood in menopausal women. *Sleep*. 1999;22(Suppl.):S224–225.

48. Cobin, R.H., et al. AACE medical guidelines for clinical practice for management of menopause. *Endocrine Practice*. 1999;5:354–366.

49. Cobin, R.H., et al. Ibid.

50. Schairer, C., et al. Menopausal estrogen and estrogen-progestin replacement therapy and breast cancer risk. *Journal of the American Medical Association*. 2000;283:485–491.

51. Rako, S. *The Hormone of Desire: the Truth about Testosterone, Sexuality, and Menopause*. New York: Three Rivers Press. 1996:33.

52. Baines, C.J., and Dayan, R. Ibid.

53. Harvey, J.A., et al. Short-term cessation of hormone replacement therapy and improvement of mammographic specificity. *Journal of the National Cancer Institute*. 1997;89:1623–1625.

54. Bernhardt, P.C., et al. Testosterone changes during vicarious experiences of winning and losing among fans at sporting events. *Physiology and Behavior*. 1998;65:59–62.

55. Hargrove, M., and Dabbs, J., Jr. Testosterone and the behavior of fraternities. Presented at American Psychological Association Annual Meeting, Toronto. 1993.

56. Blum, D. *Sex on the Brain: The Biological Differences between Men and Women*. New York: Viking. 1997:170.

57. Luboshitzky, R., et al. Relationship between rapid eye movement sleep and testosterone secretion in normal men. *Journal of Andrology*. 1999;20:731–737.

58. Roffwarg, H.P., et al. Plasma testosterone and sleep: relationship to sleep stage variables. *Psychosomatic Medicine*. 1982;44:73–84.

59. Cagnacci, A. Diurnal variation of semen quality in human males. *Human Reproduction*. 1999;14:106–109.

60. Tjoa, W.S., et al. Circannual rhythm in human sperm count revealed by serially independent sampling. *Fertility and Sterility*. 1982;38:454–459. Gyllenborg, J. Secular and seasonal changes in semen quality among young Danish men: a statistical analysis of semen samples from 1927 donor candidates during 1977–1995. *International Journal of Andrology*. 1999;22:28–36.

61. Tenover, J.L. Male hormone replacement therapy including "andropause." *Endocrinology and Metabolism Clinics of North America*. 1998;27:969–987.

62. Franchimont, P. L'andropause: medisance ou calomnie? *Revue Medicale de Liège*. 1975;30:393–396.

63. Krause, W. Brauchen wir den begriff des climacterium virile? *Fortschritte der Medizin*. 1995;113:32;35,6;39–40.

64. Testoderm Transdermal System. In Arky, R., ed., *Physicians' Desk Reference*. Montvale, N.J.: Medical Economics. 1999;53:517–520.

65. Feldman, H.A., et al. Impotence and its medical and psychosocial correlates: results of the Massachusetts Male Aging Study. *Journal of Urology*. 1994:151:54–61.

66. Karacan, Ismet, et al. The ontogeny of nocturnal penile tumescence. *Waking and Sleeping*. 1976;1:27–44.

67. Hirshkowitz, M. Sleep-related erections. *Journal of Psychosomatic Research*. 1997;42:515–516.

68. Althog, S., and Seftel, A. Evaluation and treatment of sexual dysfunction. In Friedman, R.C., and Downey, J.I., eds., *Masculinity and Sexuality. American Psychiatric Association Annual Review of Psychiatry*. 1999;18(5):55–87.

Chapter 12: Getting the Jump on Jet Lag

1. Charmane Eastman's personal communication to Lynne Lamberg. July 6, 1998, and April 23, 1999.

2. Lopez, B. On the wings of commerce. *Harper's* Magazine. October 1995:39–54.

3. Beatty, S. Lotus ads for its new Notes try to make everyone a Superman. *Wall Street Journal.* January 18, 1999:B5.

4. Monk, T.H., et al. Inducing jet lag in the laboratory: patterns of adjustment to an acute shift in routine. *Aviation, Space & Environmental Medicine.* 1988;59:703–710.

5. Aschoff, J., et al. Re-entrainment of circadian rhythms after phase-shifts of the zeitgeber. *Chronobiologica.* 1975;2:23–78.

6. Klein, K.E., and Wegmann, H.M. *Significance of Circadian Rhythms in Aerospace Operations.* AGARD monograph No. 247. Advisory Group for Aerospace Research and Development. NATO. London: Technical Editing and Reproduction, Ltd. 1980.

7. Moline, M., et al. Age-related differences in recovery from simulated jet lag. *Sleep.* 1992;15:28–40.

8. Long, M.E. What is this thing called sleep? *National Geographic.* 1987;12:787–821; Czeisler, C., and Allan, J. Acute circadian phase reversal in man via bright light exposure; application to jet lag. *Sleep Research.* 1987;16:605.

9. Oren, D., et al. *How to Beat Jet Lag: A Practical Guide for Air Travelers.* New York: Henry Holt & Co. 1993.

10. Wigler, S. Audience responds as BSO catches fire after sluggish start. *The Sun* (Baltimore). October 26, 1994:1D, 3D.

11. Wigler, S. In Taiwan, an orchestra hits its peak. *The Sun* (Baltimore). October 29, 1994:1D, 5D.

12. Boulos, Z., et al. Light treatment for sleep disorders: consensus report. VII. Jet Lag. *Journal of Biological Rhythms.* 1995;10:167–176.

13. Arendt, J., et al. Efficacy of melatonin treatment in jet lag, shift work, and blindness. *Journal of Biological Rhythms.* 1997;12:604–617.

14. Spitzer, R.L., et al. Jet lag: clinical features, validation of a new syndrome-specific scale, and lack of response to melatonin in a randomized, double-blind trial. *American Journal of Psychiatry.* 1999;156:1392–1396.

15. Graeber, R.C. Jet lag and sleep disruption. In Kryger, M.H., et al., eds., *Principles and Practice of Sleep Medicine.* Second Edition. Philadelphia: W.B. Saunders. 1994:463–470.

16. Moline, M., et al. Effects of the "jet lag diet" on the adjustment to a phase advance. *Society for Research on Biological Rhythms.* 1990:Abstract 111.

17. *International Sleep and the Traveler Survey.* Hilton Hotels/National Sleep Foundation. Washington, D.C.: National Sleep Foundation. 1996.

Chapter 13: Clockwatching at Work

1. Haynes, L. Four area teen-agers die in turnpike crash. *Sun-Journal* (Lewiston, Maine). February 5, 1994.

2. Washuk, B. A survivor's story: First car trouble, then a crash and suddenly Linda Tardif's world was never the same again. *Sun-Journal* (Lewiston, Maine). May 28, 1995:1A, 7A.; Mother drives bill enforcing trucker hours. *Journal of Commerce.* May 22, 1995:1 A, 10 A.

3. Horne, J. Vehicle accidents related to sleep: a review. *Occupational & Environmental Medicine.* 1999;56:289–294.

4. Martinez, R. Proclamation to announce the "Crashes Aren't Accidents" campaign. Washington, D.C.: U.S. Department of Transportation. 1998.

5. Machalaba, D. Schneider National to outfit trailers with tracking device to map locations. *Wall Street Journal.* May 7, 1999:A2.

6. Izer, D. Testimony on behalf of PATT before U.S. Senate Commerce Committee. Washington, D.C. September 16, 1998.

7. National Transportation Safety Board. *Fatigue, Alcohol, Other Drugs, and Medical Factors in Fatal-to-the Driver Heavy Truck Crashes.* Vol. I. PB90-917002. NTSB/SS-90/01. Washington, D.C.: National Transportation Safety Board. 1990:87.

8. *Wake-up America: A National Sleep Alert.* Report of the National Commission on Sleep Disorders Research. Vol. 1. Bethesda, Md.: National Institutes of Health. 1993.

9. Lamond, N., and Dawson, D. Quantifying the performance impairment associated with fatigue. *Journal of Sleep Research.* 1999;8:255–262; Dawson, D., et al. Fatigue, alcohol and performance impairment. *Nature.* 1997;388:235.

10. *Report of the President's Commission on the Accident at Three Mile Island.* Washington, D.C.: U.S. Government Printing Office. 1979.

11. *Marine Accident Report Grounding of the U.S. Tankship Exxon Valdez on Bligh Reef, Prince William Sound near Valdez, Alaska, March 24, 1989.* Washington, D.C.: National Transportation Safety Board. 1990:128.

12. *Report of the Presidential Commission on the Space Shuttle Challenger Accident.* Vol. II, Appendix G—Human Factors Analysis. Washington, D.C.: U.S. Government Printing Office. 1986:G-5.

13. Gianaro, C. Chernobyl's legacy. *University of Georgia Research Reporter.* 1999;28:4.

14. IAEA Conference Studies: Chernobyl A-plant accident. *Facts on File.* New York: Facts on File, Inc. August 29, 1986:634. Moore-Ede, M. *The Twenty-Four Hour Society: Understanding Human Limits in a World That Never Stops.* Reading, Mass.: Addison-Wesley. 1993:109. Polityuk, P. Solemn ceremonies, marches mark Chernobyl's 12th anniversary. AP Online. April 16, 1998.

15. Reuters. Ground water still polluted 15 years after Bhopal disaster. *The Sun* (Baltimore). December 3, 1999:28A.

16. Bureau of Labor Statistics. *Workers on Flexible and Shift Schedules.* Washington D.C.: U.S. Department of Labor, Bureau of Labor Statistics. May 1997.

17. *Plain Language about Shiftwork.* U.S. Department of Health and Human Services, National Institute for Occupational Safety and Health, Pub. 97–145.

18. Brady, D. The clocks ahead will have our own faces. *Business Week.* August 30, 1999:94–96.

19. Folkard, S. Effects on performance efficiency. In Colquhoun, P., et al., eds., *Shift Work: Problems and Solutions.* Frankfurt: Peter Lang. 1996:65–87.

20. Åkerstedt, T. *Wide Awake at Odd Hours.* Stockholm: Swedish Council for Work Life Research. 1996:23.

21. Costa, G. Effects on health and well being. In Colquhoun, P., et al., eds., *Shift Work: Problems and Solutions.* Frankfurt: Peter Lang. 1996:113–139.

22. Smolensky, M. The chronoepidemiology of occupational health and shift work. In Reinberg, A., et al., eds., *Night and Shift Work: Biological and Social Aspects.* Oxford: Pergamon Press. 1981:51–65.

23. Mardon, S. Survey finds wide range of shift premiums. *ShiftWork Alert.* 1999;4:6.

24. Åkerstedt, T. Work hours, sleepiness, and the underlying mechanism. *Journal of Sleep Research.* 1995;4(Suppl. 2):15–22.

25. Johnson, E., et al. Epidemiology of alcohol and medication as aids to sleep in early adulthood. *Sleep.* 1998;21:178–186.

26. Dumont, M. Sleep quality of former night-shift workers. *International Journal of Occupational & Environmental Health.* July 1997;3(Suppl. 2):S10–S14.

27. Landmark Communications/Searle. Survey reveals significant sleep loss among morning newscasters. Press Release. March 23, 1998.

28. Walsleben, J.A., et al. Sleep habits of Long Island Rail Road commuters. *Sleep.* 1999;22:728–734.

29. Mardon, S. Seven ways to reduce shift workers' GI problems. *ShiftWork Alert.* 1999;4(6):4–5.

30. Melbin, M. *Night as Frontier: Colonizing the World after Dark.* New York: The Free Press. 1987.

31. Knutsson, A., et al. Shiftwork and myocardial infarction: a case-control study. *Journal of Occupational & Environmental Medicine.* 1999;56:46–50.

32. Ribeiro, D., et al. Altered postprandial hormone and metabolic responses in a simulated shift work environment. *Journal of Endocrinology.* 1998;158:305–310.

33. Åkerstedt, T. *Wide Awake at Odd Hours.* Ibid.:17.

34. Mardon, S. Introducing the shiftwork index: a source of data about people who work at night. *ShiftWork Alert.* 1998;3(9):6–7.

35. Lee, K. Self-reported sleep disturbances in employed women. *Sleep.* 1992;15:493–498.

36. Moran, M. Residents in NY hospitals are still working too much. *American Medical News.* June 15 & 22, 1998:9,11.

37. Smith, L., et al. Increased injuries on night shift. *Lancet.* 1994;344:1137–1139.

38. Parks, D.K., et al. Day-night pattern in accidental exposures to blood-borne pathogens among medical residents. *Chronobiology International.* 2000;17:61–70.

39. Moore-Ede, M. *Working Nights Health & Safety Guide.* Cambridge: Circadian Information. 1998.

40. Monk, T.H., and Wagner, J.A. Social factors can outweigh biological ones in determining night shift safety. *Human Factors.* 1989;31:721–724.

41. Moore-Ede. Ibid.

42. Presser, H.B. Toward a 24-hour economy. *Science.* 1999;284:1776–1779.

43. Mardon, S. Child care company offers 24-hour service to shiftworkers in Missouri, Nevada & Iowa. *ShiftWork Alert.* 1999;4:7.

44. Monk, T.H. Shift Work. In Kryger, M.H., et al., eds., *Principles and Practice of Sleep Medicine.* Second Edition. Philadelphia: W.B. Saunders. 1994:471–476.

45. Lee, K. Prevalence of perimenstrual symptoms in employed women. *Women's Health.* 1991;17(3):17–32.

46. Labyak, S. Effects of shift work on sleep and menstrual function. *Sleep Research.* 1997;26:141.

47. Nurminen, T. Shift work and reproductive health. *Scandinavian Journal of Work and Environmental Health.* 1998;24(Suppl. 3):28–34.

48. Bisanti, L. Shiftwork and subfecundity: a European multicenter study. *Journal of Occupational and Environmental Medicine.* 1996;38:352–358.

49. Infante-Rivard, C. Pregnancy loss and work schedule during pregnancy. *Epidemiology.* 1993;4:73–75.

50. Wergeland, E., et al. Working conditions and prevalence of pre-eclampsia, Norway 1989. *International Journal of Gynaecology and Obstetrics.* 1997;58:189–196.

51. Beckett, W.S., et al. Women's respiratory health in the cotton textile industry: an analysis of respiratory symptoms in 973 non-smoking female workers. *Occupational and Environmental Medicine.* 1994;51:14–18.

52. Nurminen, T. Shift work, fetal development and course of pregnancy. *Scandinavian Journal of Work and Environmental Health.* 1989;15:395–403.

53. Bryant, K., and Zick, C. *Child Rearing Time by Parents: A Report of Research in Progress.* Ithaca: Cornell University. 1997.

54. Hochschild, A., with Machung, A. *The Second Shift: Working Parents and the Evolution at Home.* New York: Viking. 1989.

55. Gupta, S. *Time Men and Women Spend on Housework.* Ann Arbor: University of Michigan. 1998.

56. Penev, P. Chronic circadian desynchronization decreases the survival of animals with cardiomyopathic heart disease. *American Journal of Physiology.* 1998;275:H2334–2337.

57. Hilliker, N., et al. Sleepiness/alertness on a simulated night shift schedule and morningness-eveningness tendency. *Sleep.* 1992;15:430–433.

58. Miller, L. *Careers for Night Owls & Other Insomniacs.* Lincolnwood, Ill.: NTC Publishing Group. 1995.

59. Martin, S., and Eastman, C. Medium-intensity light produces circadian rhythm adaptation to simulated night shift work. *Sleep.* 1998;21:154–166.

60. Stewart, K., et al. Light treatment for NASA shift workers. *Chronobiology International.* 1995;12:141–151.

61. Mardon, S. Bright light offers huge potential benefits, but obstacles persist in the real world. *ShiftWork Alert.* 1997;2(2):6–12.

62. U.S. Congress, Office of Technology Assessment. *Biological Rhythms: Implications for the Worker.* 1991:131.

63. Mardon, S. Court upholds $400,000 award to employee who said shiftwork caused health problems. *ShiftWork Alert.* 1998;10:3,7.

64. *Plain Language about Shiftwork.* Ibid.

65. Muehlbach, M., and Walsh, J. The effects of caffeine on simulated night-shift work and subsequent daytime sleep. *Sleep.* 1995;1:22–29.

66. Morgan, D. *Sleep Secrets for Shift Workers & People with Off-Beat Schedules.* Duluth, Minn.: Whole Person Associates. 1996.

67. Carrier, J., and Monk, T.H. Effects of sleep and circadian rhythms on performance. In Turek, F., and Zee, P., eds., *Regulation of Sleep and Circadian Rhythms.* New York: Marcel Dekker. 1999:527–556.

Chapter 14: A Time to Heal

1. Friebert, E., and Greeley, A. Taking time to use medicines wisely. *FDA Consumer.* 1999;33:30–31.

2. Smolensky, M.H., and Bing, M.L. Chronobiology and chronotherapeutics in primary care. *Patient Care. Clinical Focus Supplement.* Summer 1997:1–21.

3. Smolensky, M.H., et al. Medical chronobiology: concepts and applications. *American Review of Respiratory Disease.* 1993;147(6 Pt 2):S2–19.

4. Robin, E.D. Some interrelationships between sleep and disease. *Archives of Internal Medicine.* 1958;102:669–675.

5. Gerald Sokol spoke with Lynne Lamberg, November 4 & 5, 1999.

6. Gordon Amidon spoke with Lynne Lamberg, November 4, 1999.

7. Santini, J.T., et al. A controlled-release microchip (letter). *Nature.* 1999;397:335–338.

Chapter 15: Sickness and Health from A to (Nearly) Z

AIDS

1. Darko, D.F., et al. Fatigue, sleep disturbance, disability, and indices of progression of HIV infection. *American Journal of Psychiatry.* 1992;149:514–520.

2. Groopman, J.E. Fatigue in cancer and HIV/AIDS. *Oncology.* 1998;12:335–344; discussion 345–346, 351.

3. Lee, K.A., et al. The fatigue experience of women with human immunodeficiency virus. *Journal of Obstetric, Gynecologic, and Neonatal Nursing.* 1999;28:193–200.

4. Norman, S.E., et al. Sleep disturbances in HIV-infected homosexual men. *AIDS.* 1990;4: 775–781.

5. Bollinger, R.C., et al. Risk factors and clinical presentation of acute primary HIV infection in India. *Journal of the American Medical Association.* 1997;278:2085–2089.

6. Sothern, R.B., et al. Oral temperature rhythmometry and substantial within-day variation in zidovudine levels following steady-state dosing in human immunodeficiency virus (HIV) infection. In Hayes, D.K., et al., eds., *Chronobiology: Its Role in Clinical Medicine, General Biology, and Agriculture.* New York: Wiley-Liss. 1990;(pt A):67–76.

7. Darko, D.F., et al. Sleep electroencephalogram delta-frequency amplitude, night plasma levels of tumor necrosis factor α, and human deficiency virus infection. *Proceedings of the National Academy of Sciences.* 1995;92:12080–12084.

8. Buda, F.B. High incidence of sleep disorders in symptomatic HIV positive patients. *Sleep Research.* 1997;26:544.

9. Martini, E., et al. Disappearance of CD4-lymphocyte circadian cycles in HIV-infected patients: early event during asymptomatic infection. *AIDS.* 1988;2:133–134. Bourin, P., et al. Precocious alterations of circadian rhythms in circulating B and T lymphocyte subsets in patients infected with human immunodeficiency virus (HIV). *Comptes Rendus de L'Academie des Sciences. Serie III, Sciences de la Vie.* 1989;308:431–436. Malone, J.L., et al. Abnormalities of morning serum cortisol levels and circadian rhythm of CD4+ lymphocyte counts in human immunodeficiency virus type 1-infected adult patients. *Journal of Infectious Diseases.* 1992;165:185–186. Sothern, R.B., et al. Ibid.

10. Swoyer, J., et al. Circadian rhythm alterations in HIV infected subjects. In: Hayes, D.K., Pauly, J.E., Reiter, R.J., eds., *Chronobiology: Its Role in Clinical Medicine, General Biology, and Agriculture.* New York: Wiley-Liss. 1990; (pt A):437–449.

11. Villette, J.M., et al. Circadian variations in plasma levels of hypophyseal, adrenocortical and testicular hormones in men infected with human immunodeficiency virus. *Journal of Clinical Endocrinology and Metabolism.* 1990;70:572–577.

12. Schwartz, A.G. Inhibition of spontaneous breast cancer formation in female C3H(A$^{vy/a}$) mice by long-term treatment with dehydroepiandrosterone. *Cancer Research.* 1979;39:1129–1132. Schwartz, A.G. The effects of dehydroepiandrosterone on the rate of development of cancer and autoimmune processes in laboratory rodents. *Basic Life Sciences.* 1985;35:181–191. Orentreich, N., et al. Age changes and sex differences in serum dehydroepiandrosterone sulfate concentrations throughout adulthood. *Journal of Clinical Endocrinology and Metabolism.* 1984;59:551–555.

13. Darko, D.F., et al. Growth hormone, fatigue, poor sleep, and disability in HIV infection. *Neuroendocrinology.* 1998;67:317–324.

14. Sothern, R.B., et al. Ibid.

15. Piscitelli, S., et al. Indinavir concentrations and St. John's wort (letter). *Lancet.* 2000;355:547–548.

ARTHRITIS

1. Centers for Disease Control and Prevention. Impact of arthritis and other rheumatic conditions on the health-care system—U.S., 1997. *Morbidity and Mortality Weekly Report.* 1999;48: 349–353.

2. Labrecque, G., et al. Biological rhythms in the inflammatory response and in the effects of nonsteroidal anti-inflammatory drugs. *Pharmacology and Therapeutics.* 1995;66:285–300.

3. Lamberg, L. Chronic pain linked with poor sleep: exploration of causes and treatment. *Journal of the American Medical Association* (News). 1999;281:691–692.

4. Bellamy, N., et al. Rhythmic variations in pain perception in osteoarthritis of the knee. *Journal of Rheumatology.* 1990;17:364–372.

5. Moore, J.G., and Goo, R.H. Day and night aspirin-induced gastric mucosal damage and protection by ranitidine in man. *Chronobiology International.* 1987;4:111–116.

6. Levi, F., et al. Chronotherapy of osteoarthritis patients: optimization indomethacin sustained released (ISR). *Annual Review of Chronopharmacology.* 1984;1:345–348.

7. Levi, F., et al. Timing optimizes sustained-release indomethacin treatment of osteoarthritis. *Clinical Pharmacology and Therapeutics.* 1985;37:77–84.

8. Simon, L.S., et al. Anti-inflammatory and upper gastrointestinal effects of Celecoxib in rheumatoid arthritis: a randomized controlled trial. *Journal of the American Medical Association.* 1999;282:1921–1928. Langman, M.J., et al. Adverse upper gastrointestinal effects of Rofecoxib compared with NSAIDs. *Journal of the American Medical Association.* 1999;282:1929–1933.

9. Kowanko, I.C., et al. Domiciliary self-measurements of rheumatoid arthritis and the demonstration of circadian rhythmicity. *Annals of the Rheumatic Diseases.* 1982;41:453–455.

10. Bellamy, N., et al. Circadian rhythm in pain, stiffness and manual dexterity in rheumatoid arthritis: relation between discomfort and disability. *Annals of the Rheumatic Diseases.* 1991;50:243–248.

11. Latman, N.S. Relation of menstrual cycle phase to symptoms of rheumatoid arthritis. *American Journal of Medicine.* 1983;74:957–960. Rudge, S.R., et al. Menstrual cyclicity of finger joint size and grip strength in patients with rheumatoid arthritis. *Annals of the Rheumatic Diseases.* 1983;42:425–430.

12. Singh, G., and Triadafilopoulos, G. Epidemiology of NSAID induced gastrointestinal complications. *Journal of Rheumatology.* 1999;26(Suppl. 56):18–24.

13. Huskisson, E.C. Chronopharmacology of anti-rheumatic drugs with special reference to indomethacin. In Huskisson, E.C., and Velo, G.P., eds., *Inflammatory Arthropathies.* Amsterdam: Excerpta Medica. 1976:99–105.

14. Rejholec V., et al. Preliminary observations from a double-blind crossover study to evaluate the efficiency of fluriprofen given at different times of day in the treatment of rheumatoid arthritis. *Annual Review of Chronopharmacology.* 1984;1:357–360.

15. Kowanko, I.C., et al. Time of day of prednisolone administration in rheumatoid arthritis. *Annals of the Rheumatic Diseases.* 1982;41:447–452.

16. Lamberg, L. Patients in pain need round-the-clock care. *Journal of the American Medical Association* (News). 1999;281:689–690.

17. Smyth, J., et al. Effects of writing about stressful experiences n symptom reduction in patients with asthma or rheumatoid arthritis: A randomized trial. *Journal of the American Medical Association.* 1999;281;1304–1309.

ASTHMA

1. Dethlefsen, U., and Repges, R. Ein neues therapieprinzip bei nachtlichen Asthma. *Medizinische Klinik.* 1985;80:44–47.

2. Turner-Warwick, M. Epidemiology of nocturnal asthma. *American Journal of Medicine.* 1988;85(Suppl. 1B):6–8.

3. Cochrane, G.M., and Clark, T.J.H. A survey of asthma mortality in patients between 35 and 65 years in the greater London hospitals in 1971. *Thorax.* 1975;30:300–315.

4. Weiler, J.M., et al. Asthma in U.S. Olympic athletes who participated in the 1996 Summer Games. *Journal of Allergy and Clinical Immunology.* 1998;102:722–726.

5. Mitka, M. Why the rise in asthma? New insight, few answers. *Journal of the American Medical Association* (News). 1999;281:2171–2172.

6. *Guidelines for the Diagnosis and Management of Asthma.* Expert Panel Report 2. Bethesda, Md.: National Heart, Lung, and Blood Institute. NIH Publication 98–4051, 1997:1.

7. *Practical Guide for the Diagnosis and Management of Asthma.* Bethesda, Md.: National Heart, Lung, and Blood Institute. NIH Publication 97–4053, 1997.

8. Smolensky, M.H., and D'Alonzo, G.E. Progress in the chronotherapy of nocturnal asthma. In Redfern P., and Lemmer B., eds., *Physiology and Pharmacology of Biological Rhythms.* Heidelberg: Springer-Verlag. 1997:205–249. Smolensky, M.H., et al. Chronobiology and asthma. I. Day-night differences in bronchial patency and dyspnea and circadian rhythm dependencies. *Journal of Asthma.* 1986;23:321–343.

9. Floyer, J. *A Treatise on the Asthma.* Third edition. Wilkin, R., and Innys, J., eds. London. 1726. First published in 1698.

10. Salter, H.H. *On Asthma: Its Pathology and Treatment.* London: J. Churchill. 1859.

11. Smolensky, M. Knowledge and attitudes of American physicians and public about medical chronobiology and chronotherapeutics. Findings of two 1996 Gallup Surveys. *Chronobiology International.* 1998;15:377–394.

12. *Guidelines for the Diagnosis and Management of Asthma.* Ibid.:3.

13. Martin, R.J., and Banks-Schlegel, S. Chronobiology of asthma. *American Journal of Respiratory and Critical Care Medicine.* 1998;158:1002–1007.

14. *Guidelines for the Diagnosis and Management of Asthma.* Ibid.

15. Skobeloff, E., et al. The effect of the menstrual cycle on asthma presentations in the emergency department. *Archives of Internal Medicine.* 1996;156:1837–1840.

16. *Guidelines for the Diagnosis and Management of Asthma.* Ibid.:20.

17. *American Medical Association Essential Guide to Asthma.* New York: Pocket Books. 1998.

18. D'Alonzo, G.E., Jr., et al. Circadian rhythms in the pharmacokinetics and clinical effects of beta-agonists, theophylline, and anticholinergic medications in the treatment of nocturnal asthma. *Chronobiology International.* 1999;16:663–682.

19. Helm, S.G. Diurnal stabilization of asthma with once-daily evening administration of controlled-release theophylline: A multi-investigator study. *Immunology and Allergy Practice.* 1987;11:414–419.

20. D'Alonzo, G.E., Jr., et al. Ibid.

21. Beam, W.R., et al. Timing of prednisolone and alteration of airways inflammation in nocturnal asthma. *American Review of Respiratory Disease.* 1992;146:1524–1530.

22. Reinberg, A., et al. One-month chronocorticotherapy (Dutimelan 8–15). Control of the asthmatic condition without adrenal suppression and circadian alteration. *Chronobiologia.* 1997;4:295–312.

23. Pincus, D.J., et al. Further studies on the chronotherapy of asthma with inhaled steroids: the effects of dosage timing on drug efficacy. *Journal of Allergy and Clinical Immunology.* 1997;100:771–774.

BACK PAIN

1. Pednault, L., and Parent, M. Circadian rhythm of chronic low back pain caused by discal degeneration, fusion pseudoarthritis or discoidectomy. Proceedings of the 21st Conference of the International Society of Chronobiology. Quebec, Canada. 1993:Abstract No. III–9.

2. Pednault, L., and Parent, M. Ibid.

3. Alvin, M., et al. Chronobiological aspects of spondylarthritis. *Annual Review of Chronopharmacology.* 1988;5:17–20. Reinberg, A., et al. Tenoxicam chronotherapy of rheumatic diseases. *Annual Review of Chronopharmacology.* 1990;7:293–296.

4. Alvin, M., et al. Ibid.

CANCER

1. *Cancer Facts and Figures—2000* (brochure). New York: American Cancer Society. 2000.

2. Mormont, C., et al. Mechanisms of circadian rhythms in the toxicity and efficacy of anti-cancer drugs: relevance for the development of new analogs. In Lemmer, B., ed., *Chronopharmacology: Cellular and Biochemical Interactions.* New York: Marcel Dekker. 1989:395–437.

3. Lévi, F. Chronopharmacology of anticancer agents. In Redfern, P.H., and Lemmer, B., eds., *Physiology and Pharmacology of Biological Rhythms.* Berlin: Springer. 1997:299–311.

4. *Cancer Facts and Figures—2000.* Ibid.

5. Lévi, F., et al. A chronopharmacologic phase II clinical trial with 5-fluorouracil, folinic acid, and oxaliplatin using an ambulatory multichannel programmable pump: high antitumor effectiveness against metastatic colorectal cancer. *Cancer.* 1992;69:893–900.

6. Lévi, F. Cancer chronotherapy. *Journal of Pharmacy and Pharmacology.* 1999;51:891–898. Giacchetti, S., et al. Phase III multicenter randomized trial of oxaliplatin added to chronomodulated fluorouracil-leucovorin as first-line treatment of metastatic colorectal cancer. *Journal of Clinical Oncology.* 2000;18:136–147.

7. Francis Lévi and Jean Cayzac spoke with the authors in February 1998, at the Hôpital Paul Brousse.

8. European Organization for Research and Treatment of Cancer Chronotherapy Study Group. Phase III Randomized Study of Chronomodulated Versus Nonchronomodulated Administration of Fluorouracil, Leucovorin Calcium, and Oxaliplatin as First Line Treatment in Patients with Locoregionally Recurrent or Metastatic Colorectal Cancer. Study started October 10, 1998.

9. *Cancer Facts and Figures—2000.* Ibid.

10. Hrushesky, W.J.M. Circadian timing of cancer chemotherapy. *Science.* 1985;228:73–75.

11. Touitou, Y., et al. Circadian rhythm alterations of plasma cortisol in cancer patients. *Cancer Detection and Prevention.* 1998;22(Suppl. 1):Abstract 300.

12. Rivard, G., et al. Maintenance chemotherapy for childhood acute lymphoblastic leukaemia: better in the evening. *Lancet.* 1985;2:1264–1266. Rivard, G.E., et al. Circadian time-dependent response of childhood lymphoblastic leukemia to chemotherapy: a long-term follow-up of survival. *Chronobiology International.* 1993;10:201-204.

13. Schmiegelow, K. Impact of morning versus evening schedule for oral methotrexate and 6-mercaptopurine on relapse risk for children with acute lymphoblastic leukemia. Nordic Society for Pediatric Hematology and Oncology (NOPHO). *Journal of Pediatric Hematology/Oncology.* 1997;19:102–109.

14. Ross, J.A., et al. Seasonal trends in the self-detection of breast cancer: indications from the Cancer and Steroid Hormone (CASH) study. *Breast Cancer Research and Treatment.* 1997;42:187–192.

15. Simpson, H.W., et al. Progesterone resistance in women who have had breast cancer. *British Journal of Obstetrics and Gynaecology.* 1998;105:345–351.

16. Hrushesky W.J.M., et al. Menstrual influence on surgical care of breast cancer. *Lancet.* 1989;2:949–952.

17. Hagen, A.A., and Hrushesky, W.J.M. Menstrual timing of breast cancer surgery. *American Journal of Surgery.* 1998;104:245–261. Cooper, L.S., et al. Survival of premenopausal breast carcinoma patients in relation to menstrual cycle timing of surgery and estrogen receptor/progesterone receptor status of the primary tumor. *Cancer.* 1999;86:2053–2058.

18. Hagen A.A., and Hrushesky, W.J.M. Ibid.

19. Deka, A.C., et al. Temperature rhythm—an index of tumour regression and mucositis during the radiation treatment of oral cancers. *Indian Journal of Cancer.* 1976;13:44–50.

COLDS AND FLU

1. Smith, A., et al. Diurnal variation in the symptoms of colds and influenza. *Chronobiology International.* 1988;5:411–416.

2. Cold comfort: which remedies should you choose? *Consumer Reports on Health.* 1997;9:133–137.

3. Update: Influenza activity—U.S. and Worldwide, 1998–99 season, and composition of the 1999–2000 influenza vaccine. *Morbidity and Mortality Weekly Report.* 1999;48(18):374–378.

4. Langlois, P.H., et al. Diurnal variation in responses to influenza vaccine. *Chronobiology International.* 1995;12:28–36.

COLIC

1. Weissbluth, M. Colic. In Ferber, R., and Kryger, M., eds., *Principles and Practice of Sleep Medicine in the Child.* Philadelphia: W.B. Saunders. 1995.

2. Weissbluth, M., and Weissbluth, L. Infant colic: the effect of serotonin and melatonin circadian rhythms on the intestinal smooth muscle. *Medical Hypotheses.* 1992;39:164–167. Weissbluth, M., and Weissbluth, L. Colic, sleep inertia, melatonin, and circannual rhythms. *Medical Hypotheses.* 1992;38:224–228.

3. Weizman, Z., et al. Efficacy of herbal tea preparation in infantile colic. *Journal of Pediatrics.* 1993;122:650–652.

CONSTIPATION

1. Harari, D., et al. Bowel habit in relation to age and gender. Findings from the National Health Interview Survey and clinical implications. *Archives of Internal Medicine.* 1996;156:315–320.

2. Heaton, K.W., et al. Defecation frequency and timing, and stool form in the general population: a prospective study. *Gut.* 1992;33:818–824.

3. Heitkemper, M.H., and Jarrett, M. Pattern of gastrointestinal and somatic symptoms across the menstrual cycle. *Gastroenterology.* 1992;102:505–513.

4. Kane, S.V., et al. The menstrual cycle and its effect on inflammatory bowel disease and irritable bowel syndrome: a prevalence study. *American Journal of Gastroenterology.* 1998;93:1867–1872. Heitkemper, M.H., and Jarrett, M. Ibid.

5. Corman, M.L. Management of postoperative constipation in anorectal surgery. *Diseases of the Colon and Rectum.* 1979;22:149–151.

6. Mathias, J.R., et al. Effect of leuprolide acetate in patients with moderate to severe functional bowel disease. *Digestive Diseases and Sciences.* 1994;39:1155–1162.

7. Anti, M., et al. Water supplementation enhances the effect of high-fiber diet on stool frequency and laxative consumption in adult patients with functional constipation. *Hepato-Gastroenterology.* 1998;45:727–732.

DIABETES

1. Mejean, L., et al. Circadian and ultradian rhythms in blood glucose and plasma insulin of healthy adults. *Chronobiology International.* 1988;5:227–236. Jarrett, R.J. Circadian variations in blood glucose levels, in glucose tolerance and in plasma immunoreactive insulin levels. *Acta Diabetologica Latina.* 1972;9:263–275.

2. Zimmet, P.Z., et al. Diurnal variation in glucose tolerance: associated changes in plasma insulin, growth hormone and non-esterified fatty acids. *British Medical Journal.* 1974;2:485–488. Jarrett, R.J., et al. Ibid.

3. Gibson, T., et al. Diurnal variation in the effects of insulin in blood glucose, plasma nonesterified fatty acids and growth hormone. *Diabetologia.* 1975;11:83–88.

4. Cawood, E.H.H., et al. Perimenstrual symptoms in women with diabetes mellitus and the relationship to diabetic control. *Diabetic Medicine.* 1993;10:444–448.

5. Douglas, S., et al. Seasonality of presentation of type I diabetes mellitus in children. Scottish Study Group for the Care of Young Diabetics. *Scottish Medical Journal.* 1999;44:41–46.

6. Szopa, T.M., et al. Diabetes mellitus due to viruses—some recent developments. *Diabetologia.* 1993;36:687–695.

7. Trumper, B.G., et al. Circadian variation of insulin requirement in insulin dependent diabetes mellitus, the relationship between circadian change in insulin demand and diurnal patterns of growth hormone, cortisol and glucagon during euglycemia. *Hormone and Metabolic Research.* 1995;27:141–147.

8. Tamada, J.A. Noninvasive glucose monitoring: comprehensive clinical results. *Journal of the American Medical Association.* 1999;282:1839–1844.

9. Backonja, M. Gabapentin for the symptomatic treatment of painful neuropathy in patients with diabetes mellitus: a randomized controlled trial. *Journal of the American Medical Association.* 1998;280:1831–1836.

EPILEPSY

1. Millett, C.J., et al. Seizures during video-game play and other common leisure pursuits in known epilepsy patients without visual sensitivity. *Epilepsia.* 1999;40(Suppl. 4):59–64.

2. Begley, C.E., et al. The cost of epilepsy in the United States: an estimate from population-based clinical and survey data. *Epilepsia.* 2000;41:342–351.

3. Epilepsy Foundation. *Campaign for Women's Health* (brochure). Landover, Md.: Epilepsy Foundation. 1998.

4. Duncan, S., et al. How common is catamenial epilepsy? *Epilepsia.* 1993;34:827–831.

5. Herzog, A.G., et al. Three patterns of catamenial epilepsy. *Epilepsia.* 1997;38:1082–1088. Klein, P., and Herzog, A.G. Hormonal effects on epilepsy in women. *Epilepsia.* 1998;39(Suppl. 8)S:39–S16.

6. Kilpatrick, C.J., and Hopper, J.L. The effect of pregnancy on the epilepsies: a study of 37 pregnancies. *Australian and New Zealand Journal of Medicine.* 1993;23:370–373.

7. Harden, C.L., et al. The effect of menopause and perimenopause on the course of epilepsy. *Epilepsia.* 1999;40:1402–1407.

8. Abbasi, F., et al. Effects of menopause on seizures in women with epilepsy. *Epilepsia.* 1999;40:205–210.

9. Herzog, A.G. Reproductive endocrine considerations and hormonal therapy for men with epilepsy. *Epilepsia.* 1991;32(Suppl. 6):S34–37. Herzog, A.G., et al. Testosterone versus testosterone and testolactone in treating reproductive and sexual dysfunction in men with epilepsy and hypogonadism. *Neurology.* 1998;50:782–784.

10. Autret, A., et al. Sleep and epilepsy. *Sleep Medicine Reviews.* 1999;3:201–217.

11. Nakano, S., et al. Circadian stage-dependent changes in diazepam and valproate kinetics in man: A single and repetitive administration study. *Annual Review of Chronopharmacology.* 1986;3:421–424.

12. Rosciszewska, D., et al. Ovarian hormones, anticonvulsant drugs, and seizures during the menstrual cycle in women with epilepsy. *Journal of Neurology, Neurosurgery, and Psychiatry.* 1986;49:47–51. Shavit, G., et al. Phenytoin pharmacokinetics in catamenial epilepsy. *Neurology.* 1984;34:959–961. Kumar, N., et al. Phenytoin levels in catamenial epilepsy. *Epilepsia.* 1988;29:155–158.

FIBROMYALGIA

1. Dunkin, M.A., et al. Fibromyalgia: research is providing an understanding of this common syndrome. *Arthritis Today Special Report.* September 1998:11.

2. Cote, K.A., and Moldofsky, H. Sleep, daytime symptoms, and cognitive performance in patients with fibromyalgia. *Journal of Rheumatology.* 1997;10:2014–2023.

3. Moldofsky, H., et al. Musculoskeletal symptoms and non-REM sleep disturbance in patients with "fibrocystitis syndrome" and healthy subjects. *Psychosomatic Medicine.* 1975;37:341–351.

4. Lentz, M.J., et al. Effects of selective slow-wave sleep stage disruption on musculoskeletal pain and fatigue in middle-aged women. *Journal of Rheumatology.* 1999;26:586–592.

5. Lentz, M.J., et al. Sleep and pain symptoms in women with fibromyalgia, on and off medication. Thirty-second Annual Communicating Nursing Research Conference and Thirteenth Annual Western Institute of Nursing Assembly, San Diego, California. 1999;Abstract.183.

6. Bennett, R.M. A randomized, double-blind, placebo-controlled study of growth hormone in the treatment of fibromyalgia. *American Journal of Medicine.* 1998;104:227–231.

7. Pearl, S.J., et al. The effects of bright light treatment on the symptoms of fibromyalgia. *Journal of Rheumatology.* 1996;23:896–902.

GALLBLADDER ATTACKS

1. Rigas, B., et al. The circadian rhythm of biliary colic. *Journal of Clinical Gastroenterology.* 1990;12:409–414.

GOUT

1. Harris, M.D., et al. Gout and hyperuricemia. *American Family Physician.* 1999;59:925–934.

2. Schlesinger, N., et al. Acute gouty arthritis is seasonal. *Journal of Rheumatology.* 1998;25:342–344.

3. Sydenham, T. *The works of Thomas Sydenham,* translated from the Latin by R.G. Lathan, Vol. II. London: New Sydenham Society. 1850:124.

GROWING PAINS

1. McGrath, P. Children's pain perception: impact of gender and age. Conference on Gender and Pain. Bethesda, Md.: National Institutes of Health, April 7–8, 1998. http://www1.od.nih.gov/painresearch/genderandpain/absracts.htm

2. Oster, J., and Nielsen, A. Growing pains. *Acta Paediatrica.* 1972;62:329–334.

3. Petersen, H. Growing pains. *Pediatric Clinics of North America.* 1986;33:1365–1372. Manners, P. Are growing pains a myth? *Australian Family Physician.* 1999;28:124–127.

4. Barr, R.G. Pain in children. In Wall, P.D., and Melzack, R., eds., *Textbook of Pain.* Second edition. Edinburgh: Churchill Livingstone. 1989:568–588.

HAY FEVER

1. Smolensky, M.H., et al. Twenty-four hour pattern in symptom intensity of viral and allergic rhinitis: treatment implications. *Journal of Allergy and Clinical Immunology.* 1995;95:1084–1096.

2. Reinberg, A., et al. Circadian and circannual rhythms of allergic rhinitis: an epidemiologic study involving chronobiologic methods. *Journal of Allergy and Clinical Immunology.* 1988;81:51–62.

3. Naclerio, R., and Solomon, W. Rhinitis and inhalant allergens. *Journal of the American Medical Association.* 1997;278:1842–1848.

4. Grant, A., and Roter, E. Circadian sneezing. *Neurology.* 1994;44:369–375.

5. Skoner, D. Allergies 2000: a profile of patients' treatment experiences. A survey of 4,017 adults with allergic rhinitis conducted for the Children's Hospital of Pittsburgh. 2000. Unpublished.

6. Craig, T., et al. Nasal congestion secondary to allergic rhinitis as a cause of sleep disturbance and daytime fatigue and the response to topical nasal corticosteroids. *Journal of Allergy and Clinical Immunology.* 1998;101:633–637.

7. Juniper, E.F., and Guyatt, G.H. Development and testing of a new measure of health status for clinical trials of rhinoconjunctivitis. *Clinical and Experimental Allergy.* 1991;21:77–83.

8. Smolensky, M.H., et al. Ibid.

HEADACHES

1. *Headaches: Hope through Research.* National Institute of Neurological Disorders and Stroke. NIH Publication No. 96–158, 1996.

2. Solomon, G.D. Circadian rhythms and migraine. *Cleveland Clinic Journal of Medicine.* 1992;59:326–329.

3. Hsu, L.K.G., et al. Early morning migraine. Nocturnal plasma levels of catecholamines, glucose, and free fatty acids and sleep encephalographs. *Lancet.* 1997;1:447–451.

4. Lipton, R.B., et al. An update on the epidemiology of migraine. *Headache.* 1994;34:319–328. Lipton, R., et al. Headache syndromes and their treatment. In Samuels, M., and Feske, S., eds., *Office Practice of Neurology.* New York: Churchill Livingstone. 1996:1105–1111.

5. Dalton, K. Progesterone suppositories and pessaries in the treatment of menstrual migraine. *Headache.* 1973;12:151–159.

6. Capra, Frank. *The Name above the Title.* New York: Macmillan. 1971.

7. Pareja, J.A., et al. SUNCT Syndrome: duration, frequency and temporal distribution of attacks. *Headache.* 1996;36:161–165.

8. May, A., et al. Correlation between structural and functional changes in brain in an idiopathic headache syndrome. *Nature Medicine.* 1999;5:836–838.

9. Zee, P., and Grujic, Z. Neurological disorders associated with disturbed sleep and circadian rhythms. In Turek, F., and Zee, P., eds., *Regulation of Sleep and Circadian Rhythms.* New York: Marcel Dekker. 1999:557–596.

10. Schwartz, B.S., et al. Epidemiology of tension-type headache. *Journal of the American Medical Association.* 1998;279:381–383.

11. Sachs, C., and Svanborg, E. Exploding Head Syndrome. *Sleep.* 1991;14:263–266.

12. Paiva, T., et al. Chronic headaches and sleep disorders. *Archives of Internal Medicine.* 1997;157:1701–1705. Lamberg, L. Patients in pain need round-the-clock care. *Journal of the American Medical Association* (News). 1999;281:689–690.

HEARTBURN

1. Bouchoucha, M., et al. Day-night patterns of gastroesophageal reflux. *Chronobiology International.* 1995;12:267–277.

2. Ireland, A., et al. Ranitidine 150 mg twice daily vs. 300 mg nightly in treatment of duodenal ulcers. *Lancet.* 1984;2:274–276.

3. Hatlebakk, J.G., et al. Nocturnal gastric acidity and acid breakthrough on different regimens of omeprazole 40 mg daily. *Alimentary Pharmacology and Therapeutics.* 1998;12:1235–1240.

HEART DISEASE

1. Cohen, M.C., et al. Meta-analysis of the morning excess acute myocardial infarction and sudden cardiac death. *American Journal of Cardiology.* 1997;79:1512–1516.

2. Muller, J.E., et al. Circadian variation in the frequency of onset of acute myocardial infarction. *New England Journal of Medicine.* 1985;313:1315–1322. Muller, J.E. Circadian variation and triggering of acute coronary events. *American Heart Journal.* 1999;137(4 Pt 2):S1–S8.

3. Hermida, R.C., et al. Circadian rhythm of double (rate-pressure) product in young normotensive healthy men and women. *Chronobiology International.* 2000;17, in press.

4. Deedwania, P.C., and Nelson, J.R. Pathophysiology of silent ischemia during daily life: hemodynamic evaluation by simultaneous electrocardiographic and blood pressure monitoring. *Circulation.* 1990;82:1296–1304.

5. Hansen, O., et al. The clinical outcome of acute myocardial infarction is related to the circadian rhythm of myocardial infarction onset. *Angiology.* 1993;13:185–196.

6. Cohen, M.C., et al. Ibid.

7. Rocco, M.B., et al. Circadian variation of transient myocardial ischemia in patients with coronary artery disease. *Circulation.* 1987;75:395–400. Mulcahy, D., et al. Circadian variation of total ischaemic burden and its alteration with anti-angina agents. *Lancet.* 1988;2:755–759.

8. Kuroiwa, A. Symptomology of variant angina. *Japanese Journal of Circulation.*

1978;42:459–476. Waters, D.D., et al. Circadian variation in variant angina. *American Journal of Cardiology.* 1984;54:61–64.

9. Peters, R. Circadian patterns and triggers of sudden cardiac death. *Circulation.* 1996;14:185–194.

10. Willich, S.N., et al. Weekly variation of acute myocardial infarction: increased Monday risk in the working population. *Circulation.* 1994;90:87–93.

11. Smolensky, M.H., et al. Chronobiology of the Life Sequence. In Ogata, S.I.K., and Yoshimura, H., eds., *Advances in Climatic Physiology.* Tokyo: Igaku Shoin. 1972;218–319. Peckova, M., et al. Weekly and seasonal variation in the incidence of cardiac arrests. *American Heart Journal.* 1999;137:512–515. Douglas, S., and Rawles, J. Latitude-related changes in the amplitude of annual mortality rhythm. The biological equator in man. *Chronobiology International.* 1999;16:199–212.

12. Kloner, R.A., et al. When throughout the year is coronary death most likely to occur? *Circulation.* 1999;100:1630–1634.

13. Murray, P.M., et al. Should patients with heart disease exercise in the morning or afternoon? *Archives of Internal Medicine.* 1993;153:833–836.

14. Muller, J.E., et al. Triggering myocardial infarction by sexual activity: low absolute risk and prevention by regular physical exertion. *Journal of the American Medical Association.* 1996;275:1405–1409.

15. DeBusk, R.F. Sexual activity triggering myocardial infarction: one less thing to worry about. *Journal of the American Medical Association.* 1996;275:1447–1448.

16. Ridker, P.M., et al. Circadian variation of acute myocardial infarction and the effect of low-dose aspirin in a randomized trial of physicians. *Circulation.* 1990;82:897–902.

17. Manson J.E., et al. A prospective study of aspirin use and primary prevention of cardiovascular disease in women. *Journal of the American Medical Association.* 1991;266:521–527.

18. Mevacor Tablets (Lovastatin). In Arky, R., ed., *Physicians' Desk Reference.* Montvale, N.J.: Medical Economics Co. 1999;53:1834–1838.

19. Kurnik, P.B. Circadian variation in the efficacy of tissue-type plasminogen activator. *Circulation.* 1995;91:1341–1346.

HIGH BLOOD PRESSURE

1. Meissner, I., et al. Detection and control of high blood pressure in the community: do we need wake-up call? *Hypertension.* 1999;34:466–471.

2. Burt, V.L., et al. Prevalence of hypertension in U.S. adult population: results from the third National Health and Nutrition Examination Survey 1988–1991. *Hypertension.* 1995;25:305–311. *The Sixth Report of the Joint National Committee on Prevention, Detection, Evaluation, and Treatment of High Blood Pressure.* Bethesda, Md. *Archives of Internal Medicine.* 1997;157:2413–2446.

3. Pickering, T. *Ambulatory Monitoring of Blood Pressure Variability.* London: Science Press. 1991.

4. Baumgart, P. Circadian rhythm of blood pressure: internal and external time triggers. *Chronobiology International.* 1991;8:444–450. Portaluppi, F., and Smolensky, M.H. Time-dependent structure and control of arterial blood pressure. *Annals of the New York Academy of Sciences.* 1996;Vol. 783.

5. *The Sixth Report of the Joint National Committee on Prevention, Detection, Evaluation, and Treatment of High Blood Pressure.* Ibid.

6. Freedman, S.H., et al. Some physiological and biochemical measurements over the menstrual cycle. In Ferin, M., Halberg, F., Richart, R.M., and Vande Wiele, R.L., eds., *Biorhythms and Human Reproduction.* New York: John Wiley. 1973:259–275.

7. Heintz, B., et al. Blood pressure rhythm and endocrine functions in normotensive women on oral contraceptives. *Journal of Hypertension.* 1996;14:333–339.

8. Kristal-Boneh, E., et al. Seasonal change in 24-hour blood pressure and heart rate is greater among smokers than nonsmokers. *Hypertension.* 1997;30(Pt 1):436–441.

9. *The Sixth Report of the Joint National Committee on Prevention, Detection, Evaluation, and Treatment of High Blood Pressure.* Ibid.

10. Bellomo, G. Prognostic value of 24-hour blood pressure in pregnancy. *Journal of the American Medical Association.* 1999;282:1447–1452.

11. O'Brien E, et al. Dippers and non-dippers. *Lancet.* 1998;2:397. Pickering, T. Ibid.

12. Ohkurbo, T., et al. Relation between nocturnal decline in blood pressure and mortality. *American Journal of Hypertension.* 1997;10:1201–1207.

13. O'Brien, E., et al. Ibid. Pickering, T. Ibid.

14. Kario, K., et al. Relationship between extreme dippers and orthostatic hypertension in elderly hypertensive patients. *Hypertension.* 1998;31(Pt 1):77–82. Kukla, C., et al. Changes of circadian blood pressure patterns are associated with the occurrence of lacunar infarction. *Archives of Neurology.* 1998;55:683–688.

15. Hayreh, S.S., et al. Nocturnal arterial hypotension and its role in optic nerve head and ocular ischemic disorders. *American Journal of Ophthalmology.* 1994;117:603–624. Hayreh, S.S., et al. Nonarteritic anterior ischemic optic neuropathy: time of onset of visual loss. *American Journal of Ophthalmology.* 1997;124:641–647.

16. Ayala, D.E., et al. Blood pressure variability during gestation in healthy and complicated pregnancies. *Hypertension.* 1997;30(Pt 2):611–618.

17. CLASP: a randomized trial of low-dose aspirin for the prevention and treatment of preeclampsia among 9364 pregnant women. *Lancet.* 1994;343:619–629. Dekker, G.A., and Sibai, B.M. Low-dose aspirin in the prevention of preeclampsia and fetal growth retardation: rationale, mechanisms, and clinical trials. *American Journal of Obstetrics and Gynecology.* 1993;168:214–227.

18. Hermida, R.C., et al. Time-dependent effects of low-dose aspirin administration on blood pressure in pregnant women. *Hypertension.* 1997;30(Pt 2):589–595.

19. Kokno, I., et al. Administration-time-dependent effects of diltiazem on the 24-hour blood pressure profile of essential hypertension patients. *Chronobiology International.* 1997;14:71–84.

20. Morgan, T., et al. The effect on 24 h blood pressure control of an angiotensin converting enzyme inhibitor (perindopril) administered in the morning or at night. *Journal of Hypertension.* 1997;15:205–211.

21. Product Monograph. Once at bedtime controlled onset Verelan PM. Milwaukee, Wisc.: Schwarz Pharma. 1999.

MOOD DISORDERS

1. Satcher, D., et al. *Mental Health: A Report of the Surgeon General.* Rockville, Md.: U.S. Department of Health and Human Services. 1999:244.

2. Rosenthal, N.E. *Winter Blues: Seasonal Affective Disorder; What It Is and How to Overcome It.* New York: Guilford Press. 1998:287–295.

3. Rosenthal, L., et al. Prevalence of seasonal affective disorder at four latitudes. *Psychiatry Research.* 1990;31:131–144.

4. Magnusson, A., and Axelsson, J. The prevalence of seasonal affective disorder is low among descendants of Icelandic emigrants in Canada. *Archives of General Psychiatry.* 1993;50:947–951.

5. Lewy, A.J., et al. Light suppresses melatonin secretion in humans. *Science.* 1980;210:1267–1269.

6. Kern, H., and Lewy, A. Corrections and additions to the history of light therapy and seasonal affective disorder. *Archives of General Psychiatry.* 1990;47:90–91. Lewy, A.J., et al. Bright artificial light treatment of a manic-depressive patient with a seasonal mood cycle. *American Journal of Psychiatry.* 1982;139:1496–1497.

7. Lamberg, L. Dawn's early light to twilight's last gleaming. . . . *Journal of the American Medical Association.* 1998;280:1556–1558.

8. Wirz-Justice, A. Beginning to see the light. *Archives of General Psychiatry.* 1998;55:861–862.

9. Lewy, A., et al. Morning vs. evening light treatment of patients with winter depression. *Archives of General Psychiatry.* 1998;55:890–896.

10. Sack, R.L., et al. Use of melatonin for sleep and circadian rhythm disorders. *Annals of Medicine.* 1998;30:115–121.

11. Lam, R.W., and Levitt, A.J., eds. *Canadian Consensus Guidelines for the Treatment of Seasonal Affective Disorder.* Vancouver, Canada: Clinical and Academic Publishing. 1999.

12. Wehr, T., et al. Summer depression: description of the syndrome and comparison with

winter depression. In Rosenthal, N.E., and Blehar, M.C., eds., *Seasonal Affective Disorders and Phototherapy*. New York: Guilford Press. 1989:55–63.

13. Sourander, A., et al. Mood, latitude, and seasonality among adolescents. *Journal of the American Academy of Child and Adolescent Psychiatry*. 1999;38:1271–1276.

14. Carskadon, M.A., and Acebo, C. Parental reports of seasonal mood and behavior changes in children. *Journal of the American Academy of Child and Adolescent Psychiatry*. 1993;32:264–269.

15. Low, K.G., and Feissner, J.M. Seasonal affective disorder in college students: prevalence and latitude. *Journal of American Health*. 1998;47:135–137.

16. Lam, R.W., and Goldner, E.M. Seasonality of bulimia nervosa and treatment with light therapy. In Lam R.W., ed., *Seasonal Affective Disorder and Beyond: Light Treatment for SAD and Non-SAD Conditions*. Washington, D.C.: American Psychiatric Press. 1998:193–220.

17. Kripke, D.F. Light treatment for nonseasonal depression: speed, efficacy, and combined treatment. *Journal of Affective Disorders*. 1998;49:109–117.

18. Eliot, T.S. *The Waste Land. I. The Burial of the Dead*. In *The Waste Land and Other Poems*. New York: Harcourt, Brace. 1930:29.

19. Goodwin, F.K., and Jamison, K.R. *Manic Depressive Illness*. New York: Oxford University Press. 1990.

20. Szuba, M.P., et al. Electroconvulsive therapy increases circadian amplitude and lowers body temperature in depressed subjects. *Biological Psychiatry*. 1997;42:1130–1137.

21. Kripke, D.F., et al. Bright white light alleviates depression. *Psychiatry Research*. 1983;10:105–112.

22. Kripke, D.F. Ibid.

23. Neumeister, A., et al. Bright light therapy stabilizes the antidepressant effect of partial sleep deprivation. *Biological Psychiatry*. 1996;39:16–21.

24. Berger, M., et al. Sleep deprivation combined with consecutive sleep phase advance as a fast-acting therapy in depression: an open pilot trial in medicated and unmedicated patients. *American Journal of Psychiatry*. 1997;154:870–872.

25. Duke, P., and Hochman, G. *A Brilliant Madness: Living with Manic Depressive Illness*. New York: Bantam Books. 1992:26–27.

26. Ashman, S.B., et al. Relationship between social rhythms and mood in patients with rapid cycling bipolar disorder. *Psychiatry Research*. 1999;86:1–8.

27. Kulin, N.A., et al. Pregnancy outcome following maternal use of the new selective serotonin reuptake inhibitors: a prospective controlled multicenter study. *Journal of the American Medical Association*. 1998;279:609–610.

28. Parry, B., et al. Sleep deprivation in pregnancy and postpartum depression. *American Psychiatric Association Annual Meeting Proceedings Summary*. Washington, D.C.: American Psychiatric Association. 1999:100.

29. Oren, D.A., et al. Morning light treatment for antepartum depression. *Society for Light Treatment and Biological Rhythms* (Abstract). 1999;11:7.

30. Ryan, D. Postpartum anxiety and mood disorders: effect on infant development (abstract). *American Psychiatric Association Annual Meeting Proceedings Summary*. Washington, D.C.: American Psychiatric Association. 1999:100.

31. Gregoire, A.J. Transdermal oestrogen for treatment of severe postnatal depression. *Lancet*. 1996;347:930–933.

32. Parry, B., et al. Ibid.

33. Lam, R.W., and Levitt, A.J., eds. *Canadian consensus guidelines for the treatment of seasonal affective disorder*. Ibid.:72–75.

34. Terman, M., and Terman, J.S. Bright light therapy: side effects and benefits across the symptom spectrum. *Journal of Clinical Psychiatry*. 1999;60:799–808.

35. Perlis, M.L., et al. Self-reported sleep disturbance as a prodromal symptom in recurrent depression. *Journal of Affective Disorders*. 1997;42:209–212.

36. Dagan, Y., and Lemberg, H. Sleep-wake schedule disorder as a possible side effect of CNS medications. *Chronobiology International*. 1999;16(Suppl. 1):25.

MULTIPLE SCLEROSIS

1. Davis, F.A., et al. Fluctuations of motor function in multiple sclerosis related to circadian temperature variations. *Diseases of the Nervous System.* 1973;34:33–36.

2. Namerow, N.S. Circadian temperature rhythm and vision in multiple sclerosis. *Neurology.* 1968;18:417–422.

3. Ku, Y.T. Physiologic and thermal responses of male and female patients with multiple sclerosis to head and neck cooling. *American Journal of Physical Medicine and Rehabilitation.* 1999;78:447–456.

4. Bechtel, C., et al. Keeping cool. *The Motivator.* July–August 1999:8–12.

5. Bakshi, R., et al. Fatigue in multiple sclerosis: cross-sectional correlation with brain MRI findings in 71 patients. *Neurology.* 1999;53:1151–1153.

6. King, M., et al. Facts & Issues: On fatigue. National Multiple Sclerosis Society Online. 1999. www.nmss.org.

7. Rabins, P., et al. Structural brain correlates of emotional disorder in multiple sclerosis. *Brain.* 1986;109:585–597.

8. Zorgdrager, A., and De Keyser, J. Menstrually related worsening of symptoms in multiple sclerosis. *Journal of Neurological Science.* 1997;149:95–97.

9. Kim, S., et al. Estriol ameliorates autoimmune demyelinating disease: implications for multiple sclerosis. *Neurology.* 1999;52:1230–1238.

10. Voskuhl, R. Estriol treatment for multiple sclerosis: a preliminary trial. *National Multiple Sclerosis Society Winter-Spring 1999 Research Highlights.* New York: National Multiple Sclerosis Society. 1999.

11. Smith, R., and Studd, J.W. A pilot study of the effect upon multiple sclerosis of the menopause, hormone replacement therapy and the menstrual cycle. *Journal of the Royal Society of Medicine.* 1992;85:612–613.

12. Report spurs new initiatives on sex differences in MS. Winter-Spring 1999 Research Highlights. National Multiple Sclerosis Society Online. www.nmss.org.

13. Wuthrich, R., and Rieder, H.P. The seasonal incidence of multiple sclerosis in Switzerland. *European Neurology.* 1970;3:257–265. Sibley, W.A., and Paty, D.W. A comparison of multiple sclerosis in Arizona (USA) and Ontario (Canada)—Preliminary report. *Acta Neurologica Scandinavica.* 1981(Suppl. 87); 64:61–65.

NOSEBLEEDS

1. Portaluppi, F., et al. Circadian and circannual rhythmicity in the occurrence of epistaxis. *Chronobiology International.* 1997;14(Suppl. 1):136.

OSTEOPOROSIS

1. Eastell, R., et al. Abnormalities in circadian patterns of bone resorption and renal calcium conservation in type I osteoporosis. *Journal of Clinical Endocrinology and Metabolism.* 1992;74:487–494.

2. Blumsohn, A., et al. The effect of calcium supplementation on the circadian rhythm of bone resorption. *Journal of Clinical Endocrinology and Metabolism.* 1994;79:730–735.

3. Aerssens, J., et al. The effect of modifying the dietary calcium intake pattern on the circadian rhythm of bone resorption. *Calcified Tissue International.* 1999;65:34–40.

4. Sairanen, S., et al. Nocturnal rise in markers of bone resorption is not abolished by bedtime calcium or calcitonin. *Calcified Tissue International.* 1994;55:349–352.

5. Nelson, M., and Wernick, S. *Strong Women, Strong Bones.* New York: Putnam. 2000.

6. Gertz, B.J., et al. Application of a new serum assay for type I college cross-linked N-telopeptides: assessments of diurnal changes in bone turnover with and without alendronate. *Calcified Tissue International.* 1998;63:102–106.

PEPTIC ULCERS

1. Bouchoucha, M., et al. Day-night patterns of gastroesophageal reflux. *Chronobiology International.* 1995;12:267–277.

2. Moynihan, B.G.A. *Duodenal Ulcer.* Philadelphia: W.B. Saunders. 1910:101–121. Moynihan, B.G.A. Some remarks on dyspepsia. *Dublin Journal of Medical Science.* 1910;130(No. 463, ser 3):1–15.

3. Earlam, R. A computerized questionnaire analysis of duodenal ulcer symptoms. *Gastroenterology.* 1976;71:314–317.

4. Bianchi Porro, G.B., and Lazzaroni, M. Colloidal bismuth subcitrate. In Swabb, E.A., and Szabo, S., eds., *Ulcer Disease. Investigation and Basis for Treatment.* New York: Marcel Dekker. 1991:287–319.

5. Moore, J.G., and Merki, H. Gastrointestinal tract. In Redfern, P.H., and Lemmer, B., eds., *Physiology and Pharmacology of Biological Rhythms.* Berlin: Springer-Verlag. 1997:351–373.

6. News release: Ulcers, H. pylori, and older people: you don't have to grow old with your ulcer. Atlanta: Centers for Disease Control and Prevention. October 2, 1998.

7. Howden, C.W., and Hunt, R.H. The histamine H_2-receptor antagonists. In Swabb, E.A., and Szabo, S., eds., *Ulcer Disease. Investigation and Basis for Therapy.* New York: Marcel Dekker. 1991:189–215.

8. Moore, J.G., and Merki, H. Ibid.

9. Howden, C.W., and Hunt, R.H. Ibid. Merki, H., et al. Single dose treatment with H_2-receptor antagonists: is bedtime administration too late? *Gut.* 1987;28:451–454.

10. Moore, J.G., and Merki, H. Ibid.

11. Svanes, C., et al. Rhythmic patterns in incidence of peptic ulcer perforation over 5.5 decades in Norway. *Chronobiology International.* 1998;15:241–264.

12. Devitt, J.E., and Taylor, G.A. Perforated peptic ulcer. *Canadian Medical Association Journal.* 1967;96:519–523.

13. Raschka, C., and Schorr, W. Is there seasonal periodicity in the prevalence of Helicobacter pylori? *Chronobiology International.* 1999;16:811–819.

PREMENSTRUAL SYNDROME AND PREMENSTRUAL DYSPHORIC DISORDER

1. American Psychiatric Association. *Diagnostic and Statistical Manual of Mental Disorders.* Fourth Edition. Washington, D.C.: American Psychiatric Association. 1994:715–718.

2. Schmidt, P., et al. Differential behavioral effects of gonadal steroids in women with and in those without premenstrual syndrome. *New England Journal of Medicine.* 1998;338:209–216.

3. Mortola, J.F. Premenstrual syndrome—pathophysiologic considerations. *New England Journal of Medicine.* 1998;338:256–257.

4. American Psychiatric Association. Ibid.

5. Parry, B. Light therapy of premenstrual depression. In Lam, R.W., ed., *Seasonal Affective Disorder and Beyond: Light Treatment for SAD and Non-SAD Conditions.* Washington, D.C.: American Psychiatric Press. 1998:173–191.

6. Johnson, E.O. *1998 Women and Sleep Poll.* Washington, D.C.: National Sleep Foundation. 1998:23–24.

7. Thys-Jacobs, S. Calcium carbonate and the premenstrual syndrome: effects on premenstrual and menstrual symptoms. *American Journal of Obstetrics and Gynecology.* 1998;179:444–452.

RESTLESS LEGS SYNDROME AND PERIODIC LEG MOVEMENTS

1. Willis, T. *The London Practice of Physick.* London: Basset, Dring, Harper, Crook. 1977. Reprint of 1692 edition.

2. Wilson, V.N., and Walters, A.S., eds. *Sleep Thief, Restless Legs Syndrome.* Orange Park, Fla.: Galaxy Books. 1996.

3. Allen, R.P., and Earley, C.J. Augmentation of the restless legs syndrome with carbidopa/levodopa. *Sleep.* 1996;19:205–213.

4. Hening, W., et al. Circadian pattern of motor restlessness and sensory symptoms in the idiopathic restless legs syndrome. *Sleep.* 1999;22:901–912.

5. Trenkwalder, C., et al. Circadian rhythm of periodic limb movement and sensory symptoms of restless leg syndrome. *Movement Disorders.* 1999;14:102–110.

6. Coccagna, G. Restless legs syndrome/periodic leg movements in sleep. In Thorpy, M., ed., *Handbook of Sleep Disorders.* New York: Marcel Dekker. 1990:457–478.

7. Hening, W., et al. The treatment of restless legs syndrome and periodic limb movement disorder: an American Academy of Sleep Medicine review. *Sleep.* 1999;22:970–999.

SKIN DISORDERS

1. Scheving, L.E. Mitotic activity in the human epidermis. *Anatomical Record.* 1959;35:7–20.

2. Verschoore, M., et al. Circadian rhythms in the number of actively secreting sebaceous follicles and androgen circadian rhythms. *Chronobiology International.* 1993;5:349–359. Yosipovitch, G., et al. Time-dependent variations of the skin barrier function in humans: transdermal water loss, stratum corneum hydration, skin surface pH, and skin temperature. *Journal of Investigative Dermatology.* 1998;110:20–23.

3. Stephenson, L.A., et al. Circadian rhythm in sweating and cutaneous blood flow. *American Journal of Physiology.* 1984;246:R321–324. Timbal, J., et al. Circadian variation in the sweating mechanism. *Journal of Applied Physiology.* 1975;39:226–230.

4. Gelfant, S., et al. Circadian rhythms and differences in uninvolved and involved psoriatic skin in vitro. *Journal of Investigative Dermatology.* 1982;78:58–62.

5. Rubin, N.H., and Scheving, L.E. Circadian rhythm (letter). *Journal of Investigative Dermatology.* 1983;80:79–80.

6. Pigatto, P.D., et al. Circadian rhythm of the in vivo migration of neutrophils in psoriatic patients. *Archives of Dermatological Research.* 1985;277:185–189.

7. Cormia, F.E. Experimental histamine pruitus. I. Influence of physical and psychological factors on threshold reactivity. *Journal of Investigative Dermatology.* 1952;19:21–34.

8. Mottram, J.C. A diurnal variation in the production of tumors. *Journal of Pathology and Bacteriology.* 1945;57:265–267. Frei, J.V., and Ritchie, A.C. Diurnal variation in the susceptibility of mouse epidermis to carcinogen and its relationship to DNA synthesis. *Journal of the National Cancer Institute.* 1964;32:1213–1220. Iversen, O.H., and Iversen, U.M. A diurnal variation in the tumorigenic effect response of mouse epidermis to a single application of the strong short-acting chemical carcinogen methylnitrosourea. A dose-response study of 1, 2 and 10 mg. *In Vivo.* 1995;9:117–132.

9. Ortho Tri-Cyclen Tablets. In Arky, R., ed., *Physicians' Desk Reference.* Montvale, N.J.: Medical Economics Co. 1999;53:2230.

10. McGovern, J.P., et al. Circadian and circamensual rhythmicity in cutaneous reactivity to histamine and allergenic extracts. In McGovern, J.P., Smolensky, M.H., and Reinberg, A., eds., *Chronobiology in Allergy and Immunology.* Springfield, Ill.: Thomas. 1977:79–116.

11. McGovern, J.P., et al. Ibid.

12. Cove-Smith, J.R., et al. Circadian variation in cell-mediated immune response in man and their response to prednisolone. In Reinberg, A., and Halberg, F., eds., *Chronopharmacology.* Oxford: Pergamon. 1979:369–374.

13. Lamberg, L. "Treatment" cosmetics: hype or help? *Journal of the American Medical Association.* 1998;279:1595–1596.

14. Reinberg, A., et al. Day-night differences in effects of cosmetic treatments on facial skin. Effects on facial skin appearance. *Chronobiology International.* 1990;7:69–79.

15. Bruguerolle, B., et al. Temporal variations in transcutaneous passage of drugs: the example of lidocaine in children and in rats. *Chronobiology International.* 1991;8:277–282.

16. Reinberg, A., and Reinberg, M.A. Circadian changes of the duration of action of local anaesthetic agents. *Naunyn-Schmiedeberg's Archives of Pharmacology.* 1977;297:149–159.

17. Pershing, L.K., et al. Circadian rhythm of topical 0.05% betamethasone diproprionate in human skin in vivo. *Journal of Investigative Dermatology.* 1994;102:734–739.

SLEEP DISORDERS

1. Costa e Silva, J.A., et al. Special report from a symposium held by the World Health Organization (WHO) and the World Federation of Sleep Research Societies: an overview of

insomnias and related disorders—recognition, epidemiology, and rational management. *Sleep.* 1996;19:412–416.

2. *International Classification of Sleep Disorders.* Rochester, Minn.: American Sleep Disorders Association. 1997.

3. Wiedman, J. *Desperately Seeking Snoozin': The Insomnia Cure from Awake to Zzzzz.* Memphis, Tenn.: Towering Pines Press. 1998.

4. Morris, M., et al. Sleep-onset insomniacs have delayed temperature rhythms. *Sleep.* 1990:13:1–14.

5. Lamarche, C., and Ogilvie, R. Electrophysiological changes during the sleep onset period of psychophysiological insomniacs, psychiatric insomniacs, and normal sleepers. *Sleep.* 1997;20(9):724–733.

6. Spielman, A., et al. Treatment of insomnia by restriction of time in bed. *Sleep.* 1987;10:45–56.

7. *International Classification of Sleep Disorders.* Ibid.

8. DeBeck, T. Delayed sleep phase syndrome—criminal offense in the military? *Military Medicine.* 1990;155:14–15.

9. Wagner, D. Disorders of the circadian sleep/wake cycle. *Neurologic Clinics.* 1996;14:651–670.

10. Sack, R.L., et al. Use of melatonin for sleep and circadian rhythm disorders. *Annals of Medicine.* 1998;30:115–121.

11. Campbell, S., et al. Etiology and treatment of intrinsic circadian rhythm sleep disorders. *Sleep Medicine Reviews.* 1999;3:179–200.

12. Lack, L.C., et al. Circadian rhythms of early morning awakening insomniacs. *Journal of Sleep Research.* 1996;5:211–219.

13. Léger, D. Blindness and sleep patterns (letter). *Lancet.* 1996;348:830–831.

14. Sack, R.L., et al. Melatonin entrains free-running circadian rhythms in a totally blind person. *Sleep.* 1999;22(Suppl. 1):138–139.

15. Kavey, Neil. *50 Ways to Sleep Better.* Lincolnwood, Ill.: Publications International. 1996.

16. Ancoli-Israel, S. Now I lay me down to sleep: the problem of sleep fragmentation in elderly and demented residents of nursing homes. *Bulletin of Clinical Neurosciences.* 1989;54:127–132.

17. Pollak, C., and Perlick, D. Sleep problems and institutionalization of the elderly. *Sleep Research.* 1987;16:407.

18. Pollak, C. Clinical and social consequences of disordered sleep. In *Abstracts of the NIH Consensus Development Conference on the Treatment of Sleep Disorders of Older People,* March 26–28, 1990. Bethesda, Md.: National Institutes of Health. 1990:107–109.

19. Lovell, B.B., et al. Effect of bright light treatment on agitated behavior in institutionalized elderly subjects. *Psychiatry Research.* 1995;57:7–12.

20. Schnelle, J.F., et al. The nursing home at night: effects of an intervention on noise, light, and sleep. *Journal of the American Geriatric Society.* 1999;47:430–438.

21. Roth, T. New trends in insomnia management. *Journal of Psychopharmacology.* 1999;13(4 Suppl. 1):S37–40. Lamberg, L. Sleep specialists weigh hypnotics, behavioral therapies for insomnia. *Journal of the American Medical Association* (News). 1997;278:1647–1649.

22. Nowell, P.D., et al. Benzodiazepines and zolpidem for chronic insomnia. A meta-analysis of treatment efficacy. *Journal of the American Medical Association.* 1997;278:2170–2177.

23. National Center on Sleep Disorders Research, and Office of Prevention, Education, and Control. *Insomnia: Assessment and Management in Primary Care.* National Institutes of Health Publication No. 98-4088. Bethesda, Md.: U.S. Department of Health and Human Services. 1998.

24. Morin, C.M., et al. Nonpharmacological interventions for insomnia: a meta-analysis of treatment efficacy. *American Journal of Psychiatry.* 1994;151:1172–1180.

25. Chesson, A.L., et al. Practice parameters for the use of light therapy in the treatment of sleep disorders. *Sleep.* 1999;22:641–660.

26. Zhdanova, I., et al. Melatonin: a sleep-promoting hormone. *Sleep.* 1997;20:899–907.

27. Zeitzer, J.M., et al. Do plasma melatonin concentrations decline with age? *American Journal of Medicine.* 1999;107:432–436.

28. Dagan, Y., et al. Evaluating the role of melatonin in the long-term treatment of delayed sleep phase syndrome (DSPS). *Chronobiology International.* 1998;15:181–190.

29. Lewy, A.J., et al. Melatonin shifts circadian rhythms according to a phase-response curve. *Chronobiology International.* 1992;9:380–392.

STROKES

1. Elliott, W. Circadian variation in the timing of stroke onset. A meta-analysis. *Stroke.* 1998;29:992–996.

2. Stephenson, J. Rising stroke rates spur efforts to identify risks, prevent disease. *Journal of the American Medical Association* (News). 1998;279:1239–1240.

SUDDEN INFANT DEATH SYNDROME

1. Kelmanson, I.A. Circadian variation in the frequency of infant death syndrome and of sudden death from life-threatening conditions in infants. *Chronobiologia.* 1991;18:181–186.

2. MacDorman, M.F., et al. Infant mortality statistics from the 1997 period linked birth/infant death data set. *National Vital Statistics Reports.* 1999;47(23):19.

3. Progress in reducing risky infant sleeping positions—13 states, 1996–1997. *Morbidity and Mortality Weekly Report.* 1999;48(39):878–882.

4. Gordon, A.E., et al. Cortisol levels and control of inflammatory responses to toxic shock syndrome toxin-1 (TSST-1): the prevalence of night-time deaths in sudden infant death syndrome (SIDS). *FEMS Immunology and Medical Microbiology.* 1999;25:199–206.

5. Brown, P.J., et al. Oscillations of body temperature at night. *Archives of Disease in Childhood.* 1992;67:1255–1258.

6. Schwartz, P.J., et al. Prolongation of the QT interval and the sudden infant death syndrome. *New England Journal of Medicine.* 1998;338:1709–1714.

7. American Academy of Pediatrics Task Force on Infant Positioning and SIDS. *Pediatrics.* 1992;89:1120–1126.

8. Willinger, M., et al. Factors associated with the transition to nonprone sleep positions of infants in the U.S.: the National Infant Sleep Position Study. *Journal of the American Medical Association.* 1998;280:329–335.

9. SIDS deaths reach new record low in 1997, but disparities persist for minority communities. News Release. National Institute for Child Health and Development. October 22, 1998. http://www.hhs.gov.

10. Jeffrey, H.E., et al. Why the prone position is a risk factor for Sudden Infant Death Syndrome. *Pediatrics.* 1999;104:263–269.

11. Mosko, S., et al. Infant sleep architecture during bedsharing and possible implications for SIDS. *Sleep.* 1996;19:677–684.

12. Richard, C., et al. Sleeping position, orientation, and proximity in bedsharing infants and mothers. *Sleep.* 1996;19:685–690.

13. Cohen, G.J., ed. *American Academy of Pediatrics Guide to Your Child's Sleep.* New York: Villard Books. 1999:90.

14. Firstman, R., and Talan, J. *The Death of Innocents: A True Story of Murder, Medicine, and High Stakes Science.* New York: Bantam Books. 1997.

15. Steinschneider, A. Prolonged apnea and the Sudden Infant Death Syndrome: clinical and laboratory observations. *Pediatrics.* 1972;50:646–654.

16. Lucey, J. Why all pediatricians should read this book. *Pediatrics.* 1997;100:A77.

17. Lewis, N. Across area, dozens of suspicious deaths. *The Washington Post.* September 20, 1998:A1.

TOOTHACHE

1. Pollmann, L., and Harris, P.P. Rhythmic changes in sensitivity of teeth. *International Journal of Chronobiology.* 1978;5:459–464.

2. Pollmann, L. Duality of pain demonstrated by the circadian variations in tooth sensitivity. In Haus, E., and Karat, H., eds., *Chronobiology 1982–1983.* Basel: Charger. 1984:225–228.

3. Reinberg, A., and Reinberg, M. Circadian changes of the duration of action of local anaesthetic agents. *Naunyn-Schmiedeberg's Archives of Pharmacology*. 1977;297:149–159.

4. Pollmann, L., and Hildebrant, G. Circadian profiles and circaseptan periodicity in the frequency of administration of analgesic drugs after oral surgery. *Annual Review of Chronopharmacology*. 1986;3:429–432.

5. Pollmann, L. Chronobiological considerations of aspirin and indomethacin. *Annual Review of Chronopharmacology*. 1984;1:349–352.

URINARY DISORDERS

1. Gimpel, G.A., et al. Clinical perspectives in primary enuresis. *Clinical Pediatrics*. 1998;37:23–30. Rittig, S., et al. Abnormal diurnal rhythm of plasma vasopressin and urinary output in patients with enuresis. *American Journal of Physiology*. 1989;256(4 Pt 2):F664–671.

2. Sleep enuresis. In *International Classification of Sleep Disorders, revised: Diagnostic and Coding Manual*. Rochester, Minn.: American Sleep Disorders Association. 1997:185–188.

3. Neveus, T., et al. Sleep of children with enuresis: a polysomnographic study. *Pediatrics*. 1999;103(6 Pt 1):1193–1197.

4. Desmopressin (DDAVP). *Physicians' Desk Reference*. Montvale, N.J.: Medical Economics. 2000;54:2554–2556.

5. Lackgren, G., et al. Desmopressin in the treatment of severe nocturnal enuresis in adolescents—a 7-year follow-up study. *British Journal of Urology*. 1998;81(Suppl. 3):17–23.

6. Kirkland, J.L., et al. Patterns of urine flow and electrolytes. *British Medical Journal*. 1983;287:1665–1667.

7. Donahue, J.L., and Lowenthal, D.T. Nocturnal polyuria in the elderly person. *American Journal of the Medical Sciences*. 1997;314:232–238.

8. Donahue, J.L., and Lowenthal, D.T. Ibid.

9. Saito, M., et al. Frequency-volume charts: comparison of frequency between elderly and adult patients. *British Journal of Urology*. 1993;72:38–41.

10. Clarke, H.S. Benign prostatic hyperplasia. *American Journal of the Medical Sciences*. 1997;314:239–244.

11. Sommer, P., et al. Voiding patterns and prevalence of incontinence in women: a questionnaire survey. *British Journal of Urology*. 1990;66:12–15.

12. Hirasing, R.A., et al. Enuresis nocturna in adults. *Scandinavian Journal of Urology and Nephrology*. 1997;31:533–536.

13. Burgio, K.L., et al. Nocturnal enuresis in community-dwelling older adults. *Journal of the American Geriatrics Society*. 1996;44:139–143.

14. Burgio, K.L., et al. Behavioral vs. drug treatment for urge urinary incontinence in older women: a randomized controlled trial. *Journal of the American Medical Association*. 1998;280:1995–2000.

15. *You Are Not Alone* (brochure). Baltimore, Md.: American Urological Association. 2000.

Chapter 16: Better Health in the Twenty-first Century

1. Bondmass, M., et al. Rapid control of hypertension in African Americans achieved utilizing home monitoring. *Circulation*. 1998;98(Suppl. 1):517.

2. Scott Doran spoke with Lynne Lamberg January 6, 2000.

Abbreviations Used in This Book

AACE: American Association of Clinical Endocrinologists
ACE inhibitor: Angiotensin Converting Enzyme inhibitor
ACL: Anterior Cruciate Ligament
ADA: Americans with Disabilities Act
ADHD: Attention Deficit Hyperactivity Disorder
AIDS: Acquired Immunodeficiency Syndrome
AMA: American Medical Association
APA: American Psychiatric Association
AS: Ankylosing Spondylitis
ASPS: Advanced Sleep Phase Syndrome
AZT: zidovudine
BMI: Body Mass Index
BM: Bowel Movement
BP: Blood Pressure
CDCP: U.S. Centers for Disease Control and Prevention
DHEA: Dehydroepiandrosterone
DRIs: Dietary Reference Intakes (formerly, **RDAs:** Recommended Daily Allowances)
DSPS: Delayed Sleep Phase Syndrome
DST: Daylight Saving Time
DWI: Driving While Intoxicated
DWS: Driving While Sleepy
ED: Erectile Dysfunction
F: Fahrenheit
FDA: U.S. Food and Drug Administration
FM: Fibromyalgia
HIV: Human Immunodeficiency Virus
HRT: Hormone Replacement Therapy
HPV: Human Papillomavirus

MADD: Mothers Against Drunk Drivers
MNF: Monday Night Football
MRFIT: Multiple Risk Factor Intervention Trial
MS: Multiple Sclerosis
MSLT: Multiple Sleep Latency Test
NAS: National Academy of Sciences
NASA: National Aeronautics and Space Administration
NBA: National Basketball Association
NFL: National Football League
NHLBI: National Heart, Lung, and Blood Institute
NIA: National Institute on Aging
NIH: National Institutes of Health
NIMH: National Institute of Mental Health
NREM Sleep: Non-Rapid Eye Movement Sleep
NSAID: Nonsteroidal Anti-Inflammatory Drugs
OA: Osteoarthritis
PATT: Parents Against Tired Truckers
PLMS: Periodic Limb Movements in Sleep
PMDD: Premenstrual Dysphoric Disorder
PMS: Premenstrual Syndrome
PUBMED: Public Access to National Library of Medicine
RA: Rheumatoid Arthritis
RDAs: Recommended Daily Allowances
REM Sleep: Rapid Eye Movement Sleep
RLS: Restless Legs Syndrome
SAD: Seasonal Affective Disorder
SAT: Scholastic Aptitude Test
SCN: Suprachiasmatic Nucleus
SERMs: Selective Estrogen Receptor Modulators
SIDS: Sudden Infant Death Syndrome
SRE: Sleep-Related Erection
SSRIs: Selective Serotonin Reuptake Inhibitors
TAG: Triacylglycerol
TB: Tuberculosis
TIA: Transient Ischemic Attack
TPA: Tissue-type Plasminogen Activator
UCSD: University of California at San Diego
USDA: United States Department of Agriculture

Resources for
Further Information

References for Physicians and Other Health Care Providers

Deedwania, Prakash, C., ed. *Circadian Rhythms of Cardiovascular Disorders.* Armonk, N.Y.: Futura Publishing Company. 1997.

Hrushesky, William J.M., Langer, Robert, Theeuwes, Felix, eds. *Temporal Control of Drug Delivery.* New York: Annals of the New York Academy of Sciences, Vol. 618. 1991.

Lemmer, Björn, ed. *Chronopharmacology. Cellular and Biochemical Interactions.* New York: Marcel Dekker. 1989.

Martin, Richard J., ed. *Nocturnal Asthma.* Mt. Kisco, N.Y.: Futura Publishing Company. 1993.

Portaluppi, Francesco, and Smolensky, Michael H., eds., *Time-Dependent Structure and Control of Arterial Blood Pressure.* New York: Annals of the New York Academy of Sciences, Vol. 783. 1996.

Redfern, Peter H., and Lemmer, Björn, eds. *Physiology and Pharmacology of Biological Rhythms.* Berlin: Springer-Verlag. 1997.

Touitou, Yvan, and Haus, Erhard, eds. *Biologic Rhythms in Clinical and Laboratory Medicine.* Berlin: Springer-Verlag. 1994.

Turek, Fred W., and Zee. Phyllis C., eds. *Regulation of Sleep and Circadian Rhythms.* New York: Marcel Dekker. 1999.

Chronobiology and Sleep Web Sites

American Academy of Sleep Medicine: www.aasmnet.org/
Books for Sleepless Nights: www.sleephomepages.org/books/
Canadian Sleep Society: www.css.to/
Center for Biological Timing: www.cbt.virginia.edu/
Circadian Information: www.circadian.com
European Sleep Research Society: www.esrs.org
European Society for Chronobiology: www.far.ub.es/~ crono/
KnowSleep: www.knowsleep.com
National Heart, Lung, and Blood Institute: www.nhlbi.nih.gov/health/public/sleep/index.htm
National Institute of Neurological Disorders and Stroke: www.ninds.nih.gov/patients/disorder/sleep/brain-basics-sleep.htm
National Sleep Foundation: www.sleepfoundation.org
Sleep Medicine Home Page: www.users.cloud9.net/thorpy/
SleepNet: www.sleepnet.com
Sleep Research Society (and links to sleep research societies worldwide): www.sleephomepages.org

Sleep/Wake Disorders Canada: www.geocities.com/HotSprings/1837/
Society for Light Treatment and Biological Rhythms: www.sltbr.org
Society for Research in Biological Rhythms: www.srbr.org/
Women in Sleep and Rhythm Research: www.sleephomepages.org/wisrr/
Worldwide Project on Sleep and Health: www.worldsleep.org/wpsh.html

General Health Web Sites

Healthfinder: www.healthfinder.gov. U.S. Health and Human Services Department site. Offers links to government and nonprofit agencies.

Healthweb: www.healthweb.org. A consortium of medical libraries offers links to noncommercial health sites.

Merck Manual: www.merck.com. Key features of diseases. Written for physicians.

National Institutes of Health: www.nih.gov. Access to information from federal health institutes, centers, and offices, many targeted to consumers.

National Library of Medicine: www.nlm.nih.gov. Access to articles published in more than 4,300 scientific journals, via PUBMED: www.medlineplus.gov.

Useful Library Search Terms

Biological Rhythms
Chronobiology
Chronotherapeutics
Chronotherapy
Circadian Rhythms
Sleep

News about *The Body Clock Guide to Better Health*

www.bodyclocks.com

Acknowledgments

Our editor, David Sobel, saw chronotherapy's potential to improve everyday life from the start. He kept us focused on conveying the practical implications of research findings. His able assistant, Anne Geiger, orchestrated countless details. We happily learned that she considers providing tender loving care to authors an important part of her job. Production editor Rita Quintas sharpened our language and style. Design manager Paula Szafranski helped us refine our illustrations. John Sterling, president of Henry Holt, perhaps our most critical reader, delighted us with his enthusiasm for our ideas and our approach. We are also grateful to Elizabeth Shreve, Heather Fain, Maggie Richards, Denise Cronin, and others at Holt who share our commitment to spreading the word about body time. Our agent, Vicky Bijur, served as adviser, salesperson, lawyer, cheerleader, philosopher, psychotherapist, nag, and handholder, all in one. Thanks, Vicky!

Michael thanks his wife, Nita, and children, Melissa, Brian, and Susan, who inspire his work, sustain his dedication to chronobiology, and graciously tolerate periodic disruption of their sleep/wake and social rhythms by his work schedule. He also thanks Tim Poffenbarger for preparing charts and illustrations and providing computer expertise, graphic artist Fran Holden for updating the clock illustrations, and Peggy Powell for secretarial and editorial assistance. The librarians at the Houston Academy of Medicine–Texas Medical Center and University of Texas–Houston School of Public Health helped locate required references—some hundreds of years old. Colleague Erhard Haus reviewed the manuscript, addressing issues of medical concern.

Lynne thanks her husband Stanford, a physician, for his assistance in interpreting murky medical prose, his insightful reading of early drafts, his attentiveness to news items of likely interest, and his conjuring up great dinners on her busiest nights. She thanks her daughter, Nicole, and son, Ryan, for being great listeners and for asking provocative questions. She also thanks Nicole for designing the book's Web site, www.bodyclocks.com. Writer friends Pat McNees and Robin Henig commiserated over travails of the writing process and provided sage counsel. Colleague Aaron Levin took the jacket photo. Friends Marianne Levin, Ruth Singer, Lynne Rubin, Doris Diamond, Carol Simon, and Walter Bonime offered encouragement and respite. Bonnie Oberman provided a one-client sleep-focused clipping service. Nidra Pollar translated *Observation Botanique*, the 1729 report on de Mairan's discovery of the biological clock, and Arthur Lesley translated Maimonides' twelfth-century advice to get eight hours of sleep each night.

Many specialists in sleep and chronobiology provided both information and context, often sharing preprints and data not otherwise available. Some read sections of the book and made helpful suggestions. Several individuals shared personal experiences that enliven the text. This book owes much to their generous gift of time.

Index